DIETETICS AND INTEGRATIVE MEDICINE

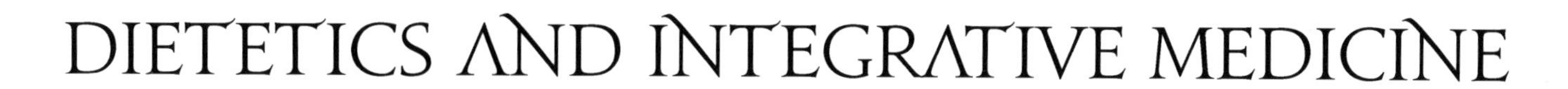

DIETETICS AND INTEGRATIVE MEDICINE

Curriculum Development Model

DIANA NOLAND, LEIGH WAGNER, RANDALL EVANS, RACHEL BARKLEY,
JEANNE DRISKO MD & DEBRA SULLIVAN PHD

Dietetics and Integrative Medicine: Principles and Guidebook

Senior Product Manager: Diana Noland, MPH RDN CCN LD, diana@diananoland.com.

ISBN-13: 9781533562289

ISBN-10: 1533562288

Printed/digital publishing in United States of America

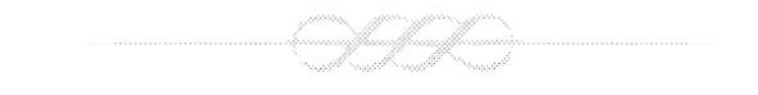

ACKNOWLEDGEMENTS

This publication was supported by an anonymous private foundation that supports grants for dietetics and nutrition students and professionals for integrative and functional nutrition education and training, as part of the larger goal of supporting human potential, social justice, health and the environment, and by the University of Kansas Medical Center Dietetics & Nutrition and KU Integrative Med Clinic without which support this document would not have been possible.

We are also grateful to Peggy Person, KU Endowment, for oversight of the financial support, and Dr. Zora DeGrandpre, MS, ND, *ZoraTech, Medical and Scientific Writing and Editing*, who significantly improved the manuscript.

We are thankful to our editors and students who provided expertise that greatly assisted the Dietetics and Integrative Medicine program.

TABLE OF CONTENTS

Acknowledgements · · · v
Definitions of Terms and Acronyms · · · xi
Introduction: Curriculum Development Model Dietetics and Integrative Medicine · · · xv

Section 1 What is Dietetics and Integrative Medicine (DIM)? · · · 1
Principles of Dietetics and Integrative Medicine · · · 2
Systems Biology and Integrative Medicine · · · 2
Introduction to Dietetics and Integrative Medicine · · · 2
An Interdisciplinary Approach · · · 2
Personalized Medicine based on Biochemical Individuality · · · 3
The role of Dietetics in Integrative Medicine (DIM) · · · 3
The Advanced Specialty of Integrative and Functional Medical Nutrition Therapy (IFMNT) · · · 4
The Specialty of Dietetics and Integrative Medicine · · · 5
Fundamentals of the Pathophysiology of Chronic Disease: The Nutritional Perspective · · · 5
The Epidemic of Chronic Disease · · · 7
The Critical Role of Nutrition in Chronic Disease · · · 7
The DIM application of the Nutrition Care Process · · · 8
Foundational Concepts of Dietetics and Integrative Medicine · · · 9
What are DIM and IFMNT? · · · 9
Tenets of Dietetics and Integrative Medicine · · · 10
Section 2 Rationale for Dietetic and Integrative Medicine Programs · · · 21
The Dietetics and Integrative Medicine Program - Rationale · · · 21
Current Need for Increased Education in Dietetics and Integrative Medicine · · · 23
Why Do We Need the DIM and IFMNT models of dietetics practice? · · · 23
The IFMNT Radial Guide · · · 23
Section 3 Dietetics and Integrative Medicine Curriculum Development · · · 25
DIM Training · · · 25
Overview · · · 25
Clinical Training · · · 26
Community Commitment · · · 26

Food Service · · · 27
DIM Accredited internships · · · 28
Option for Master's Degree · · · 28
DIM Award Program for Dietetic Interns · · · 28
DIM Graduate Certificate Online Program · · · 28
DIM-emphasis Master of Science degree programs · · · 29
Feasibility for an Academic Center · · · 31
Infrastructure, Departmental Collaboration, Regulatory Approval and Accreditation · · · 32
Foundations of Training · · · 32
Community Involvement · · · 33
Professional Development of the Faculty · · · 33
Faculty Teaching Responsibilities · · · 33
Teaching the DIM Assessment of the patient/client · · · 34
Education for the patient/client · · · 34
The Therapeutic Relationship · · · 34
Funding · · · 35
Graduate Certificate of Dietetics and Integrative Medicine · · · 36
Section 4 Curriculum · · · 39
Dietetic Internship Certificate (Total hours, 24) · · · 39
Dietetics and Integrative Medicine Graduate Certificate (Online only, 12 hours) · · · 41
Master of Science in Dietetics and Nutrition · · · 43
Criteria for M.S. Research Project of Dietetics and Integrative Medicine students/interns · · · 45
Learning Objectives and DIM Competencies · · · 46
Foundational Concepts of DIM · · · 46
Assessment and Diagnosis, Intervention, Monitoring and Evaluation · · · 46
Food Quality & Regulation · · · 47
Community Nutrition · · · 48
Expected Competencies in Computer Technology · · · 48
Section 5 Dietetics and Integrative Medicine Practicum · · · 53
Clinical Rotations: Five Module Practicum Activities and Supporting · · · 53
Introduction · · · 53
Off-site Practicum Sites · · · 53
Nutrition-related training sites · · · 55
Other Integrative training sites · · · 56
Module 1: General Orientation to Integrative Medicine Practicum · · · 57
Practicum Site, Modalities and the DIM Paradigm · · · 57
Module 2: DIM Food Preparation and Whole Foods · · · 59
Orientation to DIM food preparation: Whole Foods and Kitchen Operation · · · 59
Module 2 Activities · · · 60
Module 3: DIM Clinical Nutrition Practice · · · 63
DIM Clinical Nutrition Practice · · · 63
KU DIM Initial Nutrition Assessment Process · · · 63
Nutrition Assessment Process · · · 64

Principles of Motivational Interviewing · · · 67
OBSERVING THE PRACTITIONER (HEALTHCARE PROVIDER) · · · 67
OBSERVING THE CLIENT · · · 68
Module 4: Research · · · 70
Research from the DIM perspective · · · 70
Module 5: Community Nutrition · · · 71
DIM Community Nutrition · · · 71
Module 6: Practicum Student Assessment and Evaluation · · · 71
Introduction · · · 71
Pre and Post Evaluation for DIM Interns · · · 72
Supporting documents for Student Assessment and Evaluation · · · 72

Appendix List · · · 75
Bibliography | References Cited · · · 261

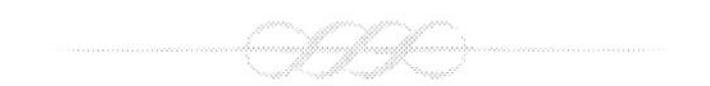

DEFINITIONS OF TERMS AND ACRONYMS

AND or "The Academy": The Academy of Nutrition and Dietetics (formerly, American Dietetic Association or "ADA")
ADIME: The AND Nutrition Care Process steps pf Assessment: Diagnosis: Intervention: Monitoring & Evaluation
AVS: After Visit Summary
DIFM: *Dietitians in Integrative and Functional Medicine* Dietetic Practice Group (DPG) of the Academy of Nutrition and Dietetics (AND)
DIM: Dietetics and Integrative Medicine
DN: Dietetics and Nutrition
EMR: Electronic Medical Record
HIPAA: The Health Insurance Portability and Accountability Act of 1996 (**HIPAA**; Pub. L. 104–191, 110 Stat. 1936, enacted August 21, 1996) was enacted by the United States Congress and signed by President Bill Clinton in 1996.
HPI: History of Present Illness
IDU: Steps for assessment of nutrition status: **I**ntake: **D**igestion & Elimination: **U**tilization of nutrients at a cellular level
IFM: Institute for Functional Medicine
IFMNT: Integrative and Functional Medical Nutrition Therapy
KU IM:: University of Kansas (KU) Integrative Medicine
KUMC: University of Kansas Medical Center
LD: Licensed Dietitian
LDN: Licensed Dietitian-Nutritionist
MAPDOM: Cellular status of **M**inerals: **A**ntioxidants: **P**rotein: **D** & fat-soluble vitamins; **O**ils/Fats; **M**ethylation Nutrients
MSQ: Medical Symptoms Questionnaire
NCP: Nutrition Care Process
PES: Problem Etiology Signs & Symptoms
PSR: Patient Services Representative
PMH: Past Medical History
RDN: Registered Dietitian-Nutritionist

Dietetics and Integrative Medicine

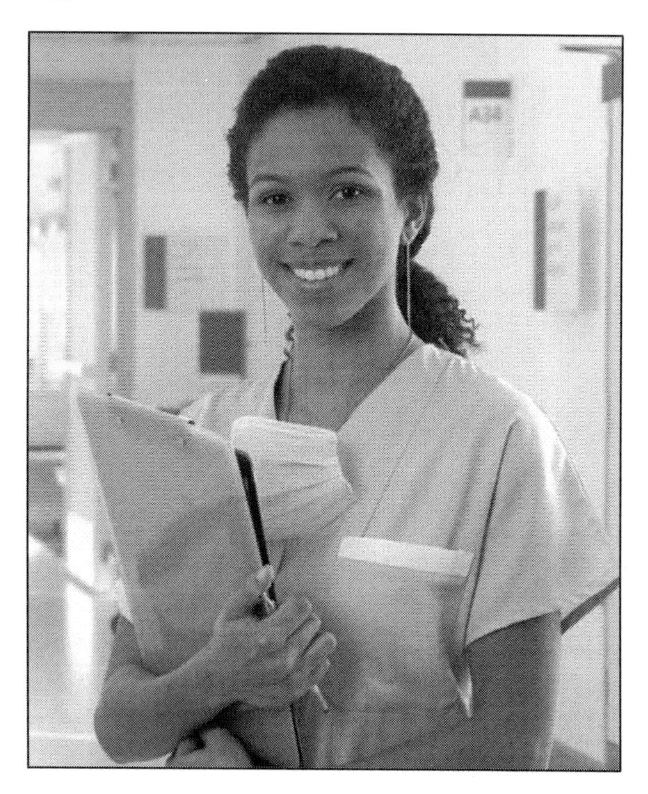

Next Generation of Dietetics for Chronic Disease

Tenets of Dietetics & Integrative Medicine

Dietetics & Integrative Medicine Curriculum Development Model

---

Introduction

CURRICULUM DEVELOPMENT MODEL DIETETICS AND INTEGRATIVE MEDICINE

Medical education continues to respond to the needs of the times, with the current challenge to all healthcare disciplines being that of the growing epidemic of chronic disease. Historically since the early 1900's when infection and injury were the common healthcare concerns, that promoted the discoveries of antibiotics, steroids and new testing modalities, medical education addressed healthcare for these conditions within every professional healthcare discipline. Dietetics began its organization in 1920 was no different, based on "acute-care" and "public health". As more understanding of the pathophysiology of chronic disease and the direct association to diet and lifestyle, the 2008 audit of the dietetics profession by the Academy of Nutrition & Dietetics, initiated recommendations for development of advanced specialties to address particular needs, with the need for solutions for chronic diseases at the top of their list. During the last several decades, a "medical transition" has been developing a new paradigm, referred to as "systems biology", which is being incorporated into the disciplines of integrative and functional medicine and others.

Systems Biology:

"Systems biology is an inter-disciplinary biology-based holistic approach considering complex interactions within biological systems to understanding and controlling biological complexity." This is the foundation of the disciplines of integrative and functional medicine.

Institute of Systems Biology 2013

Nutrition and diet are primary tools of care within the integrative medicine paradigm, and a perfect match for the advanced skill of a trained nutritionist and dietitian. Until recently, the level of advanced training in dietetics and integrative medicine (DIM) has not been available in a university setting. Rising to the occasion, the University of Kansas Medical Center, under the oversight of Dr. Deborah Sullivan, Dietetics and Nutrition, and, Dr. Jeanne Drisko, KU Integrative Medicine Clinic, set to develop an advanced level of training in DIM to begin to produce graduates trained to clinically apply the skills from an integrative medicine perspective. The following guide and principles describe the accomplishments of development over 4 years to graduate DIM professionals beginning to populate the dietetics workforce addressing the specialty needs of our chronic disease populace. This DIM eTextbook has been compiled to share the work of this DIM project as a stepping-stone for those dietetics educators desiring to add this type of program to enrich and expand their existing or new dietetics education.

This document is the first organized presentation of a model that integrates a systems biology education into an existing conventional program of medical nutrition therapy in dietetic and other healthcare professional education. It has been developed for a graduate level educational program, but is designed to be flexible enough to provide a template for undergraduate as well as graduate programs. It can be a starting point for the educational curricula of other disciplines, and is a particularly seamless approach in graduate level medical and nursing education. The vision for this DIM eText-book is to provide the momentum and energy to inject a new systems biology medical nutrition therapy model into existing conventional nutrition education programs.

In collaboration with the University of Kansas Medical Center, the Department of Dietetics and Nutrition, KU Integrative Medicine professors, doctors and nutritionists, and with the support of an anonymous private foundation, this three and half year project was a learning experience in how to successfully bring an integrative curriculum into an already existing educational program in the medical field and develop the first integrative medicine track in a dietetic program. This DIM project is an example of the collaboration necessary to build other programs in the future within existing dietetic, medical, nursing and other healthcare professions. The DIM program has become a prototype model that other interested educational institutions can learn from in developing their own programs and not having to reinvent the wheel. Each institution so inclined will be able adapt those aspects of the KUMC DIM curriculum applicable to their program.

The integrative curriculum and practicum developed are provided in order to share with other universities our research, development and implementation, so that they may teach those of the next generation of healthcare professionals who are eager to expand their knowledge of health care beyond conventional care. An anonymous private foundation generously provided the funding for this project in order to create a change driver in the hope that a more effective healthcare model will emerge to deal with the global challenge of chronic disease epidemics facing the human race. Time is of the essence.

The DIM approach is emerging as an advanced specialty within clinical nutrition that addresses the current global chronic disease epidemic by applying a holistic understanding of the unique chronic disease pathophysiology as influenced by diet, lifestyle factors, and environment.

As our bodies respond to the environment in which we live, the health of the human race is influenced by the totality of mind, body and spirit. Within that whole, the aspects of health related to the body and mind are key factors for wellness. During the 1980's the explosion of biochemical research and technology resulted in a rebirth, or a *renaissance of nutrition science.* New levels of understanding of biochemical pathways and metabolic regulation have brought about deeper understanding of the cell's function and life processes, revealing the foundational role that nutrients and water play in metabolism. They are providing a new and expanding set of tools that enable advanced application of more targeted nutrition therapy, which promotes more successful health outcomes, particularly for those living with chronic diseases.

A new awareness of the interconnectedness of the functions of body systems has produced the new discipline of *Systems Biology, or Systems Physiology,* which focuses on overall metabolism, including all biochemical reactions and effects that take place within our cells, tissues and organs. Systems Biology recognizes the holistic interdependence of each part of an organism. Ultimately, those metabolic reactions occur because of nutrient-dependent tissue structures that provide for dynamic biochemical interplay of nutrients and nutrient co-factors. Systems Biology has initiated a "medical transition", currently in an awkward phase, that is moving away from the established acute care model of medicine, where the disease is treated for and outcomes are measured by the reduction of symptoms. This transition is moving towards a systems-biology/physiology-based holistic paradigm where the individual is treated, and outcomes are measured by the state of wellness achieved by the individual. Much of the insight is gleaned from traditional medical systems like Traditional Chinese Medicine, Ayurveda and Herbology. The momentum of change is growing and signs of the establishment of a systems biology foundation for global medicine are becoming clearer and more solid.

Figure 1 illustrates the main new advances that are driving the medical transition. There is promise in the development of a model of systems based medicine that addresses the unique and newly recognized chronic disease pathophysiology currently expressed as the global epidemic of chronic disease.

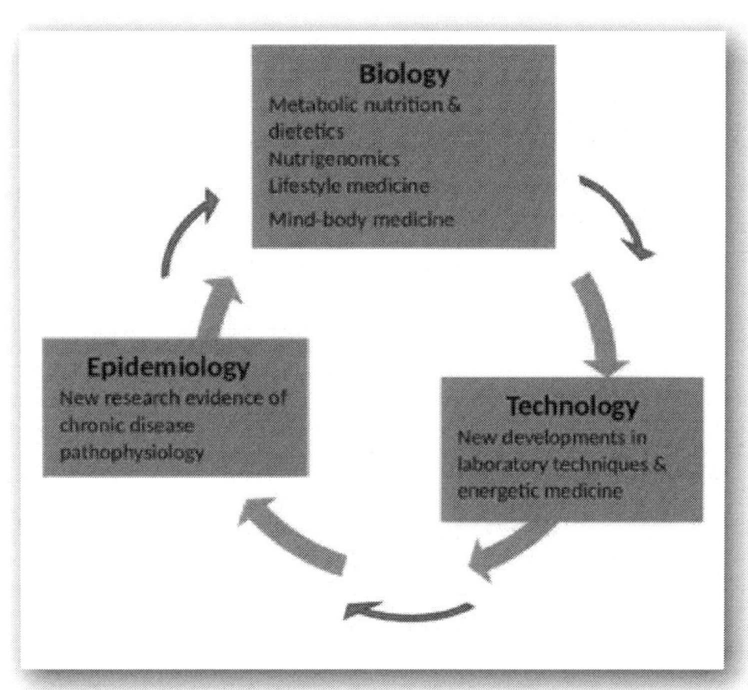

Figure 1: New Concepts in System Biology--System Cycles

The hallmark of this advanced nutrition therapy discipline is the "n of 1", the individual focus. Historically, the focus on nutrition and medical therapy has been on applying results from evidence-based, single variable population studies to an individual patient. Population study results typified by the Bell Curve in Figure 2 report the expected response of most of the population for nutritional adequacy within the 1 standard deviation. The 2nd and 3rd standard deviations of upper and lower "outliers" of nutrient needs for any particular population are not addressed in most cases[1]. However, we now, have the means by which to use the information from evidence-based science as guidelines, but also to then assess the "normal" individual as well as the "outlier" individual. We can thereby identify their unique biochemical individuality and their unique "*patient story*" so as to develop a more targeted metabolic intervention. This integrative medicine approach is then used to address the individual's complaints and condition and move them toward restoring a state of wellness.

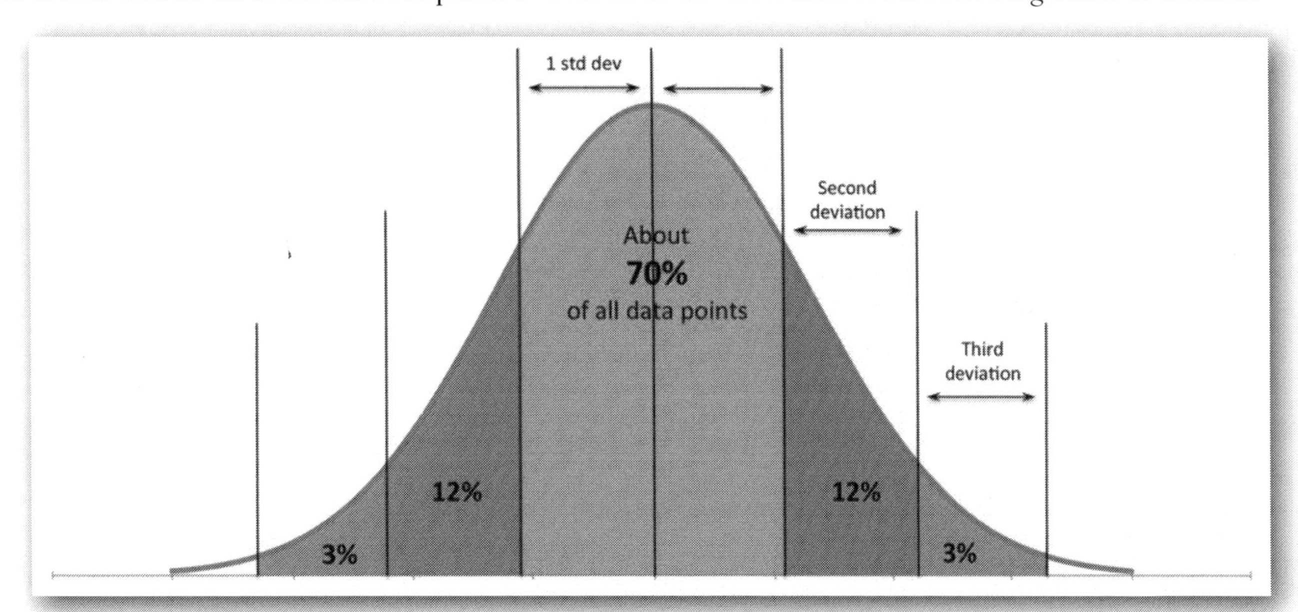

Figure 2: Normal distribution (a.k.a. "Bell Curve")

We currently have the science, technology and tools to implement this new, advanced nutrition therapy, but lack established educational training programs in which to produce systems-biology-thinking practitioners. There is a sort of *blurred image of nutrition* with which it is unclear to whom the discipline of nutrition belongs. The truth is, it belongs to multiple disciplines, and all disciplines are needed for complete health care. In the clinical practice setting, the primary focus is the education of this new paradigm of dietitian/nutritionists, medical doctors, and nurses to meet future health-care needs.

Section 1

WHAT IS DIETETICS AND INTEGRATIVE MEDICINE (DIM)?

"A blurred image of nutrition…" This has often been the image of nutrition—rather than seeing diet and nutrition as being within the central core of medical approaches to health and wellness as well as being uniquely fundamental to the prevention and treatment of the current worldwide epidemic of chronic diseases, the sciences of dietetics and nutrition have `often been relegated to a sort of secondary status in the practice of mainstream medicine. Indeed, while diet and optimal nutrition have become increasingly emphasized in many arenas, recent studies have indicated that medical schools have, perhaps counter-intuitively, been spending less time teaching the principles and practice of nutrition, with graduating medical students feeling less qualified than in previous years to deal with the nutritional needs and concerns of their patients. [1-3] Recognizing this "blurred image" (Figure 3), the University of Kansas' Program of Integrative Medicine, the KUMC Dietetics and Nutrition Department, and an anonymous family foundation dedicated to the advancement of nutritional science joined together to study the feasibility and potential implementation of continuing education, internships and award programs designed to sharpen and hone not only the image of nutritional sciences, but the incorporation of leading edge nutritional principles by practicing dieticians and nutritionists within a community setting.

The following sections will describe the need for specialists in Dietetics and Integrative Medicine, the background and the rationale for introducing a DIM educational program into dietetics and nutrition education. Graduates of the program will learn the fundamental concepts in Dietetics and Integrative Medicine (DIM) that they will be able to put into practice in their own careers and communities.

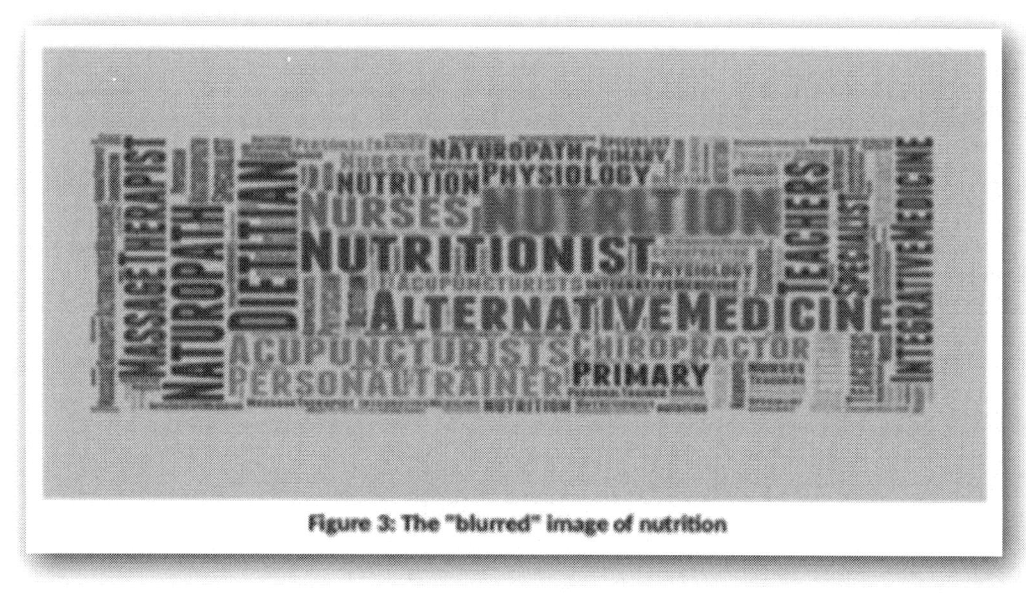

Figure 3: The "blurred" image of nutrition

PRINCIPLES OF DIETETICS AND INTEGRATIVE MEDICINE

SYSTEMS BIOLOGY AND INTEGRATIVE MEDICINE

Systems Biology incorporates the interactions of complex biological and biochemical systems, while always maintaining a holistic perspective. Integrative or functional medicine both concentrate attention on how physiological systems may become dysfunctional or unbalanced, identifying root causes of disease.

Systems biology can be described as an interdisciplinary approach that holistically focuses on complex and interrelated functions within biological systems. It seeks to discover emergent properties of cells, tissues and organisms involving metabolic networks and cell-to-cell signaling networks. Systems biology approaches seek to understand the nutritional needs and requirements of individuals by combining and integrating diverse sources of information, including genetic and molecular, so as to achieve a better understanding of cellular, tissue and organ function.

Much of modern medicine defines diseases in terms of symptoms and pathology rather than in terms of the metabolic dysfunction within an individual patient. While symptoms remain important to integrative medicine, emphasis is placed on determining the root or underlying cause, dysfunction or imbalance. This approach is clinically oriented, evidence-based and patient-centered. It uses the principles of systems biology and biochemical/genomic individuality to understand and aid in the repair or rebalancing of the system that is clinically most significant while maintaining and improving the health of the patient by maintaining and improving all of the interacting systems. *Health is not merely the absence of disease, but is instead considered to be a vital functional state* (WHO). Nutrition plays a fundamental role in these rebalancing processes since, just as nothing can be built without the proper materials, health can be neither be built nor maintained without the proper nutrients provided in proper amounts and of sufficient quality.

In dietetics, the systems biology approach focuses on the interrelationships between nutrients and genetic expression (nutrigenomics) and between nutrients and the genetic susceptibility to diseases (nutrigenetics). [4]

Nutrients can affect gene expression in a number of ways, including by functioning as ligands for transcription factor receptors, altering signal transduction pathways and by inducing or inhibiting metabolic pathways. [5-10] Nutrigenomics studies the functional implications of these interactions, while nutrigenetics studies individual risk factors for deleterious nutrient-gene interactions, with the goal of providing a personalized nutritional approach for individuals at risk for cardiovascular disease, obesity, diabetes and other disorders. [11-16]

INTRODUCTION TO DIETETICS AND INTEGRATIVE MEDICINE

Dietetics and nutritional science are evolving fields. And, while dietetics and nutrition have always been closely involved with medicine, these professions have found a natural partnership with Integrative Medicine, defined by the Consortium of Academic Health Centers for Integrative Medicine as:

> *"Integrative Medicine is the practice of medicine that reaffirms the importance of the relationship between practitioner and patient, focuses on the whole person, is informed by evidence, and makes use of all appropriate therapeutic approaches, healthcare professionals and disciplines to achieve optimal health and healing."* [4]
>
> *Developed and Adopted by The Consortium, May 2004. Edited May 2005, May 2009 and November 2009.*

AN INTERDISCIPLINARY APPROACH

Integrative medicine (IM) places the patient at the center of the healing process, addressing the patient within a holistic framework and incorporating an interdisciplinary team approach to inform a full range of physical, mental, emotional, spiritual and social or community issues. The contributions of the specialty roles within the team strengthen the informing and empowering of the patient to "take charge" of their own health and wellness.

PERSONALIZED MEDICINE BASED ON BIOCHEMICAL INDIVIDUALITY

Recognizing that no one individual physician or health care professional can completely know and understand all the unique aspects of an individual's medical, emotional and spiritual needs in addition to all aspects of an individual's environment, Integrative Medicine is an approach that welcomes other holistic healthcare providers under an inclusive umbrella of care, utilizing an interdisciplinary team to achieve the patient's optimal health and wellness.

Dietetics and Integrative Medicine combines the evidence-based approaches of medicine with a holistic view of the individual, and will utilize methodologies that can rationally be brought to bear to improve the individual's overall health and wellness.

THE ROLE OF DIETETICS IN INTEGRATIVE MEDICINE (DIM)

Integrative and functional dietetics and clinical nutrition have been defined by the Dietitians in Integrative and Functional Medicine (DIFM), an Academy of Nutrition and Dietetics (AND) Dietetic Practice Group (DPG), as:

> *"...the personalized medical nutrition therapy for prevention and treatment of chronic disease that embraces conventional and complementary therapies. Integrative and functional nutrition reaffirms the importance of the therapeutic relationship, a focus on the whole person lifestyle, biochemical individuality and environmental influences."*

The emphasis in Integrative and Functional Medicine, as well as in the integrative practice of dietetics and nutrition, is on a holistic approach that embraces all therapeutic approaches that can be utilized to achieve the individual patient's optimal health, wellness and healing. The practice of integrative and functional dietetics and nutrition, in addition, explicitly takes into account the unique inner aspects of each person (their biochemical individuality) and also their specific life experiences (physical, mental, emotional and spiritual). These are considered within the context of outside environmental influences and the effects these environmental influences, in the form of food, water, toxic environmental factors and other lifestyle factors. An effective conceptual working tool to help encapsulate all of these factors is the Functional Medicine Matrix™ (Figure 4).

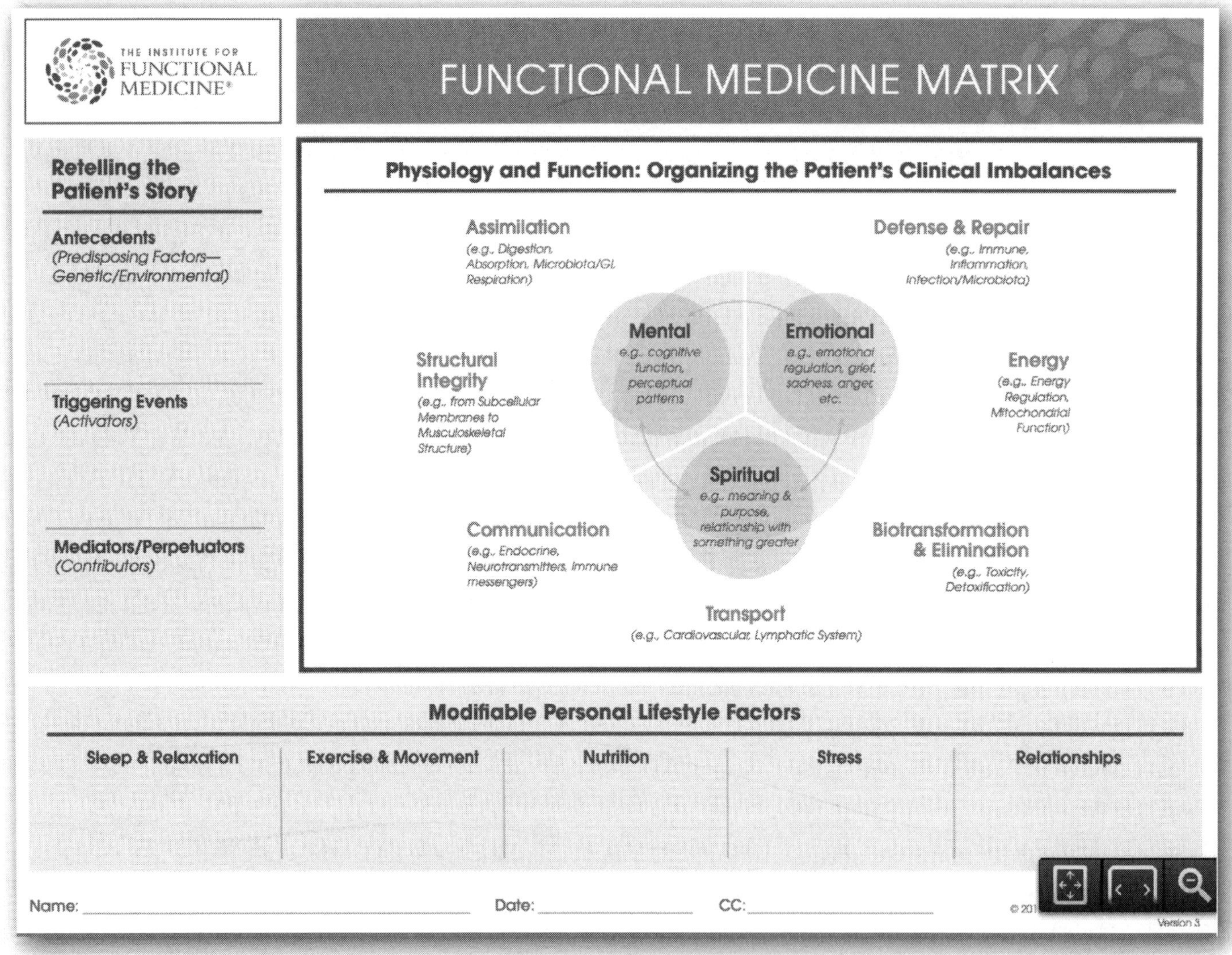

Figure 4: The Functional Medicine Matrix™

PDF available in the Appendix

Integrative and functional medicines are approaches to healthcare that can be easily incorporated by all medical specialties and professional disciplines, and by all health care systems. Its use will not only improve health care for patients, it can also enhance the cost effectiveness of health care delivery for providers and payors.[5]

THE ADVANCED SPECIALTY OF INTEGRATIVE AND FUNCTIONAL MEDICAL NUTRITION THERAPY (IFMNT)

Clinical application of dietetics as Medical Nutrition Therapy (MNT) can be described as the assessment of the nutritional status of an individual with an illness, injury or any other dietary condition with the purpose of identifying those individuals and establishing a specific, individualized nutritional and dietary plan designed to prevent the appearance or worsening of a condition, and to increase overall health while reducing health care costs.[6-9] MNT can be used in a variety of settings including home care, acute and chronic care, and includes patient education and guidance in self-management.

Medical Nutrition Therapy by nutritionists and RDNs includes:

* Implementing a comprehensive assessment (intake assessment) of an individual's nutritional status and determining a nutrition diagnosis
* Designing and implementing an evidence-based intervention
* Observing, monitoring and evaluating the patient/client's progress.

With advanced training in DIM, the nutritionist and RD gain skills in clinical application of what is being referred to by DIFM and others as "Integrative and Functional Medical Nutrition Therapy" (IFMNT) focusing on the nutritional and lifestyle needs of chronic disease. These needs are described below discussing the nutritional perspective of the pathophysiology of chronic diseases.

THE SPECIALTY OF DIETETICS AND INTEGRATIVE MEDICINE

The DIM practitioner represents an advanced level of nutrition professional. Those nutrition practitioners trained in this specialty function as a physician's primary partner on the chronic care team and is the expert in using diet and lifestyle approaches, including nutritional genomics, for preventing and managing chronic disease. The specialty knowledge and advanced skills make this practitioner unique within healthcare and able to participate within healthcare in ways never before possible.

FUNDAMENTALS OF THE PATHOPHYSIOLOGY OF CHRONIC DISEASE: THE NUTRITIONAL PERSPECTIVE

The global rise in chronic disease has been correlated with the so-called "nutrition transition", i.e. the switch from a game meat, vegetable, nut, seed and fruit-based diet to one which is high in mass-produced meat, sugar, grains, saturated fats and salt, and which uses large amounts of antibiotics, pesticides, herbicides and genetically-modified organisms to increase yields and profits. [10-14] An improved diet, tobacco cessation and increased rates of physical activity could prevent significant cases of coronary artery disease, chronic heart diseases, diabetes, metabolic syndrome, cancer, obesity and other chronic conditions[15-17] Increased stress levels, tobacco and alcohol abuse, environmental toxins and a sedentary lifestyle also can significantly impact chronic disease rates.[18-22]

Allostasis as a model of the physiological response to stress has been extensively described by McEwen and others.[23-26] Allostasis is a mechanism by which the organism responds to stress and maintain energy resources during periods of stress, ultimately seeking to maintain homeostatic mechanisms. Stress is seen to arise from both internal and external sources. *Allostatic load* describes the magnitude and sources of the stressors. There are potential scenarios that, as seen through the allostatic lens, are important to gaining an understanding of chronic disease. In one scenario, an individual is subjected to unrelenting stress from any source, be it nutritional, environmental, infectious, inflammatory or lifestyle-based, and this cumulative stress can result in an unsupportable allostatic load and the eventual collapse of one or more systems. In a second scenario, an individual encounters stress that, in theory, should be possible to adjust to, yet, potentially due to subclinical damage of one or more homeostatic systems, the individual counters with a continuous vigorous stress response, thereby damaging various interrelated systems. In a third scenario, the individual fails to respond physiologically to any stress at all. A more recent model that integrates aspects of allostasis, homeostasis and stress is called the Reactive Scope Model. It describes ranges of response to stress that include circadian and seasonal variations, toxic or threatening environmental changes, homeostatic overload and homeostatic failure.[27]

Hormesis is a toxicological term referring to the biphasic response of cells, organs, tissues and systems to an environmental toxin or other stressor. At low doses of a toxin exposed over long periods of time, there can be a detrimental effect sometimes more damaging than the toxic effects seen at acute high doses. Metabolically, this has been demonstrated in environmental low dose exposures to toxic heavy metals and toxic chemicals, like cadmium and Bisphenol A *(BPA)*. In nutrition, examples of hormesis may be found in the increased DNA damage caused by low levels of nutrients such as folate, B_6 and B_{12}, niacin, selenium and zinc; damage that is inhibited with adequate levels of the same nutrients; and again similar damaging effects when the nutrient exceeds the upper limit of safety. [28-30]

Within the models of stress response and the rise of chronic diseases, there are a number of factors significant for dietitians and nutritionists and that may be directly addressed through IFMNT. These are:

* **Inflammation**: Inflammation underlies the process of chronic disease and can be addressed by diet, targeted IFMNT and lifestyle modifications. The prostaglandin/eicosanoid pathways may be directly and specifically influenced by dietary choices, allowing for targeted non-pharmacological interventions.[31-37]
* **Immune Regulation**: The immune system is in delicate balance, and can be modulated by dietary and nutritional interventions and approaches for patients with autoimmune diseases and for those with compromised immune systems. Recent findings concerning the relationship between the health of the microbiome, the use of pro- and prebiotics, other nutritional considerations, and the effectiveness of both the innate and adaptive immune responses, hold great promise in controlling chronic disease, including autoimmune disorders as well as supporting the immune response to pathogen assault.[6,38-46]
* **Long-Latency Nutritional Deficiencies**: Many conditions develop after many years of subclinical deficiencies. These index conditions include osteoporosis (Calcium)[47,48], osteomalacia (Vitamin D)[47,49], megaloblastic anemia (folate)[50,51] and neurological/behavioral disorders (ω-3/ ω-6 essential fatty acids, iron and zinc)[50,52-57] Triage theory, originally postulated by Bruce Ames, holds that scarce micronutrients are used to support short-term survival while long-term survival may suffer. [58-62]
* **Biochemical Individuality and Genetics**: Biochemical individuality can be defined as the unique and specific dietary and nutritional needs of an individual based on their unique genome and epigenome influenced by epigenetics. This scientific field of genetics is an expanding area and offers substantial promise for individualized medical treatment and individualized integrative medical nutrition therapy. [63-72] In general, biochemical individuality is established via epigenetic changes that are influenced by environmental toxic exposures, lifestyle choices, beliefs and nutrition and are controlled at the genetic level via the processes of methylation, histone modification, acetylation and non-coding microRNAs (miRNAs).
* **Toxicity:** Both natural and synthetic toxins surround us and have been implicated in a wide variety of chronic and non-communicable diseases. [73-81] As part of the NHANES (National Health and Nutrition Examination Survey) study, the Centers for Disease Control produced the CDC Fourth National Report on Human Exposure to Environmental Chemicals where participants were tested for 212 individual compounds, metals and solvents. The majority of individuals tested positive for exposure to a variety of substances including acrylamides, trihalomethanes, bisphenol A, phthalates, chlorinated pesticides, organophosphate pesticides, pyrethroids, heavy metals, aromatic hydrocarbons, polybrominated diphenyl ethers, perfluorocarbons from non-stick coatings, and a host of polychlorinated biphenyls and solvents. [77,82] Detoxification or biotransformation of toxic molecules requires nutritional support such as key nutrient co-factors of liver metabolism (Phase I, II) and the organs of elimination (Phase III) as well as a gentle, progressive approach that takes into account the potentially harmful release of toxins stored in the adipose tissue. [69,75,76,83-88]

* **Lifestyle:** Lifestyle issues stem from family and cultural sources and include effects of the amount of rest, sleep and relaxation an individual patient experiences, as well as issues of personal satisfaction, self-esteem and mind-body concerns. In addition, it is often difficult for individuals to face the challenge of changing their eating habits and the foods they eat. Finally, issues of addiction and the use of tobacco, alcohol and various drugs, both recreational and prescribed, must be addressed, focusing on potential DINDs (Drug-induced Nutritional Deficiencies) All these issues must be viewed through the lens of the individual, the individual's biochemistry and their personal goals and motivations. [89-91] Indeed, lifestyle medicine has been called the "future of chronic disease management."[92]
* **Energy:** As food is the ultimate source of all biochemical energy, MNT and the specialist in dietetics and integrative medicine must, of necessity, understand and support the energy production of the mitochondria, cells, organs and tissues with an understanding of the systems physiology, body composition, whole foods and the genetic and epigenetic uniqueness of the individual influences by the stress and environment. [86,93,94]

THE EPIDEMIC OF CHRONIC DISEASE

Non-communicable disease (NCD) is used to describe chronic disease and includes cardiovascular disease, respiratory disease, diabetes and cancer. NCDs are a leading cause of mortality. Globally, 63% of all deaths in 2009 were due to NCDs. [95] In the US, in 2009, cardiovascular disease (including cerebrovascular diseases), cancer, chronic respiratory diseases and diabetes constituted 62% of all mortalities. Poor diet and nutrition (including a lack of fruit and vegetables couple with a high salt and saturated fat intake) and a lack of physical activity are important risk factors for NCDs. Perhaps more importantly from the public health perspective, poor diet, nutrition and physical activity are also key modifiable factors in the development of NCDs. NCDs are considered to be such a critical problem that the World Health Organization (WHO) convened a high-level meeting in 2011 to discuss policy measures and implementation plans to "prevent and control the global NCD epidemic"[96]

In addition, poor maternal health and nutrition is closely associated with increased rates of gestational diabetes, maternal obesity and long-term significant health consequences not only for their offspring, but for generations after. Maternal obesity and/or tobacco use, gestational diabetes, childhood obesity and the increase in the rates of Types 1 and 2 diabetes in childhood—and the associated socioeconomic patterns are a growing problem globally. [97-105] While a number of international organizations, including the Academy of Nutrition and Dietetics (AND, formerly known as the American Dietetic Association or ADA), have sounded the alarm, unfortunately, this situation has suffered to some extent from "malignant neglect" regarding implementation of policies. There appear to be a number of reasons for this lack of implementation—or the lack of sufficient implementation, including resistance from the food industry, or "Big Food", defined as the multination food and beverage industry, the subject of a recent PLoS Medicine series. Another concern, particularly in obesity research, has been the focus on individual behavior as opposed to population and genome-specific studies. Currently, the *Journal of Public Health Policy* actively discourage studies centered on the individual because, as the editors state, they "have come to believe that research studies concentrating on personal behavior and responsibility as causes of the obesity epidemic do little but offer cover to an industry seeking to downplay its own responsibility.'' [106]

THE CRITICAL ROLE OF NUTRITION IN CHRONIC DISEASE

Historically, medical schools have not trained physicians adequately in nutritional principles and practices. The well-known and often cited Flexner report, credited with moving medical education in the early 20th century towards a more rigorous, evidenced based and standardized approach, emphasized public health concerns, disease prevention and health promotion and the potential for academic medicine to influence public health policy. Disease prevention and health promotion as well as the more generalized public health concerns included issues of food availability and affordability, sustainable farming practices, and basic nutritional principles. These have not, however, been effectively addressed in medical school curricula. [1,2,107] In fact studies have indicated that even as the patient population is more interested and concerned about diet and nutrition, medical students have been receiving fewer than the recommended hours of training and are actually expressing less interest in nutritional approaches to public health or to chronic disease prevention and treatment.[1,2,107,108] Surveys have indicated that, in 2004 for example, only 30% of medical schools required a dedicated course in nutrition and only 38% of schools met the recommendation for 25 hours of nutritional training set by the National Academy of Sciences for nutrition education in medical school. [2] More recent surveys indicate that the situation has not improved drastically. One study found that 80% of instruction in nutrition in medical schools occurs outside of dedicated nutrition courses. [1,2] Other studies indicate that while "...Recent data support the importance of targeted nutritional therapy to reduce morbidity and mortality, yet the number of physicians interested in nutrition appears to be declining, and fewer hours of nutrition training are occurring in medical school." [1,109] In addition, both instructors and students feel that nutritional training is inadequate. The inadequacy of nutritional training for physicians is not restricted to the US—it appears to be global in scope. [109-112]

The evidence, however, indicates that public health, chronic disease prevention and treatment are in fact, significantly impacted by appropriate nutritional counseling. [113-120] Sustainable farming practices, [121,122] providing increased access to healthy foods in the community, [123-125] and an emphasis on whole foods [126,127] are approaches that are showing success on an individual and a community level.

If physicians are not being adequately trained in nutrition, sustainable farming methods, the use of whole foods to support healthy living, nutritionally-based disease prevention and disease treatment, then who is available to provide this sort of information? Recent studies and surveys indicate that there is an increasing public interest in diet, nutrition and health—and how to achieve optimal health and wellness with diet and nutrition.

For example, the Academy of Nutrition and Dietetics (formerly the American Dietetic Association), the professional organization representing registered dieticians (RDs) and the world's largest organization of food and nutrition professionals, found in the "Nutrition and You: Trends 2011" survey that an increasing number of individuals recognize the importance of healthy eating and good nutrition and try to implement healthy eating principles into their lives. 46% of respondents said they "actively seek information about nutrition and healthy eating"[17]

The Academy of Nutrition and Dietetics (AND), in its position paper entitled "The Role of Nutrition in Health Promotion and Chronic Disease Prevention" stated "...dietary intervention positively impacts health outcomes across the life span. Registered dietitians and dietetic technicians, registered *(sic)* are critical members of health care teams and are essential to delivering nutrition-focused preventive services in clinical and community settings, advocating for policy and programmatic initiatives, and leading research in disease prevention and health promotion." [17] The World Health Organization (WHO) at their 2011 conference stated that "... the global burden and threat of non-communicable diseases constitutes one of the major challenges for development in the twenty-first century, which undermines social and economic development throughout the world and threatens the achievement of internationally agreed development goals" and that nutrition, access to healthy foods, maternal and infant health and the promotion of sustainable farming methods were the "primary role and responsibility of Governments in responding to the challenge of non-communicable diseases and the essential need for the efforts and engagement of all sectors of society to generate effective responses for the prevention and control of non-communicable diseases;" [128]

THE DIM APPLICATION OF THE NUTRITION CARE PROCESS

The Nutrition Care Process (NCP) established by the Academy of Nutrition and Dietetics (AND) is referred to as ADIME and summarized as follows:

* **A**ssessment of nutritional status of an individual
* **D**iagnosis of nutritional and metabolic imbalances
* **I**nterventions of nutrition and lifestyle for improvement and resolution of diagnoses
* **M**onitoring of interventions
* **E**valuation of effectiveness and need for adjustment of interventions

Within the NCP assessment component, the KU DIM program incorporates the Institute for Functional Medicine's (IFM) Matrix Model™ [129-131] (see Figure 5 below), actively incorporating concepts of systems biology and systems physiology, antecedents or predisposing factors, and triggering or activation events, while always recognizing that an equilibrium and homeodynamics exists between and amongst the systems. The physiological systems considered throughout all tracks within the DIM program are:

* Oxidative/Reductive homeodynamics
* Detoxification and Biotransformation
* Hormone and Neurotransmitter regulation
* Psychological and Spiritual Equilibrium
* Structural and Membrane Integrity
* Digestion and Absorption
* Immune Surveillance and Inflammatory process

In addition, the IFM Matrix™ takes into account the individual's nutrition status, levels of physical activity, sleep habits, significant relationships and that individual's set(s) of beliefs and self-care principles.

FOUNDATIONAL CONCEPTS OF DIETETICS AND INTEGRATIVE MEDICINE

WHAT ARE DIM AND IFMNT?

DIM and IFMNT are positioned to be the nutritional disciplines of the future of nutrition care for chronic disease. In general, they are descriptions of a model of the advanced practice of nutrition assessment, diagnosis, intervention, and monitoring at the molecular and cellular levels that focuses on a holistic promotion of optimal health and the management and prevention of diet and lifestyle-related diseases. They are complementary to acute care medicine that excels at managing end-stage diseases, emergency and injury conditions.

DIM and IFMNT are at the core of Integrative and Functional Medicine as an integrative approach to health. The Institute for Functional Medicine (IFM) states "Functional medicine is an evolution in the practice of medicine that better addresses the healthcare needs of the 21st century. By shifting the traditional disease-centered focus of medical practice to a more patient-centered approach, functional medicine addresses the whole person, not just an isolated set of symptoms. Integrative and functional medicine practitioners spend time with their patients, listening to their histories and evaluating the interactions among genetic, environmental, and lifestyle factors that can influence long-term health and complex, chronic disease. In this way, functional medicine supports the unique expression of health and vitality for each individual."[129]

TENETS OF DIETETICS AND INTEGRATIVE MEDICINE

Dietetics and Integrative Medicine at the University of Kansas developed the *Ten Tenets of Dietetics and Integrative Medicine*. These tenets are derived from classical medical and integrative medical philosophy of nutritional science:

1. ***Individualized Integrative and Functional Medical Nutrition Therapy (IFMNT) optimizes wellness.***
2. ***Genomic uniqueness of an individual contributes to IFMNT interventions in addition to practice and evidence based medicine.***
3. ***Listening to the patient's story is the basis of the therapeutic relationships between providers and their clients to maximize health outcomes.***
4. ***"Food as epigenetic medicine" – appropriate foods and targeted nutrients—the therapeutic use of isolated or combined nutrients that can be administered as dietary supplements, medical foods, topical, cutaneous, intramuscular or intravenous injections--for an individual can act as epigenetic messages to promote wellness.***
5. ***Whole low-contaminated foods and targeted nutrients specific for the individual provide the basis of IFMNT.***
6. ***Correct nutritional insufficiencies as well as deficiencies to optimize nutrient metabolism and lower risk of chronic disease.***
7. ***Manage chronic disease inflammation through food and targeted nutrients.***
8. ***Use of targeted nutrient therapies can reduce toxin damage to metabolism.***
9. ***Beliefs and community relationships influence nutritional health (mind---body).***
10. ***Know when you are not the expert. Collaborate with other members of the integrative care team.***

Tenet 1:

Individualized Integrative and Functional Medical Nutrition Therapy (IFMNT) optimizes wellness.

Many diseases that burden Western societies are more and more identified with nutritional and lifestyle influences. Chronic diseases such as cardiovascular disease (including hypertension, cardiac conditions, and dyslipidemias)[107,132-139] ; obesity, eating disorders, diabetes (Types 1 and 2 and gestational)[139-147]; cancer[148-157]; gastrointestinal disorders[6,8,9,158-165]; compromised immune function [6,38-40,166,167]; chronic respiratory conditions, renal dysfunction[168-172]; pediatric conditions [6,173,174]; post-surgical care[175-179] and others can be powerfully impacted by nutrition insufficiencies and/or excesses. IFMNT addresses the individual in a holistic manner incorporating a systems biology assessment from the biochemical microenvironment to lifestyle to beliefs from which to base personalized interventions and monitoring. Approaching MNT through the foundation of evidenced-based nutrition science and clinical application of the lens of the "n of 1" can provide improved outcomes.

Tenet 2:

Genomic uniqueness of an individual contributes to IFMNT interventions in addition to practice and evidence based medicine.

Hearing the Patient's Story including family history can recognize genomic uniqueness. Since the discoveries of the Human Genome Project, the understanding of biochemical and genotypic individuality has progressed exponentially. For the dietitian/nutritionist the study of nutritional genomics (nutrigenomics and nutrigenetics) is developing for use in clinical application. The dietitians in integrative and functional medicine have led the front in dietetics by incorporating genomic testing into the evidence-based nutrition data considered in assessing a client. The clinical implications and potential of genomics testing related to personalized nutritional requirements holds much promise, and deepens the recognition of an individual's uniqueness.

Nutritional genomics, the study of role of genetic variations influenced by nutrients, is an emerging and exciting field in nutritional science. Each individual, with their genomic uniqueness, can be significantly affected by their internal and external environments, including by the quality, quantity and characteristics of the foods they eat—and, the foods that are recommended to them. It is important that the tenet of genomic uniqueness is recognized in the nutrition care process to increase the targeting of a client's metabolic needs. In addition, the field of *epigenetics* has provided incredible insight into the environmental influences on genomic expression, without changing the actual structure of a gene (see Tenet 4). Food is a daily, three-times-a-day, environmental message communicating with our genes impacting epigenetic alterations in the DNA.

Tenet 3:

Listening to the patient's story is the basis of the therapeutic relationships between providers and their clients

For thousands of years, physicians and healers had relatively few ancillary tools at hand with which to diagnose and treat. These healers had their own senses to detect sights, sounds, smells and sensations of signs and symptoms, but they, in addition, had to rely on listening to the patient's story in order to best understand the individual's health status. This *therapeutic relationship*, also known as the therapeutic or healing alliance, historically and traditionally has formed the basis of the healing process. [180-186]

In order to be truly successful, the therapeutic relationship in integrative medicine and dietetics should be based on genuine interest, mutual respect, and empathy. The goals of the therapeutic relationship include facilitated communication, the promotion of overall health, wellness and wellbeing, as well as self-care and independence, while maintaining professional boundaries and high standards of ethics and care.

Tenet 4:

"Food as epigenetic medicine" –appropriate foods and targeted nutrients for an individual can act as epigenetic messages to promote wellness.

Epigenomics is another emerging concept in nutritional and dietetic science. Epigenomics addresses the effects of specific nutrients on gene expression. The concept that foods and nutrients can affect gene expression has its roots in the concept that individuals have specific nutrient needs that are the expression of their unique biochemical individuality.[187-190]

Epigenetics is the study of stable, heritable changes in gene expression without involving changes in the DNA sequence. There are at least three distinct mechanisms for epigenetic changes:

* DNA methylation and other modifications such as hydroxylation and phosphorylation
* Histone modification and
* Non-coding microRNAs (miRNAs) which target specific mRNAs for suppression by affecting the mRNA stability or targeting it for degradation.[63,191,192]

These modifications are termed "epigenetic marks"

Cells have evolved over time to distinguish between periods of nutrient sufficiency and nutrient deprivation and have developed various metabolic pathways to fine-tune cellular processes so as to support continued life during periods of stress. A number of pathways, have been described that are involved in the stress pathways.[193] Aging –and the effects of caloric intake on aging, is also under the control of a number of highly conserved signaling pathways including insulin, insulin-like growth factor-1 (IGF-1), and the sirtuin pathways. Aging may by itself be implicated in the development of a number of chronic diseases. While aging itself is a normal process, addressing some of the effects of aging using specifically targeted foods and nutraceuticals is also an important component of the potential for the nutrigenomic and epigenetic approaches. On the other side of the spectrum, it is becoming increasingly clear that there is an early life origin for disease—and epigenetic factors, both in the maternal environment and in the child, can play a major role in the future development of disease. [85,86,194,195]

The levels of specific fatty or amino acids, vitamins, essential and trace minerals as well as the forms of carbohydrate or protein ingested can significantly impact gene expression and an individual's health and risk for acute or chronic disease. Equally, the rational and targeted administration of nutrients by an appropriate route can be effective in preventing and treating disease. [100,103,189,196-198]

Tenet 5:

Whole low-contaminated foods and targeted nutrients specific to the individual provide the basis of IFMNT.

IFMNT promotes the use of whole foods, foods that are minimally processed, minimally contaminated, and nutrient dense containing the maximal amounts of nutrients. In working with a client nutrition education for making wiser food choices are matched with the individual's readiness and need to change. It is the inherent nutrient density in whole foods that promotes adequate nutrient co-factor tissue levels for every metabolic function for an individual, including detoxification and elimination of various endogenous and exogenous toxic molecules.

Included in promoting a whole foods approach, IFMNT specifically seeks to expose an individual to as little contamination (in the form of various pesticides, herbicides, radiation, hormones, antibiotics, GMO, and other potential contaminants) as possible. Anecdotal and objective evidence all point to deleterious health effects from acute or chronic exposure to agricultural chemicals such as pesticides, herbicides and fungicides. For example, studies derived from the Agricultural Health Study indicated that organochlorine insecticides had an overall increased odds ratio of 1:2 for hypothyroidism among women exposed. The fungicide *benomyl* had a 3.1 odds ratio for hypothyroidism. The carbamate fungicide, *mancozeb* was associated with both hypothyroidism (OR=2.2) and hyperthyroidism (OR= 2.3)[199] Another study indicated that the use of EPTC (S-ethyl-N, N-dipropylthiocarbamate), a thiocarbamate herbicide, was associated with colon cancer and leukemia, though the authors urged caution in their interpretation. [200] A significantly increased rate of lipid peroxidation ($p<0.001$) and decreased levels of glutathione were correlated to fragmentation in DNA and changes in cellular membranes, with some proteins over-expressed and others under-expressed in the cells of carbamate-exposed workers.[201] Other studies have pointed to increased respiratory symptoms, [202-204] neurological symptoms,[205-207] cancer, [208,209] autoimmune [210-213] and other disorders.[214] The data is often limited by the complexity of variables, but overall is suggestive of sometimes subtle but potentially significant effects.

IFMNT include functional foods as part of an intervention plan when indicated. Functional foods are defined as whole foods or "fortified, enriched, or enhanced foods that have a potentially beneficial effect on health when consumed as part of a varied diet on a regular basis at effective levels based on significant standards of evidence."[215] Currently, the US Food and Drug Administration (FDA) do not have a legal definition for functional foods, but does regulate the health claims that can be made for functional foods. Medical foods may be defined as those that are evidence-based and prescribed by a physician to manage or treat a specific condition.

When nutritional insufficiencies, imbalances or genomic-nutrient specific needs are identified, a skilled IFMNT practitioner may recommend targeted nutrient therapy using dietary supplements, or Rx nutrition therapy (IV, IM) collaborating with a licensed practitioner. This targeted nutrient therapy makes use of basic nutritional knowledge as well as the expanding knowledge derived from recent and ongoing studies.

For example, prebiotics such as inulin and oligofructose increase the levels of *Bifidobacteria*, an important component of the microbiome. The increase in the levels of these bacteria results in improved insulin sensitivity, increased absorption of calcium and magnesium, and a decreased inflammatory state, and is being investigated in the treatment of inflammatory bowel diseases (IBD).[216-221]

The role of diet and nutrition in obesity, diabetes and cardiovascular disease is well known. MNT and more specifically IFMNT can be used in the treatment and prevention of these disorders, and can be fine-tuned to meet the specific needs of the patient, taking into account the patient's medical and life history as well as consideration of comorbidities, including autoimmune disorders, cancer and inflammatory conditions. [41,48,143,147,222-230]

In addition, targeted medical nutrition therapy can increasingly be genome- and epi-genome specific. For example, adequate intake of ω-3 long-chain polyunsaturated fatty acids (ω-3 LC-PUFAs), specifically docosahexaenoic acid (DHA), along with its synthesis from α-linolenic acid (ALA), is considered important in normal infant and child growth and development. The conversion rate of ALA to ω-3 LC-PUFAs is low and is dependent on the FADS (fatty acid desaturase) genotype, located on chromosome 11. A recent study in infants provided evidence that for the FADS genotype, presence or absence of breastfeeding and fish intake were responsible for up to 25% of the variation in the DHA status in the red blood cells. [231] FADS genotypes are also associated with allergic disorders in children, inflammatory processes and heart disease. [232-235] Further, post-partum depression is associated with decreased tryptophan availability and serotonin transporter gene polymorphisms that may be addressed by targeted nutrition or supplementation. [236-239] DNA methylation, an epigenetic process, can be a significant factor in the development of number of chronic, non-communicable diseases and can be programmed by both maternal factors as well as environmental factors.

DNA methylation is highly dependent on the availability of B-complex vitamins and methionine. If the maternal environment or the child's developmental environment is deficient in these factors, permanent changes predisposing to disease may ensue. [240 244] Single nucleotide polymorphisms (SNPs) in the MTHFR (methylenetetrahydrofolate reductase) gene are responsible for 1-carbon metabolism involved in a large number of important biochemical reactions, including neurotransmitter and protein synthesis, estrogen metabolism, glutathione production and homocysteine levels. MTHFR polymorphisms are related to anencephaly, homocysteinuria, neural tube defects such as spina bifida, and other congenital defects, heart disease, preeclampsia, glaucoma and some cancer, as well as potentially having roles in a large number of other conditions including migraine, autism, depression and other psychiatric disorders. It is likely that many of these conditions, in the presence of MTHFR SNPs, may be readily treated with targeted therapy including active forms of folate. [245-266]

Tenet 6:

Correct nutritional imbalances as well as deficiencies to optimize nutrient metabolism and lower risk of chronic disease.

In the US, the Institute of Medicine (IOM) and the National Academy of Sciences make recommendations in the form of Dietary Reference Intakes (DRIs), Recommended Dietary Allowances (RDAs) and Adequate Intakes (AIs) that, in theory, should be sufficient for the health of individuals. These are, in the terminology of the IOM, "estimate average requirements" (EAR) for individuals. The RDA is calculated to be the EAR plus two standard deviations of the EAR. There are a number of challenges in the use of DRIs, RDAs and AIs. [267-270] For example, none of the recently reviewed RDAs were based on the risk of chronic disease, even given the fact that nutrition is recognized as an important factor in the development of many chronic diseases. In addition, the EAR is defined as the daily intake of a particular nutrient which is estimated to be adequate in 50% of a given population or subpopulation of individuals who are apparently healthy. By this definition, 50% of that given population or subpopulation are <u>not</u> receiving an adequate intake, a situation that may be compounded for populations chronically receiving very low intake levels. In general, the risk of inadequate intake can range from 0% to 100%, based on statistical considerations and is dependent on various individual factors. [269,270] EARs have not yet been defined for a number of nutrients, including Vitamin K, pantothenic acid, biotin, choline, chromium, fluoride, manganese and others. [271] There is currently a lack of sufficient evidence for the determination of DRIs based on an endpoint of chronic disease, including cancer, diabetes, cardiovascular disease and osteoporosis, among others. [270] In addition, many DRIs are based on intake, absorption and retention data rather than bioavailability data, which, arguably, may be a more accurate determinant. [272,273]

Nutrient insufficiencies may be defined as nutrient intakes that are inadequate for optimal health for the individual. Nutrient deficiencies may be defined as nutrient intakes that are so low as to cause index disease, such as rickets (Vitamin D deficiency), pellagra (Vitamin B_3/niacin deficiency) or some forms of blindness (Vitamin A deficiency). Given the focus of dietetics and integrative medicine towards prevention and given the issues concerning the guidelines on nutrient intake, it is believed that addressing both insufficiencies and deficiencies provide the most rational approach to maintaining the health of the individual.

Tenet 7:

Manage the inflammation of chronic disease through food and targeted nutrients.

Inflammation is well recognized as one of the main underlying processes in chronic disease as well as a normal response to environmental, homeostatic (e.g. cellular debris) and pathogenic insults. [274-286] While the inflammatory response is normal and necessary, chronic and persistent systemic inflammation is the result of the lack or failure of immune regulatory mechanisms to turn off the response.

The inflammatory response can be thought of as part of the innate immune system—the evolutionarily conserved arm of the immune response. Classically, the external signs of acute inflammation are *rubor, calor, dolor* and *tumor*, but internally, inflammation can take a more chronic and destructive non-resolving course. If the cascade of biochemical, immunological and physiologic responses become dysregulated and the inflammation becomes systemic, tissues, organs and systems may be significantly damaged. [282,287,288] In addition, it is becoming clear that oxidative stress exacerbates inflammation and is, in many cases, causal. [289] Additionally, aging can be considered to be the accumulation of damage due to both inflammatory processes and the result of oxidative stress and can be ameliorated with targeted dietary and nutritional approaches. [290,291]

DIM utilizes evidence-based research indicating that diet and nutrition can have a significant effect on chronic inflammation. [292-295] Various physiologic variables such as inflammation, renal function, states of fasting, and pregnancy have been associated with biomarkers of nutritional status. [296] For example, in chronic inflammation, both water- and fat-soluble vitamin levels decrease, while ferritin, total body iron and urinary iodine levels increase.[296] Dietary intake of isoflavones (daidzein, gensitein) and lignans has been shown to be inversely related to levels of C-reactive protein, an inflammatory marker. [292,294,296] Obesity is considered an inflammatory disorder most associated with increased visceral adipose tissue (VAT) now known as an endocrine organ secreting pro-inflammatory molecules. [297,298] Weight loss has been associated with a decrease in pro-inflammatory markers, cytokines and the reported normalization of thyroid hormones. [269-273,275,280,282,284]

The list of chronic diseases that may be significantly affected by diet and targeted nutrition is long and is growing longer with expanded research in this area. Disorders and inflammatory conditions such as obesity, diabetes, cardiovascular disease, metabolic syndrome, neurological disorders and dementias, arthritis and gout, epilepsy and others have been shown to respond to targeted dietary interventions.[113,264,277,278,281,285,286,299] Including concepts of oxidative stress adds more layers to the potential targets of nutritional and dietary interventions.

Management of chronic disease is an important and growing health concern. The AND's *Council on Future Practice Visioning Report,* in 2011,[300] and again in 2015, *Change Drivers and Trends Driving the Profession: A Prelude to the Visioning Report 2017,* [301] identified the need for the Chronic Disease Management Nutrition Specialist. The roles are currently evolving and will provide unique opportunities for specially trained RDs now and in the future. Recommendation #7 (2011) of the same report supports the "continuing development of advanced practice credentials for the nutrition and dietetics profession, based on objective evidence."

> *Interprofessional Education (IPE) informs a pedagogy and curricula redesign for preparing a new health care workforce capable of optimizing health system performance in a collaborative-ready, shared decision making model. All health professions should integrate IPE into their curricula to prepare practitioners with the knowledge and skills to be effective 21st century members of the healthcare team. Professions that remain uninformed, outdated and static are at-risk of being left behind. IPE offers RDNs a significant advantage in securing a place at the "health care table."*
>
> *Change Drivers and Trends Driving the Profession: A Prelude to the Visioning Report 2017*

Tenet 8:

Use of targeted nutrient therapies can reduce toxin damage to metabolism.

Some toxins have likely always been in the human environment. Historically, the general principle in toxicology is that dose often separates a toxic material from the non-toxic material. With the newer understanding of chronic exposure of low-dose toxins called hormesis, there are types of toxins that are disadvantageous: chemicals like POPs and radiation, that could harm humans by endocrine disruption, action of chemical mixtures and susceptible populations.[302,303] For example, Arsenic, asbestos and mercury are toxic metals, and naturally occurring toxins can be found in food—hydrazines are found in raw mushrooms, and the toxin ergot produced by the mold *Claviceps purpurea* infects rye and other grains. Goitrogens are found in soybeans, nuts, millet, fruits and vegetables from the *Brassica* family—bok choy, broccoli, cabbage, cauliflower and others. Lectins are found in high levels in many seeds, grains and legumes. Aflatoxins are produced by the fungus, *Aspergillus*.

However, humans have evolved with a number of mechanisms to avoid natural toxins, including bitter taste, neutralizing enzymes, DNA repair mechanisms and toxin-induced resistance mechanisms such as increased efflux from intestinal epithelium. [304-309] On the other hand, humans have not evolved mechanisms to cope with the vast number of synthetic chemicals in our environment and used on our foods. The mass of man-made chemicals has been estimated to be over 160 billion kilograms.[310] Over 84,000 synthetic substances are registered with the US Environmental Protection Agency (EPA) yet very few have been thoroughly tested for their potential health effects, either in the short or long term. The testing process is long and, some would argue, cumbersome. For example, the assessment regarding the use of the pesticide N-methyl carbamate required 9,721 individual tolerance reassessment decisions to comply with the Food Quality Protection Act (FQPA) of 1996.[311] In addition, many of these chemicals have been protected from public review because of a classification as "Confidential Business Information", or CBI. In February of 2013, the EPA increased the public's access to this information—but, there still remain over 7,000 chemical compounds where the health and safety information is still classified as confidential. [312]

Tenets 1 and 2 of dietetics and integrative medicine emphasize the individualized approach to integrative and functional medical nutrition therapy (IFMNT) as well as the genomic uniqueness of each individual. Genomic uniqueness also presupposes unique responses to exo- and endo-toxins. Targeted and individualized nutritional therapies have the potential to aid in detoxification, support eliminatory systems, including the liver, gallbladder, kidney, skin and intestines and reduce inflammation in chronic conditions. These targeted approaches can also be utilized to prevent the rise of chronic conditions. [73,77,313-321]

Detoxification is a holistic process and should include, in addition to the use of herbs, probiotics, HCL and enzymes along with targeted foods and nutrients, minimization of exposure in the home, workplace or school. It also should include lifestyle modification where at-risk behaviors are altered to increase rest, sleep and efficiency of stress management techniques, all areas where the specialist in dietetics and integrative medicine can have an impact.

Tenet 9:
Beliefs and community relationships influence nutritional health (mind-body).

Mind-body medicine, although a relatively new understanding to western medicine, refers to the interrelationships between mental health, spiritual health and physical health. Holistic practitioners of all ancient traditions have practiced a form of mind-body medicine. Integrative medicine is bringing a renewed respect for its importance in health and disease.

Cultural, religious and societal belief systems impact nutritional health - ranging from the food choices made, how they are prepared, how and when they are eaten as well as the attitudes towards dieting, nutrition and what it means to "eat well".

Many cultures have periods of caloric restrictions or fasting. Individual attitudes toward interventions vary depending on the cultural background and belief system of the individual. For example, during the month of Ramadan, however, many physicians are reluctant to encourage their diabetic patients to fast. In other cultures, caloric restriction may be viewed less positively. Caloric restriction, however, has shown great promise for detoxification and the overall improvement of health and the treatment of diabetes, obesity and cardiovascular disease. [322-333]

Further, many disorders have a mind-body component that cannot be ignored by a nutritional specialist. Stress is an important factor in a broad range of chronic disorders and must be considered when planning nutritional strategies. [334-347]

The fields of psychoneuroimmunology and psychoneuroendocrinology are a reminder of the interrelatedness of biological systems. Homeodynamics is dependent on both endogenous and exogenous signals and how those signals are interpreted by an individual mind based on their individual life experiences. All these considerations are important—especially on an individual level—because one size definitely does not fit all.

Tenet 10:
Know when you are not the expert. Collaborate with other members of the integrative care team.

As there may be various etiologies in the health condition of a patient, all members of the healthcare team are skilled in their expertise and scope of practice, and each able to recognize when to refer to another member of the team to best address the patient's health needs. The nutritionist is sometimes the first practitioner to see a patient, and while assessing priorities may identify non-nutrition therapies that need first attention. It is the interdisciplinary appreciation of working together that provides the timing and effectiveness of therapies to facilitate the healing journey of the patient. The ethics of appropriate health care demand, in a sense, the subjugation of the individual ego for the good of the patient, recognizes the high level of functioning for patient care when working together with the expertise present in the various member of the healthcare team.

DIM Program Development

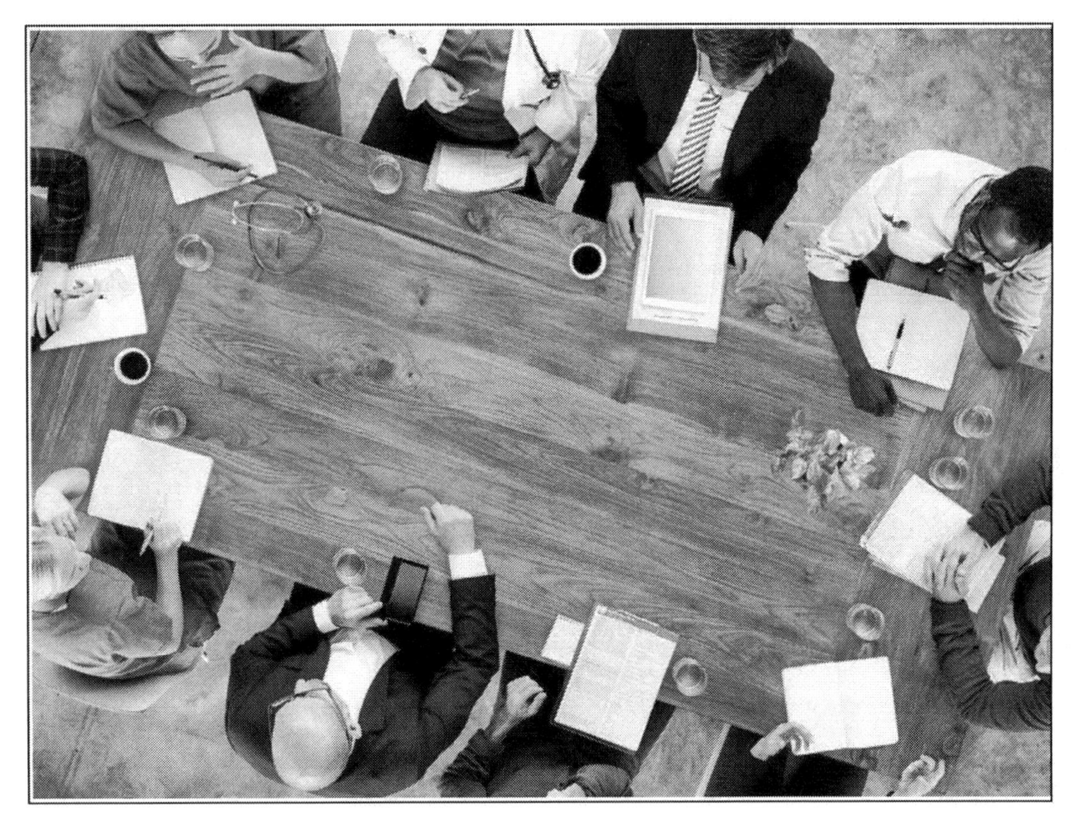

Rationale

Feasibility

Staffing

Funding

Section 2

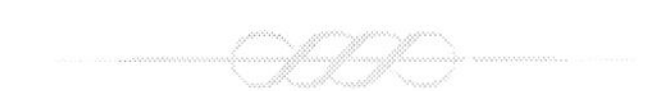

RATIONALE FOR DIETETIC AND INTEGRATIVE MEDICINE PROGRAMS

THE DIETETICS AND INTEGRATIVE MEDICINE PROGRAM - RATIONALE

In the process of deciding to create the DIM program, there were two main questions to be answered:

The **first** was whether it was feasible to create a program at the University of Kansas Medical Center (KUMC) that combined advances in the practice of dietetics and nutrition with those of Integrative Medicine?

The **second** was to provide evidence-based, practice-based and science-based rationales for this training that could then be applied to other potential programs across the country and across the world, emphasizing the central role of dietetics and nutrition in the treatment and prevention of chronic, or non-communicable, diseases.

The two main questions were vetted and deemed valid for KUMC. Each facility considering developing an integrative track in their dietetics programs will study their unique attributes and customize the basics to their needs.

At KUMC, the DIM track of the Dietetic Internship (DI) program and the Dietetic and Integrative Medicine graduate certificate program developed, were designed to allow the interested student to obtain a Master's degree in Dietetics and Nutrition along with the additional Dietetics and Integrative Medicine (DIM) graduate certificate. These programs also fulfill some of the eligibility requirements for taking the registered dietician-nutritionist (RDN) certification exam.

evidence-based:

A series of guiding statements and treatment algorithms which are developed using a systematic process for identifying, analyzing and synthesizing scientific evidence. Evidence-based dietetics practice is about asking questions, systematically finding research evidence, and assessing the validity, applicability and importance of that evidence.

Academy of Nutrition and Dietetics 2016

practice-based:

Concerns the way professionals apply their specific expertise to particular cases and synergistically use their experiences to systematically build their expertise. Practice-based use of evidence involves the synthesis of the literature and the guidance and/or recommendations for everyday practice skills from experienced dietitian-nutritionists and mentors. *The evidence-based information is combined with the dietitian's expertise and judgment and the client's or community's unique values and circumstances to guide decision-making in dietetics.*

International Federation of Dietetic Association 2010

science based:

Strong consideration in the Nutrition Care Process of the science of human metabolism and physiology by incorporating current knowledge of disease pathophysiology, potentially identified in the blood before or while experiencing symptoms, and the networking of all physiological systems to promote optimum health based on imbalances and dysfunction identified.

CURRENT NEED FOR INCREASED EDUCATION IN DIETETICS AND INTEGRATIVE MEDICINE

Given the world-wide epidemic in non-communicable diseases, the nutritional training deficit that is evident in a significant numbers of physicians, and the increasing interest from the general public as well as other health professionals, nutritionists and dietitians are well situated to provide the needed nutritional and dietetic knowledge and services.

In addition, nutritionists and dietitians who have specialized training for working as part of a team in partnership with integrative physicians are even more ideally situated to fill this need. The term coined by the Dietitians in Integrative Medicine, a DPG of the Academy of Nutrition and Dietetics, synonymous with Dietetics and Integrative Medicine, is "Integrative and Functional Medicine Nutrition Therapy" (IFMNT) as described in Figure 5.

WHY DO WE NEED THE DIM AND IFMNT MODELS OF DIETETICS PRACTICE?

* The prevalence of complex, chronic diseases is escalating globally, from heart disease and diabetes to irritable bowel syndrome, chronic fatigue, fibromyalgia, mental illness, and rheumatoid arthritis and other autoimmune disorders.
* Chronic disease is diet- and lifestyle-related disease and requires solutions in diet and lifestyle. A major strength of integrative and functional nutrition is its focus on the molecular mechanisms that underlie disease, which provides the basis for targeted, innovative solutions that can restore health.
* The current healthcare system fails to account for the unique genetic makeup of each individual or the ability of foods, toxins, and other environmental factors to influence gene expression. The interaction between genes and environmental factors is a critical component in the development of chronic disease and plays a central role in the integrative and functional nutrition approach.
* Most nutrition professionals are not adequately trained in integrating nutrition assessment at the molecular and cellular levels with emerging research in nutrition and nutritional genomics. These advanced practice skills are essential for preventing and managing today's chronic disorders.

THE IFMNT RADIAL GUIDE

The Dietitians in Integrative and Functional Medicine (DIFM) "Standards of Practice (SOP) and Standards of Professional Performance (SOPP) in Integrative and Functional Medicine" were published in the June 2011 issue of the Journal of the American Dietetic Association. The SOP address personalized nutrition care, and activities related to person-centered care. The SOPP are authoritative statements that describe a competent level of behavior in the professional role. The Integrative and Functional Medicine Nutrition Therapy (IFMNT) Radial (Figure 5) was established as an integrated conceptual framework to assist in IFMNT practice. The circular architecture of the IFMNT Radial allows for the evaluation of complex interactions and interrelationships. The Radial depicts that food is a determining factor in health and disease and is a source of biological information that influences, and is influenced by, the five key areas. The five key areas are: Lifestyle, Systems (Signs and Symptoms), Core Imbalances, Metabolic Pathways, and Biomarkers surrounding the Radial are precipitating factors that can affect the metabolism of an individual.

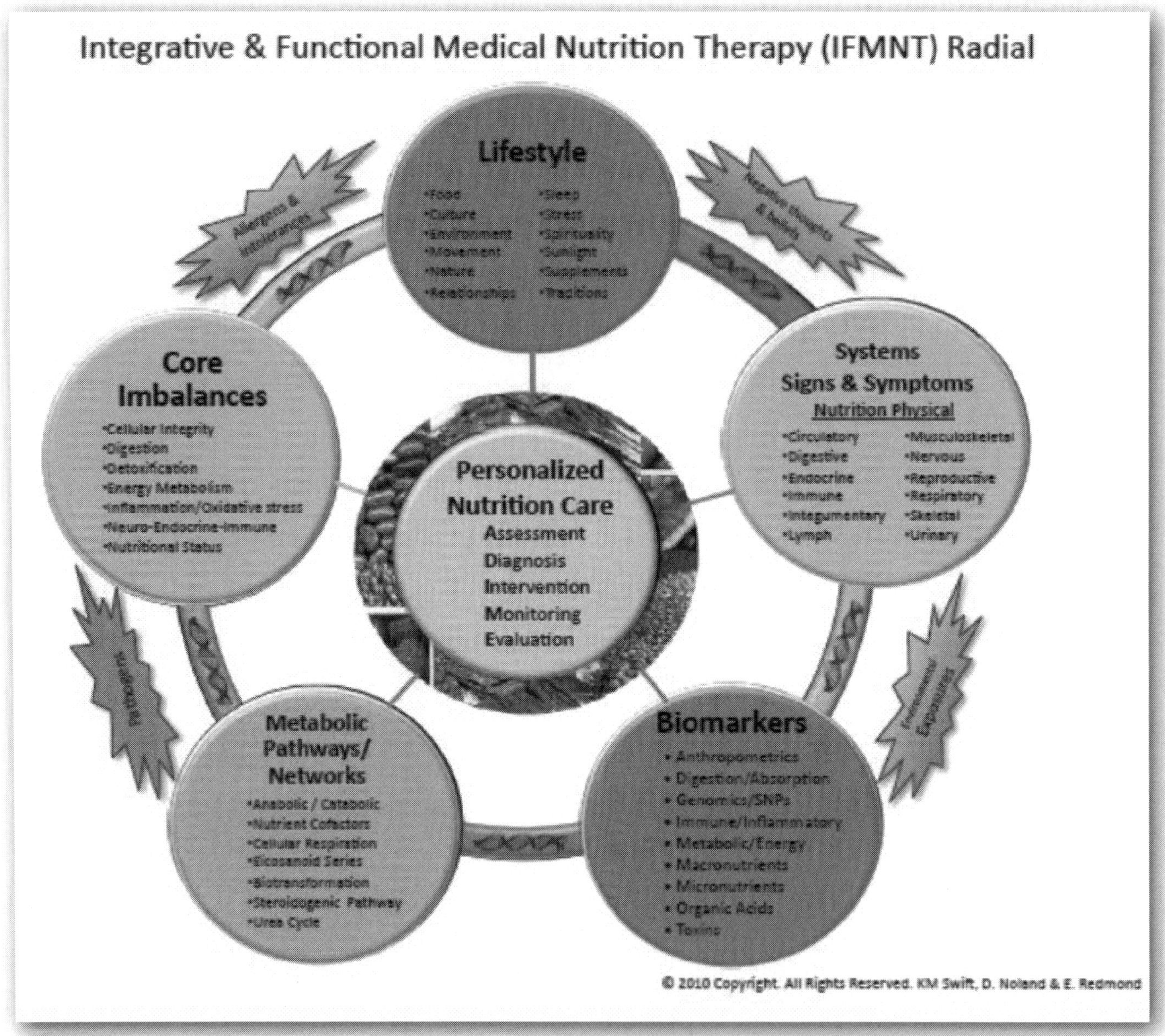

Figure 5: The IFMNT Radial

PDF available in the Appendix

Section 3

DIETETICS AND INTEGRATIVE MEDICINE CURRICULUM DEVELOPMENT

DIM TRAINING
OVERVIEW

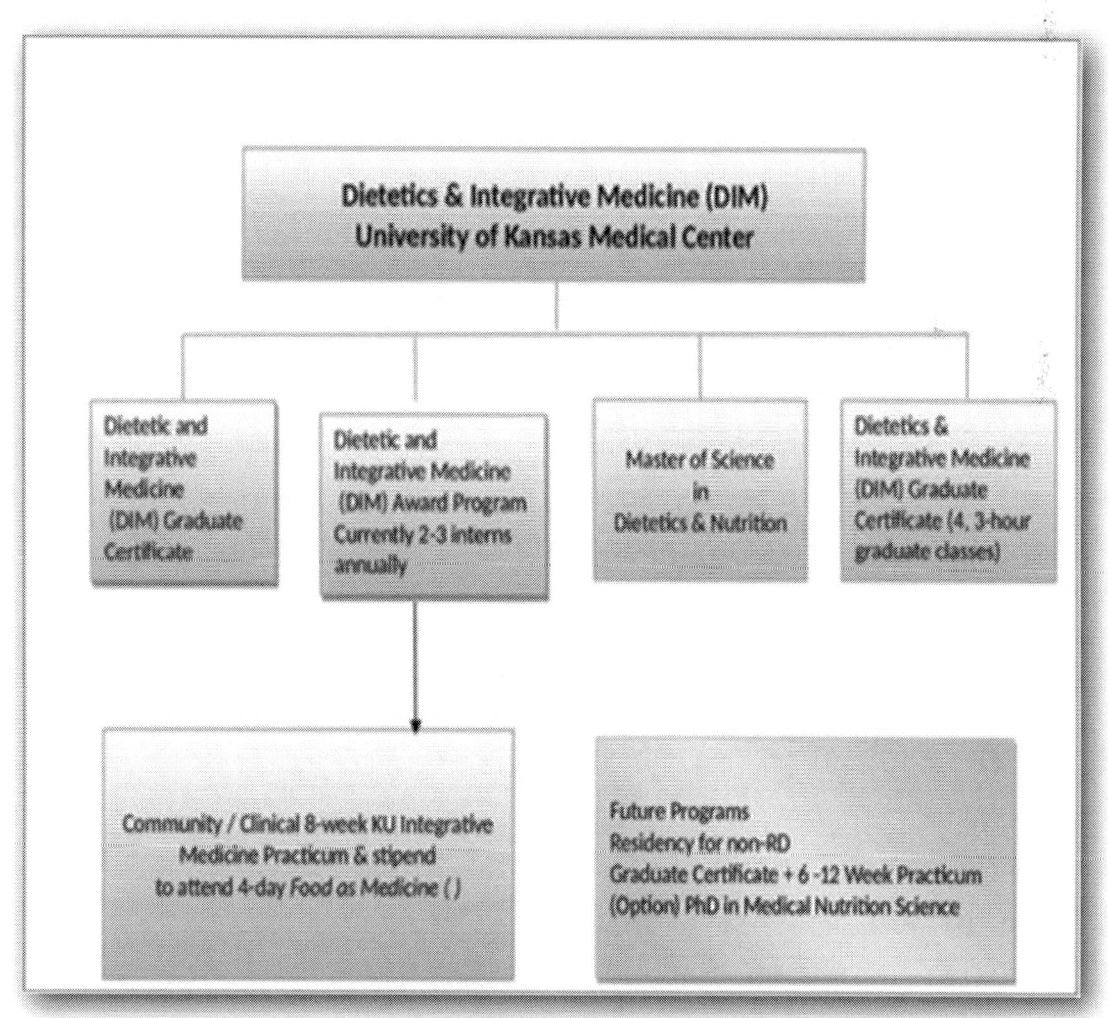

Figure 6: DIM Organization KUMC

PDF available in the Appendix

DIM practice can be complex because it focuses on the individual and attempts to identify underlying causes for symptoms or conditions. DIM patients are often in poor health and interventions require major changes in diet and lifestyle. These changes are necessary to allow for healing and to improve possible underlying metabolic causes of chronic health conditions or disease. While DIM practice can be complex, it focuses on some simple principles: the use of real, whole foods our bodies are designed to recognize and will promote optimal health, as well as identifying lifestyle factors influencing metabolic health such as sleep, activity, beliefs.

Biochemical individuality is a foundational tenet of Dietetics and Integrative Medicine (DIM); each person has a different lifestyle, family, culture, community, genetic makeup. In effect, each person has a different nutritional status. DIM interventions are specific for each individual and are based on an individual nutrition assessment. The DIM internship will provide experiences in the clinical, community and food service rotations. Individualized care is accomplished more easily in a **clinical setting**, working one on one with a client or patient.

CLINICAL TRAINING

The dietitian or nutritionist practicing in integrative medicine represents a nutrition professional skilled in practicing an advanced level of clinical nutrition in using diet and lifestyle approaches, including nutritional genomics and motivational interviewing, for preventing and managing chronic disease. This specialty knowledge and advanced skills are unique within healthcare and able to participate within healthcare in ways never before possible until current technological and scientific discoveries of the twenty years.

For nutrition-minded practitioners to achieve the necessary skill-base, clinical training in dietetics must make available the integrative approach in dietetics education. To expand current nutrition and dietetic clinical training, standards of faculty preparation, curriculum and clinic practicum sites demonstrating the integrative medicine interdisciplinary team and practices must be established. This publication describes the development of one model for which an integrative dietetic or nutrition track may be established within an already existing education program, to avoid "reinventing-the-wheel" and building on existing strong programs in the basics of nutrition science and therapeutic implementation.

KUMC was recognized in 2011 as possessing an excellent infrastructure to house the development of the first development of this envisioned model. A key component was the collaboration between the KU Integrative Medicine active clinic with the innovative Dietetics and Nutrition department within the School of Allied Professions, along with the physical infrastructure of the clinics and dietetic practicum sites. And, lastly, the clinic and faculty skills and willingness to teach and inspire the students to consider a new view of nutrition therapy. This is done by adding the more personalized assessment skills and interventions of integrative medicine to build on the existing nutritional biochemistry knowledge.

The students selected to be placed in the intense DIM Award Program training are scheduled to spend a 6- week long practicum immersed in the KU Integrative Medicine clinic shadowing the DIM Registered Dietitians and other MD, NP, and ND. They then have the option of choosing to spend their elective summer experience returning to the KU Integrative Medicine clinic for another 2-4 weeks of advanced specialty clinical training. Thus, these experiences will help the participant *think like a DIM specialist* throughout each dietetic internship rotation, including rotations in the Infusion Clinic, with medical doctors and MD fellows in the clinic, with a naturopathic physician, neurofeedback practitioners, acupuncturist, massage therapist and other outside practitioners.

COMMUNITY COMMITMENT

In the **community setting,** Dietetics and Integrative Medicine is more challenging as the DIM specialist is working with a population in which a single intervention may be appropriate only part of the time. Subsequent monitoring and evaluation of the initial intervention may prove difficult due to transient patients not being geared for return visits. Other facilities may have other community settings for practicum sites that provide less transient patients for longer term monitoring and evaluation.

FOOD SERVICE

In **food service management**, the DIM specialist prioritizes the use of the highest quality whole foods to promote healing, i.e., to use "food as medicine" in providing food for populations. Each Dietetic Internship rotation – clinical, community and food service – will emphasize and use varying degrees of the DIM tenets considering low-toxin food choices and preparation equipment as well as providing demonstrations to empower patients to incorporate these DIM tenets into their own lifestyle.

DIM ACCREDITED INTERNSHIPS

AND accredited dietetic internship (DI) programs require the completion of 24 graduate credit hours and 1,200 hours of supervised practice in a variety of practice settings. At KUMC graduate DI program, all of the 16 dietetic interns receive three intensive workshops during the 11-month internship with the emphasis on integrative medical nutrition therapy including practice experience in clinical and community nutrition, and food and nutrition management. In addition, a practice area-of-interest optional experience can be designed by the intern to meet their personal, professional and educational goals. Interns are able to choose from a variety of practice sites for each experience and are encouraged to submit ideas for new practice sites to the program director.

Students completing the dietetic internship program receive a graduate certificate from the University of Kansas. They are then eligible to apply for approval by the Commission on Dietetic Registration to take the national Registration Examination for Dietitians. KU has a proven record in producing top-level professionals, as evidenced by the first-time pass rate of 98.8% (2011-2015) by our graduates on the national Registration Examination for Dietitians. One year pass rate for five years is 100% (2011-2015).

There are more than 45 clinical education affiliations in the metropolitan Kansas City and surrounding areas as well as opportunities for international experiences. Practice sites include The University of Kansas Hospital, KU Weight Management, Children's Mercy Hospital and Clinics, VA Medical Center, KU Athletics, grocery stores, public schools, health departments, and others provide unique and flexible opportunities for the student to follow their interest while completing their internship requirements.

OPTION FOR MASTER'S DEGREE

Students are strongly encouraged to enter KU's Master of Science in Dietetics and Nutrition program upon completion of the Dietetic Internship graduate certificate program. Graduates of the dietetic internship program need an additional 16-19 hours to finish the master's degree.

DIM AWARD PROGRAM FOR DIETETIC INTERNS

Currently, there are two to three funded annual awards with a stipend available for those who qualify for the DIM internship and submit an application.

Award recipients participate in supervised practice experiences emphasizing Dietetics and Integrative Medicine along with other required dietetic internship experiences. The program provides award recipients intensive exposure to clinical, educational, and research activities in collaboration with the KUMC Integrative Medicine Department.

Those DIM award students are involved in clinical care at integrative medicine clinics, educational pursuits, and research related to Dietetics and Integrative Medicine. Students contribute to building the KU Integrative Medicine nutrition program. During the second-year, award students choosing an MS option complete the MS in Dietetics and Nutrition along with the DIM certificate. Award students are strongly encouraged to complete a thesis based on research conducted in the area of Dietetics and Integrative Medicine.

DIM GRADUATE CERTIFICATE ONLINE PROGRAM

KU's Dietetics and Integrative Medicine graduate certificate online 12-hour program offers an opportunity for working professionals or graduate students to acquire the knowledge to function as a skilled advisor to a patient and as a collaborative member of multidisciplinary health care teams. The program is open to students with bachelor's or master's degrees in dietetics, nutrition, biological sciences or other healthcare disciplines.

The program imparts DIM principles and a personalized approach to prevention and treatment of chronic disease that embraces conventional and complementary therapies. It reaffirms the importance of the therapeutic relationship, a focus on the whole person, lifestyle, biochemical individuality and environmental influences.

This is an online program only, with no campus visits required. The 12 credit hours are delivered as web-based courses, affording great flexibility to students. The curriculum includes the following four courses, with one course offered per semester:

* DN 880 Dietary and Herbal Supplements (3 hours)
* DN 881 Introduction to Dietetics and Integrative Medicine (3 hours)
* DN 882 A Nutrition Approach to Inflammation and Immune Regulation (3 hours)
* DN 980 Nutrigenomics and Nutrigenetics in Health and Disease (3 hours)

DIM-EMPHASIS MASTER OF SCIENCE DEGREE PROGRAMS

Students have the option to further their training by obtaining an MS degree. The MS degree requires an additional 19 hours for thesis students or 16 hours for non-thesis students. The DIM graduate certificate requires the completion of an additional 9-12 hours of web-based, self-paced, online courses (depending on MS electives chosen).

Admission Requirements to the DIM Programs can be viewed on the KUMC website *dietetics.kumc.edu*, : http://www.kumc.edu/school-of-health-professions/dietetics-and-nutrition.html.

A Note on the Terms Used

* **Dietetics and Integrative Medicine is the KUMC Dietetics and Nutrition Department's "umbrella" term.**
* **KUMC Dietetic Intern (DI) options: www.dietetics.kumc.edu**
  - **DIM Award Program Apply for an Award and stipend. 2-3 positions are awarded annually for dietetic interns and M.S. nutrition students.**
  - **Dietetics and Integrative Medicine Graduate Certificate (online) can be obtained by a KUMC dietetic intern, graduate nutrition student, or non-KUMC health professional. Dietetic interns can obtain the DIM certificate with an additional 12 hours of online courses. Tuition fees are in-state for KUMC Online courses.**
  - **MS in Dietetics and Nutrition – An option for dietetic interns and Award recipients with additional coursework and research. 14 hours of dietetic internship credit can be transferred to the MS degree.**
  - **PhD in Medical Nutrition Science for qualifying student after obtaining an undergraduate or a graduate degree, depending on the area of study of the degree (nutrition, biological sciences or other areas of study).**
* **DIFM (Dietitians in Integrative and Functional Medicine) is the term the Academy of Nutrition and Dietetics (AND) uses to describe the DIFM Dietetic Practice Group (DPG). www.integrativeRD.org**

FEASIBILITY FOR AN ACADEMIC CENTER

Recognizing the importance of dietetics and nutrition in integrative medicine, and the importance of continuing education in those fields, the University of Kansas' Integrative Medicine department, under the direction of Jeanne Drisko, MD, initiated a feasibility study (Phase 1), and led by Diana Noland, MPH RDN CCN LD. The goal of this study was to examine the potential for:

a) Expansion of the University of Kansas' degree and certificate programs in dietetics and nutrition
b) Incorporation of these programs into the KUMC Dietetics and Nutrition Department
c) A model of collaboration between Dietetics and Integrative Medicine departments

If achieved, these goals would fulfill a perceived need within the professional dietetic community by providing continuing professional education for those dietitians and nutritionists who would be particularly interested in combining the most recent advances in nutritional sciences with integrative and functional medical principles. These overall goals also emphasize the principles of the anonymous private foundation that generously provided funds for the DIM program and DIM Award Program as a part of its support for individuals and non-profit organizations that focus on the human potential, on issues of social justice, the environment, and health. Nutrition, particularly the relationship of nutrition to health, wellness and the prevention and treatment of chronic disease, is a high priority with the foundation, which supports both educational and training programs in integrative and functional nutrition for nutritional, dietetic and medical professionals.

The feasibility study, which was completed in 2011, answered two fundamental questions in the affirmative:

* Dietetic and Integrative Medicine Internships, Award certificates and a Master's degree program can fill an urgent and pressing need in dietetic education.
* These programs could be implemented in a practical manner, taking into account accrediting regulations, future continued collaboration between KUMC departments, potential sources of funding, prospective needs for faculty staffing and the overall time involved.

Initially, the feasibility study was undertaken with the stated goals of investigating the viability of a number of programs to be instituted through and within the University of Kansas Medical Center (KUMC), the Dietetics and Nutrition department of the School of Allied Health Professions, and with the Kansas University (KU) Integrative Medicine program. These planned programs were:

* A Dietetic Internship program (DI)
* A Dietetic and Integrative Medicine (DIM) graduate certificate program[1] (12 hours)
* A Dietetic and Integrative Medicine (DIM) Award Program (dietetic internship, DIM Grad Certificate and M.S. degree)

These three unique specialty-training tracks could lead the interested candidate to a Master of Science (M.S.) in Dietetics and Nutrition (DN), Registered Dietitian credential, and the DIM Graduate Certificate. All would focus on the DIM Ten Tenets (Part I) applied to Dietetics and Nutrition, and the role of dietetics and nutrition in the prevention and

1 The University of Kansas, Board of Regents designates non-MD graduate programs as "certificates" rather than fellowships.

treatment of a variety of chronic diseases with inflammatory and immune components, as well as chronic diseases where long-term latent nutritional deficiencies, toxic loads, lifestyle and cellular energetics play an important role.

The University of Kansas department of Dietetics and Nutrition has identified a number of areas in Dietetics and Integrative Medicine where these specially trained professionals could have a profound impact:

* Providing Integrative and Function Medical Nutrition Therapy (IFMNT) in medical clinics in cooperation with an integrative physician.
* Private practice: working under contract with health care or food companies or in their own businesses.
* Sports nutrition and corporate wellness programs, providing preventative services and educating clients about the connections between nutrition, physical activity and health.
* Food and nutrition-related business and industries working in communications, consumer affairs, public relations, marketing product development or consulting with restaurants and culinary schools.
* International Public Health Nutrition
* Research
* Education

INFRASTRUCTURE, DEPARTMENTAL COLLABORATION, REGULATORY APPROVAL AND ACCREDITATION

Full accreditation from the Commission on Accreditation for Dietetics Education of the American Academy of Nutrition and Dietetics (AND) has been in place since 1943, with recertification occurring every 7 years.

FOUNDATIONS OF TRAINING

Registered dietitians and nutritionists educate their patients and clients about the fundamentals of nutrition, assess an individual's health and dietary needs and develop appropriate meal plans, and perform evaluations regarding the success of the plans. They may work in a private practice, a hospital, the community, health-care facility, journalism, or the food industry.

Specialists in dietetics and integrative medicine take a holistic and global approach to provide a *personalized* nutrition care process including the new field of clinical application of nutrigenomics. The DIM program follows the Institute for Functional Medicine's (IFM) Matrix Model™, actively incorporating concepts of systems biology and systems physiology, antecedents or predisposing factors, and triggering or activation events, while always recognizing that an equilibrium and homeostasis exists between and amongst the systems. The physiological systems considered throughout all tracks within the DIM program are:

* Oxidative/Reductive Hemodynamics
* Detoxification and Biotransformation
* Hormone and Neurotransmitter Regulation
* Psychological and Spiritual Equilibrium
* Structural and Membrane Integrity
* Digestion and Absorption
* Immune Surveillance and Inflammatory process

In addition, the IFM Matrix™ takes into account the individual's nutritional status, levels of physical activity, sleeps habits, significant relationships, and that individual's set(s) of beliefs and self-care principles.

The specialist in dietetics and integrative medicine is also, as specified in Tenet 10, a member of a collaborative team of integrative medicine health-care professionals, wherein the input and knowledge of team members can inform the nutritional approach. The DIM specialist is involved in the advanced practice of nutrition assessment (including at the cellular and molecular levels), diagnosis, intervention, and monitoring (also at the molecular and cellular levels) that focuses on the promotion of optimal health and the management and prevention of diet- and lifestyle-related diseases.

COMMUNITY INVOLVEMENT

The KU Dietetics and Integrative Medicine – or DIM– certification program also involves active work in Community Supported Agriculture (CSA) and sustainability programs that are based on the belief that optimal nutrition starts with sustainably grown foods. A CSA is a program of "community of individuals who pledge support to a farm operation so that the farmland becomes, either legally or spiritually, the community's farm, with the growers and consumers providing mutual support and sharing the risks and benefits of food production. Typically, the members, or "share-holders", of the farm or garden pledge in advance to cover the anticipated costs of the farm operation and farmer's salary. In return, they receive shares in the farm's bounty throughout the growing season, as well as the satisfaction gained from reconnecting to the land and participating directly in food production. Members also share in the risks of farming, including poor harvests due to unfavorable weather or pests. By direct sales to community members, who have provided the farmer with working capital in advance, growers "receive better prices for their crops, gain some financial security, and are relieved of much of the burden of marketing."[348]

Another component of the community practicum is the concept of the Healing Kitchen, where program participants and members of the community learn the practical aspects of the whole foods principles, advancing the use of nutritious, unprocessed foods, community involvement, environmental stewardship to prevent, treat and heal. The exposure to and use of the Healing Kitchen housed within the KU Integrative Medicine clinic during the Dietetics and Integrative Medicine Practicum are critical elements in the training of specialists in dietetics and integrative medicine.

Finally, this community involvement extends to concerns of public health and the community-wide effects of obesity, diabetes, cardiovascular disease, depression and other chronic conditions that impact the individual, the family, the community and the nation. The DIM community influence involves integration with local and state public policy-legislative regulations regarding food and dietetics/nutrition practice laws. Upon certification, the individual will be armed with the tools to "spread the word" around their communities and in their daily practice.

PROFESSIONAL DEVELOPMENT OF THE FACULTY

FACULTY TEACHING RESPONSIBILITIES

Proper staffing of all aspects of the DIM-related educational experiences determines the quality and depth of education the students will receive during their time spent in the DIM program. As an educational institution embarks on developing a program track of teaching an integrative medicine based in systems biology, it is fundamental to the success of the program to acquire professional faculty and assistants that embrace and support the concepts described in the Ten Tenets of DIM. To ensure perpetuity of any DIM program, a document titled "*Standards of Dietetics and Integrative Medicine for Preceptors/Instructors*" was developed to describe basic requirements for the primary faculty and instructors involved in the program. Without a commitment to these standards there is a risk the original developers of the DIM program with be replaced as time goes on by those not retaining and envisioning the concepts of DIM.

TEACHING THE DIM ASSESSMENT OF THE PATIENT/CLIENT

Integral to the DIM and IFMNT assessment approach is a holistic understanding of an individual's past and current dietary habits in addition to a complete medical history (including family history) and current and past recreational drug and medication use (necessary to determine potential drug-induced nutrient deficiencies (DINDs)). The assessment may include food records (diet diary), questionnaires regarding food frequencies, allergies and sensitivities, aversions and cravings. The assessment also includes a detailed biochemical profile, a physical examination emphasizing signs and symptoms of nutrient deficiencies noted in the eyes, skin, nails, mouth and tongue, and physical measurements of body height, weight, BMI, and percentages of body fat. Macro- and micro-nutrient assessment can also be determined through assessing all the nutrition data collected including nutritional imbalances identified through biochemical testing

Other data is also evaluated as part of a holistic practice, including individual and family attitudes toward food and eating, cultural and/or religious and spiritual practices and behaviors, financial resources, history of toxic exposures, and the patient's overall understanding of basic nutritional principles.

This information is compiled, along with a history of physical exercise and activity levels, to develop a comprehensive overview of the individual's macro- and micro-nutritional needs, deficiencies, strengths, weaknesses and potential nutritional and dietetic approaches to dietary modifications, supplementation, specialized diets, and specific modes of administration including by enteral or parenteral (e.g. IV infusion) means.

A critical and unique aspect of the IFMNT approach central to these graduate programs is the incorporation of concepts derived from functional medicine and systems biology. The individual's unique genomic and epigenomic background, detoxification and energy balance, inflammatory load, and the overall function of their immune system are all considered in order to form a more complete patient story.

EDUCATION FOR THE PATIENT/CLIENT

Education is a critical component in any integrative and functional medical nutrition therapy. The educational approach can range from the didactic—the presentation of basic nutritional information, to the practical—cooking classes or tours of local healthy food stores, for example. In addition, the educational process may be counselor-led or self-paced, depending on the patient's particular needs and goals.

THE THERAPEUTIC RELATIONSHIP

It is much more important to know what sort of a patient has a disease than what sort of a disease a patient has.

William Osler

The *therapeutic relationship* is a concept within integrative medicine derived from many of the traditional medical disciplines like Traditional Chinese medicine *(TCM),* Ayurveda, Shamanism, and others. All recognize the importance of the practitioner understanding the patient's experience of his/her illness. A therapeutic relationship starts between the practitioner and client by eliciting all of their concerns. Recently it was described by Allen as "the cornerstone of practice" in the nursing profession.[349] It begins by creating a partnership to facilitate and empower the patient toward wellness. Research on doctor-patient interactions over the past twenty years indicates that doctors who fail to pay attention to the patient's concerns miss important clinical information.[350] In listening to the patient's story one discovers what underlies symptoms, signs, and pathophysiology. The therapeutic relationship is an integral part of the practice of dietetics and integrative medicine. Integrative medicine continues to strengthen this part of healing that recognizes the therapeutic relationship. There is a concern by the practitioner with the mediation needed to achieve peace and balance and, perhaps understanding the ultimate cause of the condition. Illness is viewed as an imbalance rather than a battle between "good genes" and "bad genes" or "good cholesterol" and "bad cholesterol". Genes and cholesterol are neither good nor bad—they simply are. As we are learning, however, we can influence the expression of these genes to positively impact the overall health and wellness of the patient. The practitioner who looks at and understands the possibilities of healing in a holistic way can benefit the process rather than force the process.

In developing a therapeutic relationship with a client, the action is the condition or illness, and the reaction should be the result of conscious choice and informed nutritional knowledge from the healer and the healed, rather than a reflexive attempt to "save" a patient. Balance is again the key. Both the specialist in dietetics and integrative medicine and the patient/client can learn from the experience. Everyone's experience of illness is different and is based on their experience with life. The therapeutic relationship, is above all, based on a respect and consideration of that person's experience with life as it is reflected in their physical, mental, emotional and spiritual selves.

Mindfulness, compassion, intent, love, acceptance, self-cultivation and intuition are all vital tools for the healer-practitioner. Ultimately, it is the patients' choice to be healed. A cure may or may not be possible, depending on the particular situation, and this must be faced, accepted and honored. Finally, an integrative practitioner must always be aware of the inherent healing power in the patient/client and the ultimate role that the patient's own choices have to play in their healing process. Accepting that as their patient's choice respects the patient so they are able to best deal with that choice. A non-judgmental stance, respecting the individuals' choices without having to agree with them will prove effective.

Often, those in the health professions are warned not to get too "involved" with the patient because of the perceived detriment to both the patient and the practitioner. This warning however, may be better applied to noting the difference between empathy and compassion for the patient which is a healing process and allows the patient dignity and freedom of choice as opposed to sympathy and enabling the patient which treats the patient as an object of pity and conversely limits dignity and choice.

FUNDING

The development of the KUMC DIM Internship, DIM Graduate Certificate, and DIM Award Program were funded by the generous donation of an anonymous private foundation. In developing a Dietetic and Integrative Medicine educational program, the necessary funding and in-kind costs should be identified during the feasibility study.

GRADUATE CERTIFICATE OF DIETETICS AND INTEGRATIVE MEDICINE

The graduate certification in DIM is an on-line program offered as a one year or 4 semester certificate with one class in fall, spring and two in summer semesters. No campus visits are required and all students receive in-state tuition.

The program consists of 4 courses (3 credit hours each, totaling 12 hours) covering dietary and herbal supplements, an introductory course on DIM, nutritional approaches to inflammation and immune regulation, and the growing fields of nutrigenomics and nutrigenetics in human health and disease. The courses are recommended to be taken in the order of DN 881, DN 882, and DN 980. DN 880 can be taken in any order.

Curriculum

Dietetics and Integrative Medicine

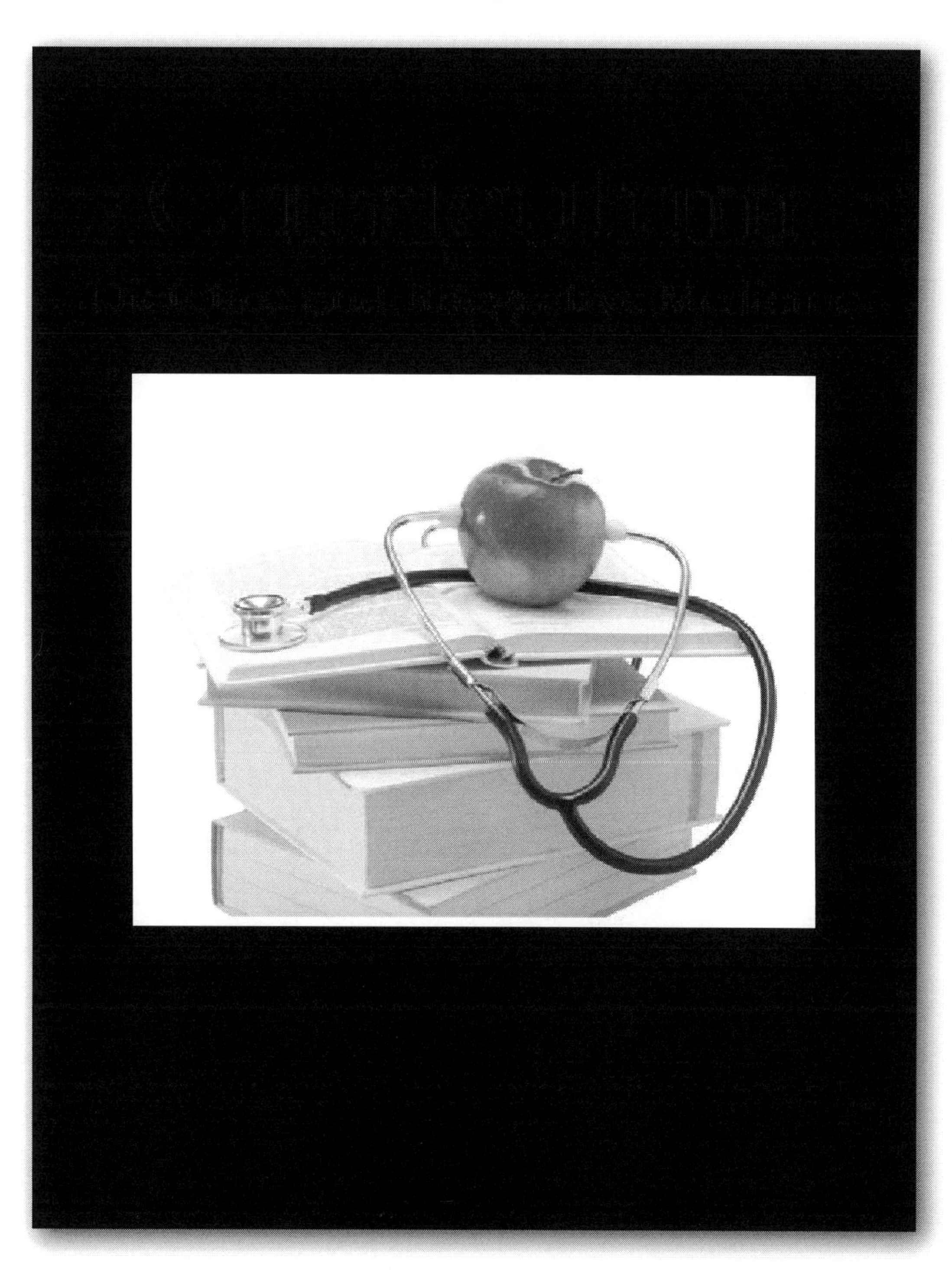

Section 4

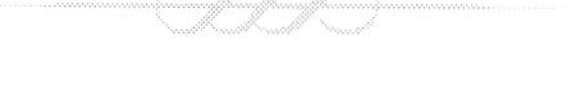

CURRICULUM

DIETETIC INTERNSHIP CERTIFICATE (TOTAL HOURS, 24)

As part of the School of Health Professions, the KU Department of Dietetics and Nutrition is located on the University of Kansas Medical Center campus in Kansas City, Kansas. where students benefit from the opportunity to interact with a large number of health care professionals and leading researchers. Dietetics and Nutrition was first established at KU in 1943 at the KU Medical Center as an ADA-approved dietetic internship program.

The following KUMC curriculum is the strong clinical and medical nutrition educational program in the Dietetics and Nutrition department that has reached out to include training for an advanced specialty in integrative medicine dietetics.

Course	Hours
DN 825 Medical Nutrition Therapy I	**3**
DN 826 Medical Nutrition Therapy II	3
DN 822 Management Dietetics and Nutrition I	2
DN 823 Management Dietetics and Nutrition II	2
DN 841 International Nutrition	1
DN 842 United States Public Health Nutrition	1
DN 817 Seminar in Dietetics and Nutrition I	1
DN 818 Seminar in Dietetics and Nutrition II	1
DN 827 Practicum: Process in Clinical Dietetics	10

- **DN 817 Seminar I** (1 hour)
  - Seminar designed to promote effectiveness of professional written and oral communication, increase knowledge of research, and review content information in selected topics in dietetics.
- **DN 818 Seminar II** (1 hour)
  - To promote effectiveness of professional written and oral communication, to increase knowledge of research, and to review content information in selected areas in dietetics.
- **DN 822 Management in Dietetics & Nutrition I** (2 hours)
  - Managerial skills in health care quality improvement and food service are practiced. Students are typically enrolled in DN 827 Practicum supervised practice experiences associated with the dietetic internship. Prerequisite: food service systems or commensurate practical experience.

- **DN 823 Management in Dietetics & Nutrition II** (2 hours)
    - Managerial style is related to food policy, financial benchmarking and applied nutrition practice. Students are typically enrolled in DN 827 Practicum supervised practice experiences associated with the dietetic internship. Prerequisite: food service systems or commensurate practical experience.
- **DN 825 Medical Nutrition Therapy I** (3 hours)

Course content introduces the student into the concepts of an intermediate study of nutritional therapy of disease. Course content includes evidence based practice in prevention and nutritional management of diseases. Patient assessment and medical chart documentation are covered. Elements of pathology and biochemistry of the nutrition related problems are integrated into course topics. This course is designed for students enrolled in the dietetic internship but students from other departments may enroll with consent of instructor. Prerequisite: Undergraduate coursework in nutrition, diet therapy, biochemistry and physiology or consent of instructor.

- **DN 826 Medical Nutrition Therapy II** (3 hours)

Course content includes current nutrition theory and evidence based practice in prevention and treatment of disease. Advanced therapies and patient management in nutrition support will be discussed. Course topics include pediatric nutrition, obesity, cardiovascular disease, diabetes, cancer, renal disease, and gastrointestinal diseases. Elements of pathology and biochemistry of the nutrition related problems are integrated into course topics. This course is designed for students enrolled in the dietetic internship but students from other departments may enroll with consent of instructor. Prerequisite: Undergraduate coursework in nutrition, diet therapy, biochemistry and physiology, DN 825 or consent of instructor.

- **DN 827 Practicum** (10 hours) DIM track

Due to the donation of an anonymous private foundation, KU Integrative Medicine is fortunate to house a Healing Foods Kitchen to use for cooking demonstrations and to teach patients how to carry out recommendations on how to use Food as Medicine. This class provides the practical application of the theoretical background the student is acquiring, using real, whole and predominantly local and sustainably farmed foods.

The Practicum takes the student through all the steps of food preparation, including"

- Compiling recipes,
- Checking kitchen inventory and compiling a list of needed ingredients,
- Obtaining the necessary ingredients from the KUMC Community Supported Agriculture (CSA) share, Prairie Birthday Farms and Fair Share Farm CSA if available or in season and obtaining the remainder of the ingredients.
- Food preparation
- Composting and clean up

Sample DIM Intern Practicum Independent Projects

- Review charts, compile and organize data related to food sensitivities
    - Relate to diabetes or pre-diabetes: Gluten sensitivity/Celiac Disease related to diabetes.
    - Relate to Medical Symptoms Questionnaire
    - Relate food sensitivities and gluten/dairy sensitivities
    - Other ideas related to food sensitivities
- BIA phase angle related to:
    - Neurofeedback data
    - RBC fatty acids
    - Minerals/electrolyte levels
    - Cancer prognostic markers and survivorship
- Work with one of the KU IM doctors and/or fellows on research projects

* DN department projects/activities
* Review literature using the Nutrition EBL on a desktop and web program for file management

* **DN 841 International Nutrition** (1 hour)

A study of global public health and nutrition concerns in various nations, assessment of nutritional status of diverse populations, international health and nutrition organizations, policies, and interventions. We explore the roles of dietitians, nutritionists, and others in creating and implementing international public health and nutrition policies and interventions. To enroll in the course you must be a student in the Graduate Certificate Dietetic Internship Program, the Dietetics and Nutrition Master of Science Program, the Great Plains IDEA, or have the consent of the instructor. Cross-listed with DIET 841.

* **DN 842 United States Public Health Nutrition** (1 hour)

A study of U.S. public health and nutrition concerns in diverse U.S. populations, assessment of nutritional status in communities, health communication, nutrition policies and community based nutrition interventions; exploration of the roles of dietitians, nutritionists, and others in developing and delivering nutrition policies and interventions in U.S. communities. Prerequisite: Must be a student in the Graduate Certificate Dietetic Internship Program, the Dietetics and Nutrition Master of Science Program, the Great Plains IDEA, or have the consent of the instructor.

DIETETICS AND INTEGRATIVE MEDICINE GRADUATE CERTIFICATE (ONLINE ONLY, 12 HOURS)

* **DN 880 Dietary and Herbal Supplements** (3 hours online)

Develop skills to partner with patients in making dietary supplement decisions. Explore the safe, efficacious use of botanicals and supplements in nutritional support of aging, maternal health and wellness. Discussions on supplementation in the prevention and treatment of chronic disease include: arthritis, cancer, cardiovascular, diabetes, digestive, mood and renal disorders. Prerequisite: Human physiology is advisable. Course offered each year, usually summer.

* **DN 881 Introduction to Dietetics and Integrative Medicine** (3 hours online)

Introduction to principles guiding the practice of integrative and functional medical nutrition therapy; clinical application of the nutrition care process (assessing, diagnosing, intervening, monitoring, and evaluating) toward restoring function for an individual client; lab interpretation; focusing on the unique nutritional imbalances characteristic of chronic disease pathophysiology; principles of detoxification; supporting individuals with persistent symptoms; preventing chronic disease; DIM interventions including food and dietary supplements along with lifestyle recommendations. Prerequisites: Introductory genetics, medical nutrition therapy, or consent of instructor. Course offered annually, usually fall.

* **DN 882 A Nutrition Approach to Inflammation and Immune Regulation** (3 hours online)

Inflammation and immune dysregulation is common in chronic disease. The course presents the integrative medicine approach to identify the underlying causes of inflammatory and immune-related conditions and associated nutritional influences; advanced assessment protocols including lab interpretation and nutrition physical exam; applies individualized food and dietary supplement interventions as powerful modulators of the pathophysiology of inflammatory and immune responses. Prerequisites: Medical nutrition therapy, genetics or consent of instructor. Course is offered once a year, usually spring.

* **DN 980 Nutrigenomics and Nutrigenetics in Health and Disease** (3 hours online)

A review of nuclear receptors and their mechanisms of action with specific examples of regulation by nutrients (essential nutrients, retinoids, fatty acids), amino acid control of gene expression, lipid sensors (PPARs), selenoprotein expression, and functional genomic studies (atherosclerosis, cancer, obesity, metabolic syndrome, Type 2 diabetes mellitus, inflammation) with relationships to nutrient intake and polymorphisms. Prerequisite: introductory genetics, DN 836, 895 or 896 or permission of instructor. Course offered each year, usually summer.

The University of Kansas Medical Center
Department of Dietetics and Nutrition

Graduate Certificates: Dietetic Internship & Dietetics and Integrative Medicine
Dietetics and Nutrition Master of Science Degree, Thesis Option

Year 1 – End of year 1 dietetic intern completes DI certificate & eligible to take RD exam

Fall Semester 2013 – 11 hours	Spring Semester 2014 – 11 hours	Summer Semester 2014 – 6 hours
DN 817 Seminar in Dietetics & Nutrition I – 1 hr.	DN 818 Seminar in Dietetics & Nutrition II – 1 hr.	**DN 880 Dietary & Herbal Supplements – 3 hr.***
DN 825 Medical Nutrition Therapy I – 3 hr.	DN 826 Medical Nutrition Therapy II – 3 hr.	DN 819 Scientific Writing for Nutrition – 1 hr.
DN 822 Management in Dietetics & Nutrition I – 2 hr.	DN 823 Management in Dietetics & Nutrition II – 2 hr.	
DN 841 International Nutrition – 1 hr.	DN 842 US Public Health Nutrition – 1 hr.	
DN 827 Practicum – 4 hr. (graded S/U) 496 hours supervised practice	DN 827 Practicum – 4 hr. (graded S/U) 496 hours supervised practice	DN 827 Practicum – 2 hr. (graded S/U) 248 hours supervised practice

Year 2 – End of year 2 graduate student completes MS degree and DIM certificate

Fall Semester 2014 – 10 hours	Spring Semester 2015 – 10 hours	Summer Semester 2015 – 4 hours
DN 881 Introduction to Dietetics and Integrative Medicine – 3 hr.*	**DN 882 A Nutrition Approach to Inflammation and Immune Regulation – 3 hr.***	**DN 980 Nutrigenomics and Nutrigenetics in Health and Disease – 3 hr.***
DN 895 Macronutrients & Integrative Metabolism – 3 hr.	DN 896 Micronutrients & Integrative Metabolism – 3 hr.	
DN 834 Methods of Research in Nutrition – 3 hr.	BIOS Principles of Statistics in Public Health – 3 hr.	
DN 899 Thesis – 1 hr.**	DN 899 Thesis – 1 hr. **	DN 899 Thesis – 1 hr.**
**Non-thesis replace 3 hr. DN 899 with DN 854 in fall or spring semester	Non-thesis option requires additional 3 hour elective course	52 graduate hours completed over 2 years for thesis option; 55 hours for non-thesis option

***Required courses for DIM Certificate** **Updated May 8, 2013**

Figure 7: KUMC DIM Graduate Certificate and M.S. Class Schedule

PDF available in the Appendix

MASTER OF SCIENCE IN DIETETICS AND NUTRITION

Table 1

Required Courses		Thesis Non-Thesis
DN 834 Methods of Research in Nutrition		3
Biostatistics (700-800 level)		3
DN 895 Advanced Macronutrients and Integrated Metabolism		3
DN 896 Advanced Micronutrients and Integrated Metabolism		3
DN 817 Seminar in Dietetics and Nutrition I		1
DN 818 Seminar in Dietetics and Nutrition II		1
DN 819 Scientific Writing for the Nutritional Sciences		1
Research (DN 899 Thesis or DN 854 Special Problems in Dietetics and Nutrition)		3 (minimum)
*Electives	Thesis 12 hours	Non-Thesis 15 hours

The coursework includes:

* **DN834 Methods of Research** (3 hours)
  - A study of basic research terminology and designs commonly used in nutrition research. Topics include: research on animals, tissue culture and human subjects; qualitative, quantitative and outcomes research; ethical issues in research; dissemination of research findings; and appropriate use of research findings. Prerequisite: Consent of instructor.
* **DN 895 Advanced Macronutrients & Metabolism** (3 hours)
  - Energy-containing macronutrients and fiber presented from the perspective of their importance in human nutrition. Structural properties, digestion, absorption and metabolism are emphasized. Fuel utilization in response to food intake and exercise, cellular and whole-animal energetic and energy balance integrate metabolism. Students take an active role in presenting and discussing and exhibit advanced skills in analysis and presentation. Prerequisite: Biochemistry
* **Biostatistics (700-800 level)** (3 hours): Course options include:
* **BIOS 704: Principles of Statistics in Public Health** (3)
* **BIOS 714: Fundamentals of Biostatistics** I (3)
* **BIOS 715: Statistical Computing in Research** (2)
* **BIOS 717: Fundamentals of Biostatistics II** (3)
* **BIOS 720: Analysis of Variance** (3)
* **BIOS 725: Applied Nonparametric Statistics** (3)
* **BIOS 730: Applied Linear Regression** (3)
* **BIOS 735: Categorical Data and Survival Analysis** (3)
* **BIOS 740: Applied Multivariate Methods** (3)
* **BIOS 806: Special Topics in Biostatistics: Biostatistical Programming** (3)
* **BIOS 810: Clinical Trials** (3)
* **BIOS 820: Statistical Computing/SAS Base L1** (3)
* **BIOS 825: Nonparametric Methods** (3)

- **BIOS 830: Experimental Design** (3)
- **BIOS 835: Categorical Data Analysis** (3)
- **BIOS 840: Linear Regression** (3)
- **BIOS 871: Mathematical Statistics** (3)
- **BIOS 872: Mathematical Statistics II** (3)
- **BIOS 890: Linear Models (**3)
- **BIOS 898: Collaborative Research Experience** (3)

- **DN 896 Advanced Micronutrients & Metabolism**(3 hours)
  - Vitamins and minerals presented from the perspective of their requirements as nutrients for normal human physiological functions with emphasis on their underlying roles in structure, function and metabolism. Students take an active role in selecting, presenting and discussing recent published research and to exhibit advanced skills in analysis and presentation. Prerequisites: Biochemistry.
- **DN 817 Seminar in D&N I** (1 hr)
  - Seminar designed to promote effectiveness of professional written and oral communication, increase knowledge of research, and review content information in selected topics in dietetics.
- **DN 818 Seminar in D&N II** (1 hr)
  - To promote effectiveness of professional written and oral communication, to increase knowledge of research, and to review content information in selected areas in dietetics.
- **DN 819 Scientific Writing for the Nutritional Sciences** (1 hr)
  - Research proposal preparation and / or scientific manuscript writing experience. This course will provide the student with an overview of the steps used in proposal writing and/or the steps in preparation of a scientific manuscript for publication.
- **Electives**
  - Up to 6 hours may be outside the D&N program. However, students completing the dietetic internship and the MS program will have limited hours available for electives due to courses required for the internship program
- **Research**
  - For MS with thesis option: DN 899. The research can take place over several semesters and involves writing a research proposal and well as the collection and analysis of data. The student will have a thesis committee, consisting of faculty members with an interest in the research proposal. The research is written in the form of a thesis, which is then presented to the department and followed by questions from the thesis committee and any interested attendees. The thesis option also requires a 30-minute oral examination.
  - For MS non-thesis option: DN 854. This is a project completed during a single semester and may include one or more of the following options:
    - Writing an intensive review of the literature on a given topic.
    - Participation with a faculty member in the development of a research proposal or grant.
    - Participation with a faculty member in conducting a pilot project.
    - Participation with a faculty member in the design, implementation, or evaluation of a program in a specialized area of dietetics practice.
    - Collection and/or analysis of data in conjunction with a faculty member engaged in research.
      - Additional requirements:
        - A 2- to 5-page written proposal and write-up of the project and a 30-minute oral presentation to the department.
        - A 1-hour general oral examination

CRITERIA FOR M.S. RESEARCH PROJECT OF DIETETICS AND INTEGRATIVE MEDICINE STUDENTS/INTERNS

While choosing a thesis research topic during the Master of Science year, DIM Students at KU Medical Center review the available research topics and ask a research question or questions that investigate, in depth, one of the seven principles of nutrition and dietetics listed below from an integrative medicine perspective. An easy way to ensure an integrative topic is including at least one of these DIM principles:

1. Biochemical Individuality
2. Chronic Disease Pathophysiology
3. Nutritional influence on Inflammation
4. Nutritional influence on Immune Regulation
5. Long Latency Nutrient Insufficiencies
6. Nutritional Toxicology and Epigenetics
7. Energy Metabolism: Cell to Body Composition
8. Lifestyle: Diet, Physical Activity/Exercise, Sleep, Beliefs, Community/Relationships, Environment

Each of the above can be expanded upon and outlined/supported with the following articles/publications.

- Augustine MB, Swift KM, Harris SR, Anderson EJ, Hand RK. Integrative Medicine: Education, Perceived Knowledge, Attitudes, and Practice among Academy of Nutrition and Dietetics Members. J Acad Nutr Diet. 2016 Feb;116(2):319-29.
- Wagner LE, Evans RG, Noland D, Barkley R, Sullivan DK, Drisko J. The Next Generation of Dietitians: Implementing Dietetics Education and Practice in Integrative Medicine. J Am Coll Nutr. 2015;34(5):430-5. Epub 2015 May 11.
- Ford, D., Raj, S., Batheja, R. K., Debusk, R., Grotto, D., Noland, D., Redmond, E., et al. (2011). American Dietetic Association: standards of practice and standards of professional performance for registered dietitians (competent, proficient, and expert) in integrative and functional medicine. *Journal of the American Dietetic Association*, *111*(6), 902–913.e1–23. doi:10.1016/j.jada.2011.04.017
- Jones DS, Hofmann L, Quinn S. 21st century medicine: A new model for medical education and practice. Gig Harbor, WA:The Institute for Functional Medicine, 2009;p1-35. (Consortium of Academic Health Centers for Integrative Medicine definition of Integrative Medicine), http://www.imconsortium.org
- Sears, B., & Ricordi, C. (2011). Anti-inflammatory nutrition as a pharmacological approach to treat obesity. *J Obes*, *2011*. doi:10.1155/2011/431985
- McCann, J. C., & Ames, B. N. (2009). Vitamin K, an example of triage theory: is micronutrient inadequacy linked to diseases of aging? *Am J Clin Nutr*, *90*(4), 889–907. doi:10.3945/ajcn.2009.27930
- Heaney, R. P. (2012). The nutrient problem. *Nutr Rev*, *70*(3), 165–169. doi:10.1111/j.1753-4887.2011.00469.x
- Diamanti-Kandarakis, E., Bourguignon, J.-P., Giudice, L. C., Hauser, R., Prins, G. S., Zoeller, R. T., & Gore, A. C. (2009). Endocrine disrupting chemicals. *Endocirine reviews.*
- Lacey, K., & Pritchett, E. (2003). Nutrition Care Process and Model: ADA adopts road map to quality care and outcomes management. *Journal of the American Dietetic Association*, *103*(8), 1061–72. doi:10.1053/jada.2003.50564
- Heaney, R. P. (2003). Long-latency deficiency disease: insights from calcium and vitamin D. *The American journal of clinical nutrition*, *78*(5), 912–9. Retrieved from http://www.ncbi.nlm.nih.gov/pubmed/14594776

LEARNING OBJECTIVES AND DIM COMPETENCIES
FOUNDATIONAL CONCEPTS OF DIM

* **Define and describe** the role systems physiology plays in dietetics and integrative medicine using the *Institute for Functional Medicine Matrix*™. (Consider the complex interaction between genetics, the environment and lifestyle overtime and resulting health). **(Clinical, Community)**
* **Give 2 examples** of the health and nutritional influence of stress or beliefs (thoughts, feelings, culture, religion, spirituality, other) on a patient's/client's health. **(Clinical, Community)**
* **Describe** the meaning of "Structure equals function" in relation to nutritional status and health. **(Clinical, Community)**
* **Identify** three (3) textbook references for Dietitians and healthcare practitioners in Integrative Medicine **(Clinical, Community)**

ASSESSMENT AND DIAGNOSIS, INTERVENTION, MONITORING AND EVALUATION

Assessment and Diagnosis

* Clearly state three (3) distinguishing aspects of a nutrition assessment from the perspective of Dietetics and Integrative Medicine Assessment compared to a conventional acute care nutrition assessment. Describe how they are similar and how different from conventional dietetics. **(Clinical, Community)**
* List five (5) of the many signs of nutritional deficiency or insufficiency that can be noted upon administering a Nutrition-Focused Physical Exam. **(Clinical)**
* **List** three (3) companies that are commonly used for outside nutritional testing or laboratory assessments. **(Clinical)**
* **Name** three (3) conventional and three (3) functional nutritional laboratory assessments that are useful in performing a successful nutritional assessment within the context of Dietetics and Integrative Medicine. Be able to discuss why and under what circumstances they might be most useful.**(Clinical)**
* Using a Bioelectric Impedance Analysis (BIA) device, **analyze** body composition of a patient/client. Discuss the differences between BIA, Bod Pod, DEXA and other body composition devices. Describe what is being measured by each assessment and the advantages or disadvantage of each. Be able to discuss why and under what circumstances they might be most useful. **(Clinical)**
* Within the context of the patient's individual story, **analyze** a food diary for content and quality of **(Clinical)**:
  - Fat, Protein, Carbohydrate, Fiber, Liquid (water/other), Phytonutrients
  - Sunlight exposure with emphasis on residence (location, latitude) and Vitamin D food intake
  - Meal Timing and Snacking
  - Supplements
  - Medications
  - Toxic load
* **Assess** patient lifestyle factors that contribute to nutritional status (sleep, physical activity/inactivity, beliefs, etc.). **(Clinical, Community)**
* Regarding other aspects of lifestyle (in addition to dietary intake), **describe** the impact of the following lifestyle factors and how these may affect nutritional status **(Clinical, Community)**:
  - Sleep and sleep quality, circadian rhythm

  - o Community and family/friend support
  - o Food access, preparation or other limits on a healthy nutrition lifestyle
  - o Belief system regarding: health, religion/spirituality, cultural or other
- * **Describe** nutritional influences on the following aspects of Dietetics and Integrative Medicine (**Clinical, Community**):
  - o Inflammation
  - o Immune regulation or dysregulation
  - o Long Latency Nutritional Insufficiencies (aka "Long Latency Deficiency Disease")
  - o Epigenetics/gene expression
  - o Body Composition
- * Using the Natural Medicines Comprehensive Database, be able to check interactions or drug-induced nutrient depletions (DINDs) for medications, dietary supplements, herbal supplements, etc. (**Clinical**)
- * List at least two (2) common Nutrition Diagnostic Statements used to diagnose nutrition problems that are often used in Dietetics and Integrative Medicine (E.g. Altered gastrointestinal function; altered nutrition-related laboratory values; altered nutrient utilization; etc.) (**Clinical**)

Intervention, Monitoring and Evaluation

- * Be able to describe, verbally or in written form, the factors considered in recommending an elimination diet and the purpose of the timing and removal of a specific food or foods. (**Clinical**)
  - o List three (3) different types of elimination diets (FODMAPs, comprehensive elimination, Histamine, Nightshades, Gluten, Casein, etc.)
  - o Describe how to schedule and monitor the reintroduction or challenge of eliminated foods.
- * Describe or define when nutritional supplementation is appropriate and outline key parameters to monitor for a patient or client. Explain instances when it would be inappropriate to recommend supplementation. (**Clinical, Community**)
- * Have the capability to effectively and efficiently search the scientific literature to support interventions for patients or clients. (**Clinical, Community**)
- * Discuss the physiological, biological and scientific basis of various "diets" (Consistent Carbohydrate, "Cardiac" Diet, Modified Elimination, Ketogenic, other). Discuss the appropriate application of each to populations versus individuals. (**Clinical**)
- * Discuss the importance of monitoring individualized nutrition interventions. Give 2-3 strategies (action steps) for monitoring a patient. (**Clinical**)

FOOD QUALITY & REGULATION

- * Describe the importance of soil quality, mineral/nutrient content, and its effect on nutritional recommendations. (**Community**)
- * Describe Endocrine-Disrupting Chemicals (EDCs) and list 2 common substances or groups of substances that would be considered EDCs. Name ways to avoid EDCs through food or lifestyle efforts. (**Clinical, Community**)

* Describe instances where food quality would be higher or lower when produced: locally, organically, conventionally, in various growing conditions. State other reasons you might consider nutritional quality, or content of carcinogenic and endocrine-disrupting chemicals. **(Clinical, Community)**
* Participate in public policy to influence food and nutrition laws **(Community)**
* Describe five (5) key aspects of a successful local food system. Describe the differences and similarities from hospital or other foodservice experience(s) you have had. **(Community, Management)**
* Be able to independently plan, organize and prepare for a cooking demonstration in the Healing Foods Kitchen or in another cooking demonstration venue. **(Community, Management)**
* Be able to write a recipe: correctly listing ingredients, describing instructions and altering ingredients to meet needs of those with food sensitivities/allergies, those avoiding excess sodium, and other specific dietary needs. **(Community, Management)**

COMMUNITY NUTRITION

* List general nutrition recommendations that can be given in a group setting. (E.g. Whole foods and minimally-refined foods are optimal for most people; many people benefit from a primarily plant-based diet; Low-toxin food optimizes health) NOTE: Dietitians in Integrative Medicine must do an individualized nutrition assessment to determine a patient's/client's nutrition status). **(Community)**
* List or name various community-based organizations and/or websites that could help dietitians, healthcare practitioners or the lay public to access whole, real, minimally-refined foods. **(Community, Clinical)**

EXPECTED COMPETENCIES IN COMPUTER TECHNOLOGY

The student shall exhibit sufficient competence in computer technology to:

* Receive electronic mail communications from the course instructor.
* Open electronic mail attachments.
* Use research databases and explore internet web sites.
* Download computer slide presentation files provided for class session notes.
* Own, purchase and install, or be willing to access through the Instructional Technology Center at the University of Kansas Medical Center, Microsoft Power Point® and Microsoft Word® computer applications.

KUMC Master of Science in Dietetics and Nutrition

Table 2

Year 1	All-Student Activities	Practicum Activity	Coursework
Fall Term	**Early Fall (August)** Workshop: Introduction to Dietetics and Integrative Medicine	Clinical Rotation with KU Hospital	General Dietetics and Nutrition Curriculum
Spring Term	**Early Spring (January)** Workshop: *Evidence for Dietetics and Integrative Medicine practice*, Nutrition Care Process, clinical applications, Nutrition Physical Exam, Case Studies, Clinical Scenario)	**8-weeks (248 hours)**: Community Rotation (KU Integrative Medicine) **8-weeks (248 hours)**: Management Rotation (various sites/locations)	General Dietetics and Nutrition Curriculum
Spring Term	**Late Spring (April)** DI Workshop: Entrepreneurship in nutrition practice / Business aspects of nutritional supplements	Students switch after each 8 week rotation (Community and Management rotations)	General Dietetics and Nutrition Curriculum
Summer Term	**None**	**8-weeks (248 hours)**: • Area of Interest Rotation (KU Integrative Medicine) • Center for Mind-Body Medicine "Food as Medicine"	DN 880 Dietary and Herbal Supplements (2-3 credits) May start writing literature review for thesis to begin fall semester
Year 2	**Graduate Assistanceship**	**Research Activities**	**Coursework**
Fall Term	16-20 hours weekly: work as a Graduate Research Assistant (GRA) or Graduate Teaching Assistant (GTA) with DN Faculty on relevant work or teaching.	**Masters' Thesis**: With an advisor from Dietetics and Nutrition Department, work on research project through the lens of Dietetics and Integrative Medicine	General Dietetics and Nutrition Curriculum DN 881 Introduction to Dietetics and Integrative Medicine (3 credits)
Spring Term	16-20 hours weekly: work as a Graduate Research Assistant (GRA) or Graduate Teaching Assistant (GTA) with DN Faculty on relevant work or teaching.	**Masters' Thesis:** With an advisor from DN Department, work on research project through the lens of Dietetics and Integrative Medicine	DN 882 A Nutrition Approach to Inflammation and Immune Regulation
Summer Term		**Masters' Thesis:** Complete research, write thesis and defend thesis with oral defense.	DN 980 Nutrigenomics and Nutrigenetics in Health and Disease (3 credits)

DIETETICS EDUCATION
A NEW LENS FOR CHRONIC DISEASE

DIM PROGRAMS
PRACTICUM

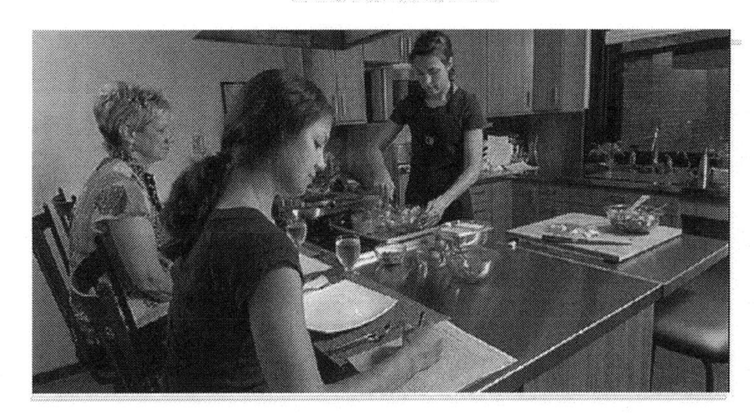

Integrative and Functional
Medical Nutrition Therapy (IFMNT)

PERSONALIZED NUTRITION
NUTRIGENOMICS

TARGETED NUTRIENTS
DIET AND LIFESTYLE

Section 5

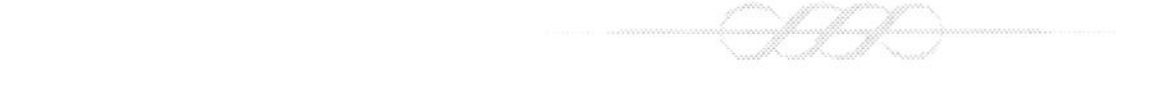

DIETETICS AND INTEGRATIVE MEDICINE PRACTICUM

Two-three nutrition or dietetic interns each year are awarded the desired opportunity to immerse their dietetic education in the DIM Practicum with concentrated assignments in the KU Integrative Medicine Clinic under the preceptorship of the IFMNT RDs and nutritionists. The following Modules describe the foundation of their DIM training in addition to the working relationships with the entire integrative medicine medical team.

CLINICAL ROTATIONS: FIVE MODULE PRACTICUM ACTIVITIES AND SUPPORTING INTRODUCTION

The Dietetics and Integrative Medicine educational objective is to impart to nutritional-dietetic students the working knowledge required to effectively practice as an integrative clinical nutrition practitioner. The key foundation of this training is the time spent with experienced integrative medicine interdisciplinary team members in an integrative or functional medicine clinic or healthcare delivery setting. During the DIM Track in the dietetic internship, M.S. program or DIM Award Program, the mentoring that takes place as part of the integrative practicum experience has proven to be a vital component of ensuring the DIM award recipients with a solid paradigm of the clinical nutrition of integrative medicine. For an effective integrative practicum experience, the mentoring preceptors must be qualified in the basic tenets of Dietetics and Integrative Medicine. A *Standards of Dietetic and Integrative Medicine Preceptors/Instructors* document is included with the Appendix material to reference the staff qualifications. If fully trained individuals are not available to teach a particular program, the Standards document includes a provision for introducing new instructors and preceptors to the *Ten Tenets of Dietetics and Integrative Medicine* as well as suggested concurrent DIM training.

The following five Practicum Modules were developed at the University of Kansas Medical Center KU Integrative Medicine clinic for the DIM Award Program and provides an example for practicum curriculum that can be adapted to any nutrition-related health professionals program (medical, nursing, dietetics, physical therapy, pharmacy, and others). Please refer to the Appendix Practicum Curriculum documents and websites: www.dietetics.kumc.edu, and, integrativemed.kumc.edu.

OFF-SITE PRACTICUM SITES

There are a number of training sites located within or near the Kansas City area that provide supervised practice experience. These include hospitals, clinics, community health care agencies and other practice settings in which dietetics and nutrition services are provided. Each location will need to seek out practicum sites emphasizing individualized clinical therapies including whole clean foods, lifestyle education, low-toxin environmental choices, etc.

Student training sites should primarily be food and nutrition-related. However, it is important for students to obtain the full breadth of the integrative medicine paradigm. Students should be encouraged to shadow, volunteer and participate in a wide variety of opportunities. Here are some ideas of modalities and/or integrative health professionals that could benefit a future DIM practitioner.

NUTRITION-RELATED TRAINING SITES

Table 3

Nutrition Service	Provider or Site
Medical Nutrition Therapy	Integrative RDN
Mindful Eating	Integrative RDN; Psychologist (PhD)
Whole food preparation	Chef; Chef Educator; Whole Foods Markets or similar stores with "Healthy Eating Specialist";
Low-toxin food production and preparation	Organic farm Organic restaurant
Local food production and/or sale	Community garden Farmers market Community Supported Agriculture (CSA) Local restaurant (sourcing local foods)

OTHER INTEGRATIVE TRAINING SITES

Table 4

Service	Provider/Preceptor/Site
Acupuncture	Acupuncturist (LAc)
Biofeedback/Neurofeedback	Advanced Practice Registered Nurse (APRN); Certified Neurofeedback Technician
Chiropractic Consultation	Doctor of Chiropractic (DC)
Fitness Assessment	Exercise Physiologist (MS)
Guided Imagery	Physician (MD); Health Psychologist (PhD); Psychotherapist (LPC, LPA)
Health Coaching	Masters level health professionals with training in coaching and integrative medicine
Healing Touch	Nurse (RN); CHTP
Herbal/Botanical Medicine	Physician (MD); Naturopathic Doctor (ND)
Homeopathy	Naturopathic Doctor (ND)
Hypnotherapy	Health Psychologist (PhD) or Psychotherapists (LPC, LPA)
Infusion Therapies	Physician (MD); Registered Nurse (RN); Advanced Practice Registered Nurse
Integrative Consultations	Physician (MD); Advanced Practice Registered Nurse (APRN)
Lifestyle Change Consultations	Physician (MD); Advanced Practice Registered Nurse (APRN); Registered Nurse (RN); Registered Dietitian Nutritionist (RDN)
Massage and Body Work	Certified Massage Therapist (CMT)
Musculoskeletal/Structural Assessment	Doctor of Chiropractic (DC); Physician (MD)
Naturopathy	Naturopathic Doctor (ND)
Nutrition	Registered Dietitian Nutritionist (RDN)
Pediatric Integrative Consultation	Physician (MD – Pediatrician); Registered Dietitian Nutritionist (RDN)
Personal Training	Exercise Physiologist (MS)
Physical Therapy	Physical Therapist (PT)
Psychotherapy and/or Health Psychology	Health Psychologist (PhD); Psychotherapists (LPC, LPA); Social Worker (LCSW)
Reiki	Reiki specialist, "master"
Tai Chi	Certified Tai Chi Instructor
Yoga Therapy	Certified Yoga Teacher

MODULE 1: GENERAL ORIENTATION TO INTEGRATIVE MEDICINE PRACTICUM
PRACTICUM SITE, MODALITIES AND THE DIM PARADIGM

Module 1 Activities

Reference: DIM Tenets: Introduction to the Tenets of DIM

* Orientation to Integrative Medicine site
* Introduction to DIM Nutrition Care Process (specific for various sites)
* Complete Pre- and Post-Evaluation for DIM Practicum Experience
* Case Studies: Practitioner can share cases in a presentation or go through charts or records for examples.
* Video: The Blood Sugar Solution by Dr. Mark Hyman – DVD
* DIFM Archived Webinar Lectures
* DIM: What, Why and How?
* Rotate with other Integrative Medicine practitioners:
    - Infusion Nurse and Advanced Practice Registered Nurse (APRN) in the Infusion Clinic
    - Medical Doctors
    - Naturopathic Doctor
    - Neurofeedback technicians
    - Other modalities: Acupuncture, Reiki, chiropractor, massage therapy, biological dentistry, and others.

Supporting Documents for Module 1

* Pre- and Post-Evaluation DIM Practicum Experience
* Orientation to Integrative Medicine Practicum Site
* Ten Tenets of Dietetics and Integrative Medicine (DIM)
* IFMNT Radial Conceptual Diagram
* IFM Matrix
* How to think like a Dietetics and Integrative Medicine (DIM) specialist
* DIM from an Intern's Perspective

Pre and Post Evaluation for DIM Interns

* What is an Elimination Diet?
* What is the purpose of an Elimination Diet?
* Name 5 of the 10 top food sensitivities/allergens?
* What does it mean to have "increased intestinal permeability" or "leaky gut"? How might it be measured?
* Give one example of the signs and/or symptoms of a specific nutrient deficiency
* What is the function of the "IDU" nutrition assessment tool?
* What does "*MAPDOM*" stand for?
* List as many possible ways you can think of to cook/prepare vegetables.
* Why might organic food be emphasized in an individual's nutrition intervention plan?

* Although DIM emphasizes an individual nutrition assessment, what are some general nutrition recommendations that would be appropriate for all people?
* Please list and describe the *Ten Tenets of DIM*.
* List one way that a person's genetics or family history could affect the way you counsel a patient or create an individual's nutrition intervention.
* Describe some differences between the conventional Nutrition Care Process (NCP) and that from a DIM perspective

Orientation to Integrative Medicine Practicum Site

Preceptors may want to provide a formal Orientation to the clinic, including background, a tour with introductions to team members and general guidelines for the student to follow throughout the rotation, including:

* Days & Hours of Operation
* Department meetings, Grand Rounds or "Chart Review" Sessions
* Dress code
* **How to address team members:** Some Integrative teams prefer to go by first name and some prefer specific titles. It is important that students know how to address the preceptor and the team.
* **Healing Foods Kitchen**: If your site has a demonstration kitchen or has access to a demonstration kitchen, orient the student to the kitchen etiquette.
* **Integrative Medicine Modalities:** Describe the different modalities offered at your site. This will vary greatly. Those offered at KU Integrative Medicine include:
  - Medical Consultations
  - Naturopathic Medical Consultations
  - Nutrition Consultations
  - Cooking Demonstrations
  - Biofeedback, including Neurofeedback Therapy
  - Intravenous and Intramuscular Nutritional Therapies
  - Outpatient Nutritional Pharmacy (associated with KU Hospital)
* **Integrative Medicine Modalities:** Describe services that you refer to often. For example:
  - Acupuncture
  - Chiropractic
  - Massage Therapy
  - Biological Dentistry
  - Physical Therapy
  - Conventional Medical Specialties: Surgery, Oncology, Radiation, Nephrology, Gastroenterology, etc.
  - Energy healing: Attunement, Reiki, other
  - Therapeutic Breath work Practitioner
  - Others, as needed

WHOLE FOODS

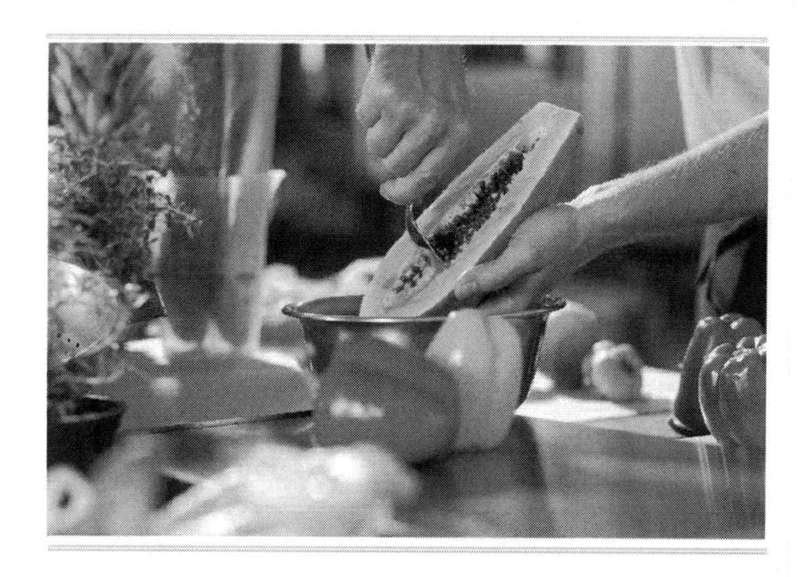

NUTRIENT DENSE

LOW TOXIN

LOW PROCESSED

MODULE 2 ACTIVITIES

Reference: DIM Tenet(s): 1, 2, 4, 5, 6, 7, 8

* Assist with acquisition of food products, grocery shopping, and/or possible communication with food delivery service.
* Rotate with a RDN who teaches whole foods-based cooking classes or demonstrations
* Prepare for and assist with Healing Foods Kitchen Demonstration in the KU Integrative Medicine Healing Foods Kitchen

Healing Foods Kitchen Guide

KU Integrative Medicine is fortunate to house a Healing Foods Kitchen within the clinic to teach patients, staff, students and the public how to cook the healthy, whole foods that we recommend: teaching people how to use Food as Medicine. This document outlines the student's role in the kitchen after the preceptor has determined the content of the cooking class. However, it is possible to delegate to the student the task of formulating or deciding on class recipes and content. The following assumes the preceptor has determined class content and recipes.

Interns' or Students' Role in the Kitchen

The week prior to the cooking class:

Recipes: At least a week or more before class, the preceptor or student(s) should choose appropriate recipes for the cooking class. When determined, the recipes can be formatted appropriately. Please see "Recipe Format & Instructions" Document, "Example Recipe Format – Chicken Breast with Tomato and Coconut" document for Recipe-writing instructions and guidance.

Ingredient Inventory: Based on the recipes, a shopping list is developed. Upon completing the shopping list, check the current kitchen inventory to determine which ingredients are available and which are needed for the cooking class. Record amounts needed or mark/check-off the items already in stock. Check with a faculty advisor for possible substitutions. Please see the "Grocery Shopping Template" for guidance.

Grocery List: Based on the Recipes, Ingredient Inventory and local, whole and organic food availability, create a shopping list to submit to take with you to the grocery store or to send to the grocery delivery service.

Grocery Shopping: If you are tasked with doing the grocery shopping, take reusable bags and try to envision how the groceries can be organized based on recipes for ease of assembly and preparation. Complete grocery shopping at least by the morning or early afternoon of the day before class.

Grocery Delivery Service: If there is a grocery delivery service available in your area, it may be economical to have an outside service shop for and deliver the groceries for cooking classes. If so, contact them with the grocery list and specifics to the email address provided for their services about a week before the cooking class. Groceries should be delivered by 1 pm the day before class to give ample preparation time and to identify any last-minute or missing items.

Week of the class / Evening before or morning before cooking demonstration:
Food Acquisition: Food can be acquired a variety of ways: CSA pickup, farmer drop-off and/or grocery shopping or grocery delivery service. When the groceries arrive, place them in the proper storage area, (refrigerator, freezer, cabinet). By 1 pm the day before cooking class, all ingredients should be accounted for. Any missing ingredients will need to be purchased for class.

Food Preparation: The day prior to and the morning of cooking class, most foods should be cleaned, cut, measured, prepared for the cooking class. Leave some of the produce items to be "demonstrated" for the cooking class. Each recipe should be measured and assembled separately and either stored in the refrigerator or on the counter. Please use baking sheets, plates, bags or other equipment to keep all ingredients for a single recipe together.

Read recipes ahead of time: It will be important to understand the flow of the cooking to supply the teacher with the ingredients for upcoming recipes, as needed.

* Keep a portion of the foods (produce, herbs, spices, etc.) to be demonstrated and used as examples for students to observe. This is the purpose of the class!
* Using recipes, note foods to be prepared during class (Most foods and ingredients are precut and measured but often-small portions are reserved for demonstration in class).
* Keep a compost bag available (in a bowl) for waste when prepping foods.
* Items can be placed in bowls covered with cellophane and labeled.
* When portioning place items for each recipe on a separate cooking tray to keep them together.
* Note on each recipe foods that are prepped and ready for the class.
* If portioning foods the day before the class – process only the foods that can keep overnight.

Morning of Cooking Demonstration
Class Preparation: Finish preparing remaining foods and ingredients. Clean the kitchen floor and counter for the class.

Class Food Organization: Ingredients should be labeled with name and amount of ingredient, as the recipes will be assembled or completed in the order of the class. As much as possible, organize the class recipes from left to right (or right to left), so that you can move as systematically as possible. Place the ingredients for each recipe in the order they will be used starting with the first ingredients used closest to where the teacher will stand. Note: Some recipes will need to remain on trays in the refrigerator or to the side because space is limited.

Place Settings: The Patient Service Representatives have a "final attendance" list at the front desk of KU Integrative Medicine. Place table settings for the number of attendees enrolled for the class. Left side of plate is for forks, right side of plate is knife with blade facing plate and spoon on the outside. Glasses are filled with water on the top right side of the place setting. Recipes and note pages should be printed and placed under the place mats on the right side of the place setting. Pens should be provided for notes.

During Cooking Class:
Equipment: Please prepare for use of blender, immersion blender, food processor, or other kitchen gadgets and equipment. Because space is limited, you may only need to be aware of the time these need to be ready for use during the class.

Turn on the light in the exhaust hood (over the range top). Also, if the oven will be used in class, please turn it on to the correct temperature at the beginning of class.

Classes: Classes move pretty quickly and can be a little hectic if there are a lot of questions from the audience.

As the assistant, it is important to focus on what the teacher is doing to anticipate things she may need or help with cooking (listen for questions) as she works on many recipes at one time. The RDN will teach nutrition while cooking, so it will be helpful to assist her while somewhat limiting interaction with the audience to avoid confusion, as time is limited.

As recipes are started help with removing the covers from the ingredients and remove empty containers as they are used to clear the cooking space

Smaller items can be set in the sink while larger items can be loaded on the dish washer trays

* The preceptor may ask you to help by cleaning appliances or other cooking utensils (like the food processor) if they are to be used for more than one recipe
* As items are prepared you will serve them to the audience

After Class

* **Clean up**: You can run most of the cooking equipment and dishes through the washer. As one load is washing you can load the second rack to be washed and continue rotating. When dishes come out of the washer they can be put away, if they are still wet they should be dried with a towel then put away. Clean the counters and run the disposal (check for small measuring spoons in the disposal) and finish by sweeping the floor.

Supporting Documents for Module 2

(no supporting documents)

MODULE 3: DIM CLINICAL NUTRITION PRACTICE

DIM CLINICAL NUTRITION PRACTICE

Reference: DIM Tenet(s): 1-10

The preceptor and DIM student(s) should arrange mutually convenient time to "shadow" him or her.

Activities

*See below and appendices for relevant documents

* Review the KU DIM Initial Assessment Process.
* Orientation to DIM Clinic, Tools of the Trade, and general assessment tools
* Read and view Motivational Interviewing (MI) Document and watch web videos on MI basics from "Heart Foundation Australia" (publicly available online).
* Utilize the *Dietitians in Integrative and Functional Medicine* (DIFM) www.integrativeRD.org website for member-only access to:
    - Natural Medicine Comprehensive Database
    - Archived webinars
    - Newsletters
    - Locate DIFM members and practitioners nationwide
* Read *Consultation Guidelines* document. It is important for the preceptor to maintain rapport with patients and for students not to interrupt the developing therapeutic relationship.
* Read KUMC Nutrition Physical Exam Checklist
* Review Table of Specialized Diets
* Review GI Tract Assessment Table
* Refer to GI Nutrient Absorption Sites
* Observe and work with the RDN as he/she sees clients:
    - Nutrition Care Process: Assessment, Diagnosis, Intervention, Monitoring and Evaluation
    - Nutrition Intake Forms: Review forms completed by clients. May refer to IFM Matrix, Health History Timeline or other integrative framework reference.
    - Nutrition Physical Exam
    - Body composition assessment using Bioelectric Impedance Analysis (BIA)
* Refer to Natural Medicines Comprehensive Database (available on DIFM DPG website as a member benefit) to learn about nutritional supplements

KU DIM INITIAL NUTRITION ASSESSMENT PROCESS

Background

The initial nutrition assessment at KU Integrative Medicine (KU IM) is based on the Nutrition Care Process established by the Academy of Nutrition and Dietetics (The Academy), and is summarized as follows: Assessment, Diagnosis, Intervention, Monitoring, Evaluation

Appointment Preparation

In preparation for the initial DIM Nutrition Assessment, charts can be prepared using the

* Nutrition Intake Form
* Nutrition Charge Sheet
* Supplement order form/Supplement contact information
* References for assessment of patient nutrition status

Initial Assessment – Dietetics and Integrative Medicine

The DIM Practitioner:

Introduce yourself, welcome and ask how the person prefers to be addressed.

Invite patient to sit in designated chair in "safe" counseling area.

If family or friend with client wanting to accompany session, privately ask client for permission.

Privately request permission of the patient if an RD-intern might observe the appointment.

Patient Services Representative (PSR) Photograph: Take a photograph of the patient to place in the chart. This will be used for ease of recognition, better recall of patient story, and team approach to care.

* Notice of Privacy Practices (PSR)
* HIPAA Authorization (PSR)
* Diet Prescription or specific KU IM Referral form (pink or blue form)
* Integrative Nutrition Intake Form (self or physician-referred)
* Diet Diary (1 to 3-day history)
* Fats and Oils Questionnaire
* Medical Symptoms Questionnaire (MSQ)

NUTRITION ASSESSMENT PROCESS

Background and explanation of assessment

Upon referral or scheduling an appointment with a patient, explain what they may expect during an appointment with an integrative nutrition practitioner. It may be helpful to share the handout "Working with a Dietetics and Integrative Medicine Practitioner". This may be provided in the form of a letter to the patient after being referred by one of the physicians, or it may be handed to the patient when he/she arrives at the appointment by the PSR.

Direct appointment with Integrative Nutrition Practitioner without a physician-referral:

* Provide handout, "Working with a Dietetics and Integrative Medicine Practitioner", to scheduled patient by the PSR.
* Ask client to state the most important goals during the session – be sure to address them during the session and in the Summary
* Briefly explain the nutrition assessment process
* In-office assessments (BIA, weight, waist circumference, nutrition physical exam (refer to PDF "KU PHY EXAM CHECKLIST"), etc.)
* Review Intake Forms (major concerns, history, nutrition habits, review Medical Symptoms Questionnaire (MSQ) thoroughly, family history/genomics)
* Ask patient to sign MSQ
* Review Diet Diary (1-3 or more days provided. If not available, take a brief typical day dietary intake: 24-hour recall) and Fats and Oils Survey.

* Develop intervention of a nutrition action plan and supplement plan
* Summarize intervention plan and ask if any question.
* Determine the follow up plan including next appointment and any other tasks for patient

In-office assessments and measurements

* In-office assessments in the following order (if applicable)
    - Nutrition Physical Exam (completed throughout appointment's entirety)
    - Height and weight (hallway)
    - BIA Measurement (BIA assessment room/Acupuncture table)
    - Waist Circumference (BIA assessment room/Acupuncture table)
    - Hand Grip dynamometer (BIA assessment room)

Other assessments/measurements not currently used in KU DIM

* Other circumferences (Pediatric: Head; Sports: bicep; Muscle injury: atrophy of specific muscle(s); Amputation)
* Frame Size
* 0_2 Saturation (consult room) (Respiratory issues)
* Blood Pressure and Pulse (matched with capacitance; high pulse)
* Zinc Tally Taste Test
* Iodine Patch Test
* Urinary pH
* Urinary Ascorbic Acid
* Review forms with patient/client

DIM Nutrition Intake Form (Initial Comprehensive or Brief Follow-Up Form)

* Fill in blanks and ask questions in areas needing clarification or expansion
* Ask additional questions, if necessary
* Diet Diary
* Review important findings in lab work / note labs needing to be monitored / retested and timeline
* Review BIA results and other measurements

Develop & discuss priorities & nutrition action plan

References: original-patient & educational Handouts/copy-client records

* Review most important nutrition/lifestyle changes to accomplish goals within anticipated compliance
* Review supplement recommendations for understanding, tolerance, manageability
* Discuss important lifestyle changes (exercise, sleep, stress management, food preparation, procurement)

* Discuss whether further testing (laboratory) is recommended (Refer to "Systemization of Laboratory Evaluation")
* Set measurable goals for next appointment

Review other recommendations

* Explain if further testing is recommended from physician, nutritionist or home tests
* Schedule follow-up, "Touch Base" (phone call within a week for 10-15 minutes to answer questions and monitor progress of Nutrition Action Plan).
* Plan time for follow-up visit: 1-8 weeks

Documentation and Follow-up

* After appointment, be sure chart is in order and action items are followed-up and completed (email articles, "to-dos", recipes, etc.)
* Dictate note; and subsequently edit, print and sign note; to be submitted to attending physician to review and sign
* Compose and print the nutrition and supplement plan, if necessary
* What should be done prior to the next visit, (Labs, diet diary, etc.)
* Document treatment goal for patient
* Develop Nutrition Care Process documentation statement(s), Nutrition **P**roblem, **E**tiology, Signs & Symptoms (PES) based on assessment

KU DIM Consultation Etiquette

1. It is important to understand DIM consultations:
   a. Patients are often very sick and in many cases making difficult nutrition and lifestyle changes at a time when they do not feel well.
   b. Patients often have a good understanding of basic nutrition principles.
   c. A DIM RDN's style of nutrition therapy adapts to each patient and evolves during the consultation based on each patient's knowledge, understanding, willingness to change and specific medical conditions.
2. Before the appointment try to become familiar with the patient's chart. (See *Chart Orientation* document.)
3. Allow the RDN to introduce you to the patient.
4. Let the RDN introduce you and just respond with brief "hello, nice to meet you" statement. Keep introduction brief to allow more time for the RDN and the patient.
5. Be prepared for the consultation by understanding how the consult is conducted for new patients and returning patients. (See *KU Integrative Nutrition Care Process* document).
6. Do not speak unless the RDN asks you to (or patient asks, but do not encourage). Be ready during the consult to assist the RDN when asked. Limit your interaction with the patient so the RDN can efficiently conduct the consult.
7. Ask questions to build and maintain rapport.
8. Use feedback to make appropriate nutrition recommendations based on answers, new labs, symptoms and concerns, etc.

9. If necessary, assist the RDN in: finding papers, labs, handouts, and make copies at the front desk.
10. During the consultation, remain silent, or "like a fly on the wall". Stay engaged in the consultation, as the preceptor may request you look up manufacturer information, assist her with copies, or help with clinic communication.
11. At the end of the consult, remember to thank the patient, assist them in checking out, gathering paperwork, remaining handouts, BIA, etc.
12. Over time, you will be trained in conducting the BIA assessment.
13. The flow of each patient consult is different, so although it is preferable to do the BIA right away, it is often important to sit down and build trust/rapport with the patient to move smoothly to the next step in the Nutrition Assessment process.
14. It may be beneficial to take notes and follow the preceptor's patient interview anticipating questions and responses to questions, considering how you might respond if presented the same situation.

PRINCIPLES OF MOTIVATIONAL INTERVIEWING

Motivational Interviewing (MI) is "a collaborative person-centered form of guiding to elicit and strengthen a person's motivation for change." It is a counseling technique that is a patient-centered and goal-oriented. Integrative Nutritionists and other practitioners use motivational interviewing mainly in the clinical setting when working one-on-one with patients or clients. The following document, based on a Five-Part Series on MI from the Australian Heart Association (February 2012), summarizes some of the key principles of MI. During Week 2 of the Practicum, the intern is to take note of MI in practice while observing an integrative RD. Listed on page 2 are some questions and prompts to take note during patient-practitioner consultations.

Working with patients/clients with chronic disease means practitioners often are working toward behavior change. In MI, ***ambivalence*** is a foundational challenge. In MI, ambivalence refers to both the desire to change and the desire to maintain the status quo.

As you watch the video and as you shadow other healthcare practitioners, refer to page 2 for reflections while observing the practitioner and patient. Start by asking these questions:

- Who is making the argument for change?
  - Patient? Practitioner? Parent? Child? Spouse? Other?
- Is the encounter patient-centered?
- Is the encounter goal-directed?

OBSERVING THE PRACTITIONER (HEALTHCARE PROVIDER)

Does the practitioner...

- MSQ - Use open questions?
- Practice "Reflective Listening"?
- Show the "Righting Reflex"?
- Fall into the "expert trap"?

OBSERVING THE CLIENT

Does the patient demonstrate ambivalence (the desire to change with the desire to remain the same)?

Do you notice the patient using "change talk"?

* **Desire for change**: What are the patient's desires, preferences and wishes for change?
* **Ability to change**: If the patient were to change, what strategies would he or she use to achieve change? *How* would the patient change?
* **Reasons for change**: Most predictive of an actual change made by patient/client. E.g. Get in shape, reduce risk of disease, for kids, etc.
* **Need for change:** Visceral/emotional reasons for change. Values-based.

Do you notice the patient/client using "commitment language"?

* Patient/client's statements of commitment to actual change

Do you notice the patient/client using "sustain talk"?

Patients'/clients' own reasons against change. Desire for status quo, inability for change.

4 Principles of Motivational Interviewing

Expressing empathy: Reflective Listening
Developing discrepancies: How certain behaviors fit with who the patient wants to be?
Rolling with Resistance: ↑ resistance, ↓ likely change, validate
Supporting self-efficacy: Build confidence and hope

Motivational Interviewing Spirit

Collaborative: Patient and Practitioner working together to set goals & formulate solutions
Evocation: The practitioner inspires or elicits motivation from the client or patient
Respect: The practitioner respects the client/patient's choices, resources, ability to follow-through to change, and decision *not* to change, if that is a result of the session.

O.A.R.S. SKILLS of Motivational Interviewing

Open Questions: To elicit evocative spirit and avoid yes/no questions
Affirmations: Affirm the client/patient's strengths and efforts. *Sincerity is important
Reflections: Reflections of what the client/patient wants, needs or feels
Summary: Summarize what the patient believes. Repeat a summary of a compilation of what the patient needs or wants in terms of behavior change or non-change.

Figure 8: Motivational Interviewing

PDF available in the Appendix

MODULE 4: RESEARCH

RESEARCH FROM THE DIM PERSPECTIVE

Reference: DIM Tenet(s): 1-10

Activities

* Learn the system categories of Dietetics and Integrative Medicine (Organ Dysfunction, Cardiometabolic, Cancer, Immune System, etc.) and catalogue/categorize articles that are unfiled in the file management system used at the assigned facility.
* Rotate with designated clinician doing clinical trials if available (at KU Integrative Medicine clinical trials are in cancer related to IV nutritional therapies and outcomes).
* Rotate with designated faculty and learn about the facility Evidence Based Library on their file management software.

MODULE 5: COMMUNITY NUTRITION

DIM COMMUNITY NUTRITION

Reference: DIM Tenet(s): 1-10

The DIM Community rotation will vary widely between practicum sites. *Localharvest.org* is a helpful website to connect preceptors and students to local, organic farms, community supported agriculture farms (CSAs) or farmers markets. Kansas City is home to a healthy Food Policy Coalition or "Greater Kansas City Food Policy Coalition" that can be a great way to network and create contacts for students to rotate and help out and learn from the food community. Community nutrition from a DIM perspective focuses on nutrient density, creating community to support healthy food choices and learn why low-toxin food is important for agricultural sustainability.

Module 5 Activities

* Shadow an RD at a health food store or grocery outlet that emphasizes whole, real foods. This could be a Hy-Vee grocery store RD or a Whole Foods "Healthy Eating Specialist".
* Shadow an RD who gives healthy eating shopping tours. For example: Gluten-Free Shopping Tour, Healthy Foods Shopping Tour, Healing Foods Cooking Class
* Rotate at a farm that emphasizes soil restoration, minimal use of pesticides, herbicides or other "endocrine-disrupting compounds".
* Rotate with a restaurant that purchases from and prepares low-toxin, local and/or seasonal foods.
* Observe, help prepare and/or assist with community presentations and activities.
* The preceptor may give community presentations or group presentations on-site.
* Locate an RD that gives presentations to the community about low-toxin, local or seasonal eating.
* Some non-profit organizations or healing community centers are great locations to find integrative-focused community presentations or small groups. Examples: "Gilda's Club" or "Turning Point" (Kansas City-specific) or others

Supporting Documents for Community Experiences

* Orientation to KU Healing Foods Kitchen
* Grocery List Template
* Recipe Format & Instructions
* Example Recipe Format – Chicken Breast with Tomato and Coconut
* KU Healing Foods Kitchen Cooking Class Calendar

MODULE 6: PRACTICUM STUDENT ASSESSMENT AND EVALUATION

INTRODUCTION

The pre- and post-evaluation tool should be administered to students prior to starting their DIM Practicum and at the completion of the practicum period. The evaluation tool can (and should) be altered based on the specialty of the clinic or practicum setting. The tool covers items outlined in the Practicum Objectives, which should be adjusted, again, to the specialty of the practicum site.

PRE AND POST EVALUATION FOR DIM INTERNS

* What is an Elimination Diet?
* What is the purpose of an Elimination Diet?
* Name 5 of the 10 top food sensitivities/allergens?
* What does it mean to have a leaky/permeable gut?
* What is the function of the "IDU" Nutrition Assessment Tool?
* What does MAPDOM stand for?
* List as many possible ways you can think of to cook/prepare vegetables.
* Although Integrative Dietetics and Nutrition really emphasizes the Individual Nutrition Assessment, what are some general dietary recommendations that would be appropriate for all people?
* Please list and describe the Ten Tenets of Integrative Nutrition.
* Be able to discuss the following areas:
  - Triglyceride levels are more likely associated with simple CHO intake not cholesterol intake
  - General dietary guidelines
  - Describe a simple way to explain how to eat healthy... whole foods
  - Identify healthy fats and oils, clean protein, sources of complex carbohydrates
  - Name two ways genetics affect nutrition recommendations or health
  - Name two ways the methylation cycle impacts health
  - What is/are the most common underlying cause(s) for most chronic health conditions
  - Briefly describe the difference between conventional nutrition therapy and Integrative Dietetics and Nutrition therapy
  - Treating symptoms versus treating root causes

SUPPORTING DOCUMENTS FOR STUDENT ASSESSMENT AND EVALUATION

* Pre and Post Evaluation for DIM Interns

APPENDIX

PROGRAM DEVELOPMENT

CURRICULUM DEVELOPMENT

PRACTICUM GUIDE

SUGGESTED RESROUCES

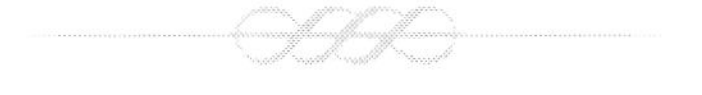

APPENDIX LIST

All documents described in the text can be found in downloadable and printable forms on the following website: www.dieteticsandintegrativemedicine.com

General:

* DIM Award Application Fall 2015
* DIM Graduate Certificate Curriculum
* DIM Organization Chart KUMC
* Standards of Dietetics and Integrative Medicine for Preceptors/Instructors
* Workshop Program: Intro to DIM
* Workshop Program: DIM NCP
* Workshop Program: DIM Business and Dietary Supplements

Module 1: General Orientation to Integrative Medicine

* 1. What is DIM
* 2. Dietetics and Integrative Medicine – What, Why and How
* 3. Ten Tenets of Dietetics and Integrative Medicine
* 4. DIM Learning Objectives
* 5. How to Think Like an Integrative RD
* 6. Orientation to KU Integrative Medicine
* 7. KU DIM Assessment Process
* 8. Tools of the Trade for Clinical Nutrition Assessment
* 9. IFMNT Radial
* 10. IFM Matrix
* 11. What is BIA ?
* 12. Nutritional Supplementation Needs Assessment
* 13. Practicum Overview Table - DIM
* 14. Example of an 8 week Practicum

* 15. DIM Practicum Guidelines - Community
* 16. Time Sheet
* 17. Pre and Post Evaluation for DIM Interns
* 18. DIM Intern Check List
* 19. Text and Electronic References for DIM
* 20. Reading Assignment Reflections Form

Module 2: DIM Food Preparation and Cooking Classes

* 1. Orientation to KU HFK and Student Responsibilities
* 2. Cooking Class Outline – Intern Orientation
* 3. Cooking Class Outline Template
* 4. Kitchen Checklist
* 5. Recipe Format and Instructions

* 6. Example Recipe Format – Chicken and Coconut Milk
* 7. Grocery List Template

Module 3: DIM Clinical Nutrition Practice

* 1. KU DIM Nutrition Care – Assessment Process
* 2. Motivational Interviewing
* 3. Consultation Guidelines
* 4. **I**ntake|**D**igestion|**U**tilization (IDU) Nutrition Status Assessment
* 5. How to Prepare to Observe a Nutrition Consult
* 8. KU Nutrition Intake Forms – New Patient
* 9. KU Nutrition Intake Forms – KU IM Referral
* 10. IFM Matrix
* 11. IFM Timeline of Health History
* 12. GI Tract Assessment Table
* 13. Dental Assessment
* 14. Medical Symptoms Questionnaire (MSQ)
* 15. Fats - Oils Questionnaire
* 16. GI Nutrient Absorption Sites
* 17. Nutrition Assessment Form (blank)
* 18. Nutrition Assessment Questionnaire (Short)
* 19. KUMC Nutrition Physical Exam Checklist
* 20.Specialized Diets for GI Healing
* **Patient Handouts:**
  - A – Protein Servings
  - B – Carbohydrate Servings
  - C – Fats and Oils Servings

- D – Diet Diary and Instructions
- E – Diet Diary Form (blank)
- F – Dietary Withdrawal and Challenge Guidelines
- G – Plate Meal – Menu Guide

Module 4: DIM Research

- **Criteria for Student Research Projects for DIM**
- **Research Projects for Interns**

Module 5: DIM Community Nutrition (see Module 2)

- **Community Nutrition Resources and Websites**

Module 6: Practicum Student Assessment and Evaluation (no supporting documents)s

Distributed at the Dietetics and Integrative Medicine Workshop for Dietetics Interns
On October Fall Semester
Updated October 7, 2015 by Rachel Barkley, DI Program Director

The University of Kansas Medical Center
Department of Dietetics and Nutrition
Dietetics and Integrative Medicine Award

Application Guidelines for Dietetic Interns
Awards for 2016

Application Deadline: 3 weeks

The University of Kansas Medical Center (KUMC) Dietetics and Nutrition Department annually offers two awards for dietetic interns completing the Dietetics and Integrative Medicine Graduate Certificate. The award supports selected students as they complete the Dietetic Internship (DI) graduate certificate and Master of Science (MS) degree in Dietetics and Nutrition along with the additional Dietetics and Integrative Medicine (DIM) graduate certificate.

The Department of Dietetics and Nutrition invites applications from dietetic interns. Completion of the 45 graduate hours for the 2 certificate programs along with the MS degree requires 2 full years of work on the KUMC campus. If a student already has a Master's degree they complete the DI and DIM certificates only. The application deadline is November 2, 2015 and selected fellows are notified in December 2015.

Students are provided financial assistance during the second year of study in the summer semester of 2016. Funding is provided by the Esperance Family Foundation to cover some travel costs and fees to approved conferences, educational expenses, and/or practice experiences. For the past summer semester of 2015 each recipient received a $2,000 award used to support registration and travel expenses to the Food As Medicine conference.

Additionally, a student stipend may be offered by the Department of Dietetics and Nutrition during the second year of graduate study based on availability of graduate research or teaching assistantships. The assistantships provide tuition assistance along with a salary for 16 hours work weekly with the assigned DN faculty. Students apply for the assistantship positions during the spring 2016 semester and assistantships awarded start in the fall 2016 semester.

The DI graduate certificate is a three semester program consisting of 24 graduate credit hours and 1,200 practicum hours, accredited by the Accreditation Council for Education in Nutrition and Dietetics. The DI graduate is eligible to take the national certification examination for registered dietitians immediately after finishing the DI. Degree-seeking students in the DI graduate certificate transfer 14 hours (excluding DN 827 Practicum hours) toward the MS degree. The MS degree requires an additional 16 hours for thesis students or 19 hours for non-thesis students. The Dietetics and Integrative Medicine graduate certificate requires the completion of an additional 12 hours of web-based courses. The 4 additional courses required for this certificate are DN 880 Dietary and Herbal Supplements (summer semester), DN 881 Introduction to Dietetics and Integrative Medicine (fall semester), DN 882 A Nutrition Approach to Inflammation and Immune Regulation (spring semester), and DN 980 Nutrigenomics and Nutrigenetics in Health and Disease (summer semester, prerequisite of genetics).

Dietetic interns who receive the awards participate in supervised practice experiences emphasizing Dietetics and Integrative Medicine along with other required dietetic internship experiences during the spring and summer semesters. They are involved in clinical care at integrative medicine clinics, educational experiences, and research related to Dietetics and Integrative Medicine. During the second-year students complete the MS in Dietetics and Nutrition along with the DIM certificate. Students receiving the award are encouraged to complete research conducted in an area related to Dietetics and Integrative Medicine. They are also expected to contribute to dietetics and integrative medicine training and workshops offered to dietetic interns and graduate students during and after completion of the fellow experiences. It is anticipated that they serve as preceptors after graduation from the graduate programs.

Criteria Assessed for Selection of Awards

1. Degree: A bachelor's degree from a didactic program in dietetics accredited by the Accreditation Council for Education in Nutrition and Dietetics is required for admission. The degree must be from a regionally accredited U.S. university or college. Accredited programs are listed on The Academy of Nutrition and Dietetics web site (www.eatright.org). Degrees earned outside the United States must be evaluated for equivalency (see the Accreditation Council for Education in Nutrition and Dietetics International Fact Sheet at www.eatright.org).

2. Graduate Record Examination Score: A valid score on the Graduate Record Examination general test is required. Recommended scores to be competitive are combined scores for Verbal Reasoning and Quantitative Reasoning of 300 or higher and Analytical Writing of 4 or higher (new GRE scoring system). For the prior GRE scoring system combined of 1000 for Verbal Reasoning and Quantitative Reasoning and 4 for Analytical Writing.

3. Grade Point Average: A cumulative undergraduate grade-point average of 3.0 on a 4.0 scale for college course work is required.

4. Successful completion of a 3 credit hour genetics course prior to starting the graduate certificate program. The course may be at the undergraduate or graduate level.

5. The Selection Process: The following criteria are considered when selecting individuals for the awards.

    - Academic performance*
    - Graduate Record Examination scores*
    - Work and volunteer experience*
    - Leadership*
    - Recommendations*
    - Essay*
      *Obtained from DICAS application
    - Submit a letter of interest that demonstrates educational, work, volunteer or other

experiences related to dietetics and integrative medicine along with other documents or references that show you are an excellent candidate for the award.

Submit applications to Rachel Barkley via email attachment at rbarkley@kumc.edu. You do not need to include DICAS information that has an asterisk (*) by it as the Department of Dietetics and Nutrition has DICAS application files. You do need to submit the letter of interest and other documents or references you want the committee to review.

Letter of interest content

After reviewing "Introduction to Dietetics and Integrative Medicine" and "Dietetics and Integrative Medicine for Chronic Disease", describe your experiences along with your visions of future practice and research interests. Provide examples of specific educational and work experiences related to dietetics and integrative medicine, e.g., participation in coursework, training, conferences, projects, research, and practice, you have completed that make you an excellent candidate. If you have not completed an introductory genetics course (3 hours at the undergraduate or graduate level) describe where and when you plan to complete the course.

Application Review

The applications are evaluated by a committee consisting of members of Department of Dietetics and Nutrition (DN) faculty and Integrative Medicine (IM) RDN from the University of Kansas Medical Center. The top candidates complete an interview with DN faculty and IM RDN. Two students are selected and notified in December of the award.

Introduction to Dietetics and Integrative Medicine

The graduate certificate program offers an opportunity for graduate students with bachelor's or master's degrees in dietetics, nutrition, biological sciences or health professions to acquire the knowledge to function as a skilled advisor to the patient and a collaborative member of interdisciplinary health care teams; professionals who work effectively with integrative and conventional medical practitioners. The graduate certificate is for academically qualified students and professionals interested in pursuing health careers emphasizing medical nutrition therapy for treating the unique needs of ambulatory clients with chronic diseases.

The definition used by the Dietitians in Integrative and Functional Medicine (DIFM), an Academy of Nutrition (AND) and Dietetics Dietetic Practice Group (DPG), is a starting point to describe this evolving advanced specialty of dietetics and nutrition. The approach of dietetics and integrative medicine arose from the challenges of the global epidemic of chronic disease and is built upon many of the principles of traditional medical practice.

> **Integrative nutrition**: *Personalized medical nutrition therapy for prevention and treatment of chronic disease that embraces conventional and complementary therapies. Integrative and functional nutrition reaffirms the importance of the therapeutic relationship, a focus on the whole person, lifestyle, biochemical individuality and environmental influences. (*From the Dietitians in Integrative and Functional Medicine DPG: American Dietetic Association Meeting. April 25. 2010. Buena Park, CA.)
>
> Resources:
> www.integrativeRD.org
> www.integrativemed.kumc.edu
> www.imconsortium.org

Registered Dietitians have the knowledge of food and the body's metabolism that allows them to effectively utilize areas of nutrition science and newer technologies in nutritional biochemistry important in caring for people with chronic disease conditions. The following principles are priorities in the practice of Dietetics and Integrative Medicine.

Biochemical individuality/nutrigenomics: Assessing and developing interventions based on personalized assessment, diagnosis, intervention and monitoring/evaluation. Included in the integrative nutrition toolbox is the emerging field of nutrigenomics that provides information for interpreting the nutrition-related associations of known polymorphisms.

1. *Chronic disease physiology:* Skill in assessment and intervention for the core clinical imbalances common to all chronic disease conditions, with the understanding of critical nutrient regulatory co-factors:
   - *Inflammation* - consideration of the key role essential fatty acids and bioflavanoids play in maintaining optimum inflammatory response.
   - *Immune regulation* - consideration of the key role phytonutrients and nutrition status play in immune strength and function.
   - *Long latency nutritional insufficiencies* - consideration of the long latency nutrient insufficiencies involved in the pathophysiology of chronic disease and nutritional biochemistry to fully understand long latency effects and how to assess and intervene to treat illnesses.

- *Energy metabolism* - consideration of all aspects of energy metabolism from the cellular/mitochondrial energy production to body composition and how to assess and intervene to promote wellness.
- *Environmental nutritional toxicology and epigenetics* - consideration of internal and external environmental toxic factors that influence metabolic interactions and genetic expression, including heavy metals, pollutant chemicals, food allergens or sensitivities, biotoxins, electromagnetic frequencies (EMF), stress and others. Sustainable, organic, and/or toxin-free foods and food preparation recommendations are also considered.

2. *Integrative nutrition assessment and intervention:*
   - *Whole foods, dietary supplements and IM/IV nutrition therapies:* Skill in the use of whole foods, nutraceutical and herbal therapies, medical foods and nutritional consultations on therapeutic intramuscular and intravenous nutrient (IV/IM) therapies when indicated.
   - *Lifestyle:* Skill in assessment of diet, food security and other lifestyle and environmental factors within the framework of physiological systems that are known factors in development of chronic disease, including timeline of antecedents, mediators and triggers.
   - *Conventional and functional laboratory testing:* Familiarity with, and skilled in, reviewing biochemical, functional and genomic data that can give information on the functions of metabolic pathways or networks, skill in investigating and identifying trajectories toward nutritional imbalance within the clinical context.
   - *Integrative collaboration with chronic care team*: Skill in integrating client care with physicians (MD, DO, ND), chiropractors, physician assistants, nurse practitioners, nurses, physical therapists, psychologists, other specialty dietetic professionals (e.g., eating disorders, metabolic, genetics, renal, pediatrics, etc.), as well as other practitioners (e.g., acupuncture, homeopathy, massage, etc.).
   - *Business model for integrative nutrition private practice and medical group*: Familiarity with a business model for the operation of a private practice and contractual relationship in a medical group setting. Includes management of a nutritional pharmacy. Training includes contractual, legal and ethical implications of practice.

Dietetics and Integrative Medicine for Chronic Disease - An Emerging Need

According to the U.S. Bureau of Labor Statistics, employment of Registered Dietitians is expected to rise due to greater emphasis on disease prevention, the growing elderly population, and expanded public interest in nutrition. Chronic lifestyle diseases are a leading cause of premature death and are one of the greatest challenges faced globally by health care professionals. Diet is important lifestyle factor in relation to chronic disease prevention. Industrialized countries are undergoing a "nutrition transition" as populations eat more unhealthy foods that may include toxic and metabolic disruptors that exacerbate chronic disease. Other lifestyle factors, e.g., physical inactivity and the consumption of tobacco and alcohol products also contribute to an unprecedented rise in chronic diseases worldwide. The need to educate and train nutrition experts skilled in working with ambulatory chronic disease patients is both a looming challenge and opportunity.

The Academy of Nutrition and Dietetics (AND, previously ADA) published key recommendations for dietetics education to provide for advanced specialty training in the

Report of the Phase 2 Future Practice & Education Task Force (March 2008).

- *Recommendation 5*: Faculty of dietetics education programs continue to implement a variety of flexible quality education models including opportunities created for new models in response to current trends. All of health care is being challenged with the global epidemic of chronic diseases with trends emerging toward training specialists to deal with unique chronic disease needs.
- *Recommendation 8:* The professional organization continues to recognize specialty practice areas in dietetics and provide support for additional appropriate education and credentialing opportunities. Future specialty areas were identified, including Health Promotion/Disease Prevention. Within each broad specialty practice area, there might be sub-specialty areas such as Integrative Nutrition.

Additional recommendations were presented in the *Report of the Phase 2 Future Practice & Education Task Force (2010).*

- *Recommendation 7:* The Task Force recommends that ADA continue to recognize specialty practice areas in dietetics and provide support for additional appropriate education and credentialing opportunities.
- *Recommendation 8:* The Task Force recommends that ADA define and recognize advanced practice specialties. Advanced practitioners will be supported with educational programming and the appropriate credentials.

The *Council on Future Practice Visioning Report* (2011) identified the following Specialist RD roles but not further developed. The roles are currently evolving and will provide unique opportunities for RDs now and in the future.

- Chronic Disease Management Nutrition Specialist (addresses treatment/management of diseases such as cardiovascular disease, obesity, diabetes and includes palliative care)
- Genomics Specialist

Graduates of the Dietetics and Integrative Medicine Graduate Certificate have the capacity to work in a variety of areas such as:

- Medical clinics providing medical nutrition therapy with conventional and integrative medicine physicians;
- Private practice working under contract with health care or food companies or in their own business;
- Sports nutrition and corporate wellness programs, offering preventative services and educating clients about the connection between nutrition, physical activity and health;
- Food and nutrition-related business and industries working in communications, consumer affairs, public relations, marketing product development or consulting with restaurants and culinary schools;
- Public health, assessing the nutritional health of communities, implementing interventions and monitoring health outcomes;
- Academia, conducting research as well as professional and medical education.

The University of Kansas Medical Center
Department of Dietetics and Nutrition

Dietetics and Integrative Medicine Award

Interview Questions

What experiences influenced your interest in dietetics and integrative medicine?

Tell us why you want a position and what makes you a good candidate for a position?

What are your research interests related to dietetics and integrative medicine?

Describe the practice setting you want to work in after completing your studies.

How will the dietetics and integrated medicine fellow experience impact your future practice?

DIM AWARD APPLICATION 2015 - EXAMPLE

Name of interviewed applicant____

Rubric for Assessing DIM Award Interview Responses

	Developing	Adequate	Accomplished
Clarity of responses	The responses were disjointed and hard to follow	Some of the responses were clear	The responses used language that enhanced comprehension
Focus of response	There were some points made in responses, but they were not put into a framework	Some of the points used in responses were specific to the questions	The points were very specific and focused on the questions
Elaboration of points	There was little elaboration used in each response	Some responses contained an elaboration using examples from experience or evidence	Most responses contained an elaboration using examples from experience or evidence
Thoughtfulness	The responses showed little thoughtfulness or reflection	The responses contained some personal reflections	The responses were appropriately reflective and contained some personal references
Enthusiasm	The responses showed little enthusiasm	The responses indicated modest interest	The responses showed a high level of enthusiasm
Body language	The interviewee seemed uncomfortable in the interview	The interviewee was prepared and comfortable during the interview	The interviewee seemed very self-confident throughout the interview process

Comments:

Name of Interviewer____

The DIM Graduate Certificate

The KUMC Dietetics and Integrative Medicine graduate certificate program offers an online educational opportunity for working professionals or graduate students where they can acquire the knowledge to function as a skilled Dietetics and Integrative Medicine Practitioner, acting as an advisor to the patient and as a collaborative member of multidisciplinary health care teams. The program is open to students with bachelor's or master's degrees in dietetics, nutrition, biological sciences or other healthcare professions.

The KUMC DIM program is a leader in online and self-paced educational opportunities, exploring a personalized approach to prevention and treatment of chronic disease that embraces conventional and complementary therapies. It reaffirms the importance of the therapeutic relationship, a focus on the whole person, lifestyle, biochemical individuality and environmental influences.

This is an online program only, with no campus visits required. The 12 credit hours are delivered as web-based courses, affording great flexibility to students. The curriculum includes the following four courses, with one course offered per semester:

DN 880 Dietary and Herbal Supplements (3 hrs online)

Develop skills to partner with patients in making dietary supplement decisions. Explore the safe, efficacious use of botanicals and supplements in nutritional support of aging, maternal health and wellness. Discussions on supplementation in the prevention and treatment of chronic disease include: arthritis, cancer, cardiovascular, diabetes, digestive, mood and renal disorders. Prerequisite: Human physiology is advisable. Course offered each year, usually Summer semester.

DN 881 Introduction to Dietetics and Integrative Medicine (3 hrs online)

Introduction to principles guiding the practice of integrative and functional medical nutrition therapy; clinical application of the nutrition care process (assessing, diagnosing, intervening, monitoring, and evaluating) toward restoring function for an individual client; focusing on the unique nutritional imbalances characteristic of chronic disease pathophysiology; supporting individuals with persistent symptoms; preventing chronic disease. Prerequisites: Introductory genetics, medical nutrition therapy, or consent of instructor. Course offered each year, usually Fall semester.

DN 882 A Nutrition Approach to Inflammation and Immune Regulation (3 hrs online)

Inflammation and immune dysregulation is common in chronic disease. The course presents the integrative medicine approach to identify the underlying causes of inflammatory and immune-related conditions and associated nutritional influences; applies individualized nutritional interventions, as powerful modulators of the pathophysiology of inflammatory and immune responses. Prerequisites: Medical nutrition therapy, genetics or consent of instructor. Course offered once a year, usually Spring semester.

DN 980 Nutrigenomics and Nutrigenetics in Health and Disease (3 hrs online)

A review of nuclear receptors and their mechanisms of action with specific examples of regulation by nutrients (essential nutrients, retinoids, fatty acids), amino acid control of gene expression, lipid sensors (PPARs), selenoprotein expression, and functional genomic studies (atherosclerosis, cancer, obesity, metabolic syndrome, Type 2 diabetes mellitus, inflammation) with relationships to nutrient intake and polymorphisms. Prerequisite: DN 836, 895 or 896 or permission of instructor. Course offered each year, usually Summer semester.

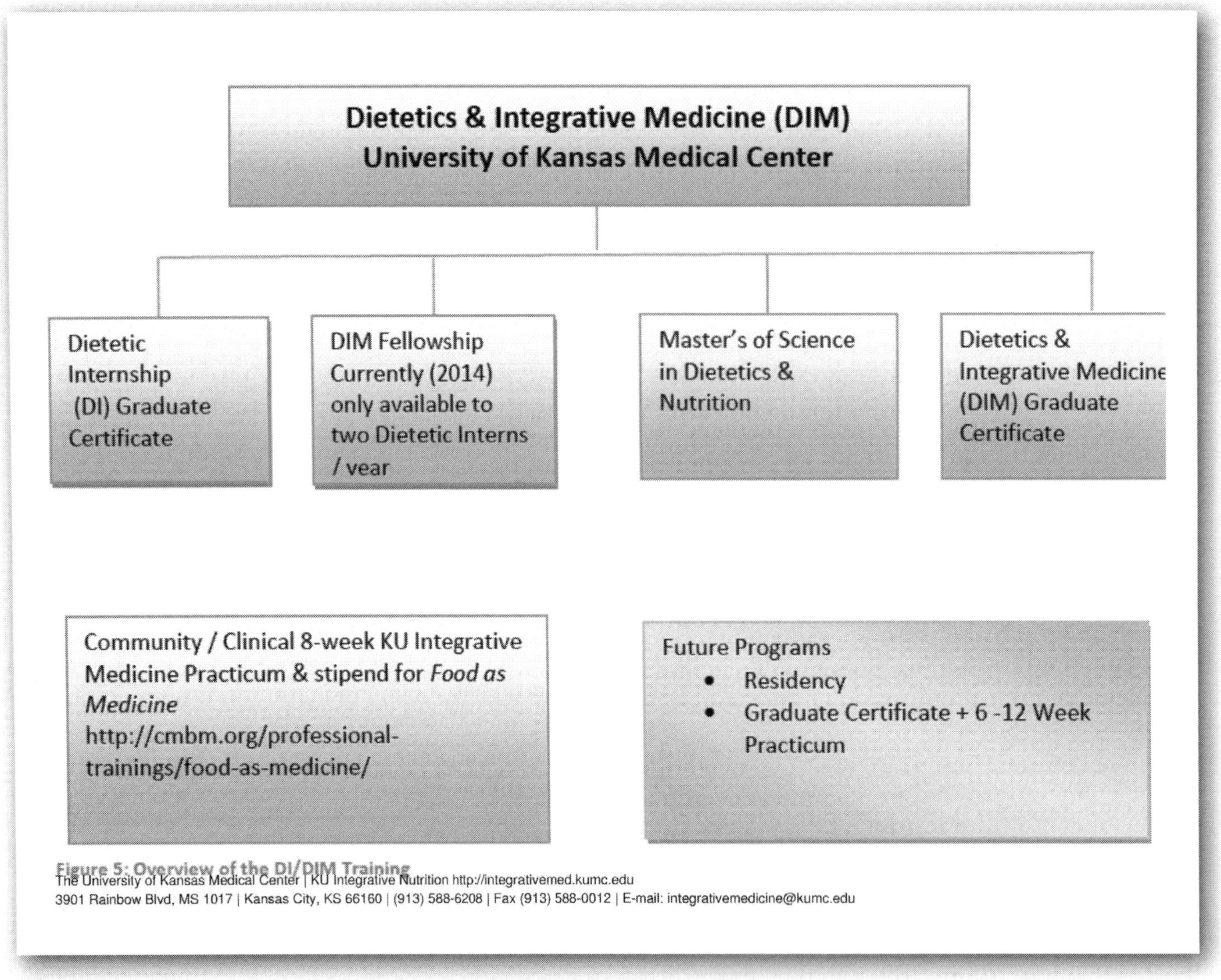

Dietetics & Integrative Medicine (DIM)
University of Kansas Medical Center

Dietetic Internship (DI) Graduate Certificate

DIM Fellowship Currently (2014) only available to two Dietetic Interns / year

Master's of Science in Dietetics & Nutrition

Dietetics & Integrative Medicine (DIM) Graduate Certificate

Community / Clinical 8-week KU Integrative Medicine Practicum & stipend for *Food as Medicine*
http://cmbm.org/professional-trainings/food-as-medicine/

Future Programs

- Residency
- Graduate Certificate + 6 -12 Week Practicum

Figure 5: Overview of the DI/DIM Training

The University of Kansas Medical Center | KU Integrative Nutrition http://integrativemed.kumc.edu
3901 Rainbow Blvd, MS 1017 | Kansas City, KS 66160 | (913) 588-6208 | Fax (913) 588-0012 | E-mail: integrativemedicine@kumc.edu

Standards of Dietetics and Integrative Medicine for Preceptors/Instructors

Dietetics and Integrative Medicine (DIM) describes a new and advanced-specialty dietetic discipline that employs a novel approach to nutritional medicine therapies that is applicable to all healthcare professions. DIM is a unique specialty discipline that addresses the early pathophysiologic alterations leading to chronic disease that occurs over the individual's lifespan, and incorporates a new paradigm based on concepts described in systems biology. This approach complements the acute care model of western conventional medicine that effectively addresses end-stage chronic disease as well as emergency medicine. The DIM training involves a paradigm that represents an added challenge standing in contrast to the process of incorporating new protocols and procedures into an existing model. Thus, the education of a student by a healthcare professional experienced in clinical application of the new paradigm is of utmost importance.

Because the primary application of DIM medical nutritional therapy is within the profession of dietetics and nutrition, the standards described below are presented in the terms of the field of dietetics, but can be translated to standards within other health professions.

Each primary practicum preceptor and/or Dietetics and Integrative Medicine program instructor must meet the following Standards of Dietetics and Integrative Medicine.

DIM Preceptor/Instructor Standards

1. Working knowledge of the *Ten Tenets of Dietetic and Integrative Medicine* / interview by DIM Team
2. CV with previous training, education and experience in integrative or functional medicine approaches (evaluated on individual basis)
3. If no previous training, potential preceptor or instructor to develop and submit a plan for concurrent DIM training to be approved by KUMC DN and KU IM over an academic year
4. Review basics of DIM before beginning preceptor or instructor assignment:
   - Ten Tenets of Dietetics and Integrative Medicine
   - Curriculum Development of DIM (eTextbook), read and schedule discussion with a KU IM staff
   - Watch video *What is Integrative Medicine?* https://www.youtube.com/watch?v=pAOdB2Appe0 Duke University Interview about integrative medicine and the doctor-patient relationship.
   - Shadow a KU IM RD for one or more patients / schedule at (913) 588-0012
   - Attend a Friday-Patient-Chart Review session in KU IM Clinic / arrange with KU IM RD
5. For those preceptors or instructors new to DIM, the DIM Team will provide an advanced integrative RD contact-mentor available for oversight and reference during the first offering of their assigned training program.

Programs at the University of Kansas Medical Center requiring preceptors and/instructors to meet these standards are:

Dietetics and Nutrition Department, School of Allied Health Professions

DIM Graduate Certificate Program (12 hours)

- DN 880 Dietary and Herbal Supplements (3 hours-online)
- DN 881 Introduction to Dietetics and Integrative Medicine (3 hours-online)
- DN 882 A Nutritional Approach to Inflammation and Immune Regulation (3 hours-online)
- DN 980 Nutrigenomics and Nutrigenetics in Health and Disease (3 hours-online)

DIM Dietetic Internship (DI) Workshops

- DI Orientation Week: Introduction to Dietetic and Integrative Medicine (August)
- DI DIM application to the Nutrition Care Process (January)
- DI DIM Business/Entrepreneurial Workshop (April)

KU Integrative Medicine

Community / Clinical Practicum Site

- 6-week Community and Clinical Practicum, KU Integrative Med Nutrition Dept., Spring Semester
- Summer Practicum 4-week (option),
  - KU Integrative Med Nutrition Dept.
  - Other arranged DIM practicum site

8/18/14 Dietetics and Integrative Medicine Project Standards

Dietetics & Nutrition Dietetic Internship Orientation Workshop
"Introduction to Dietetics & Integrative Medicine (DIM)"

Attendees: All KUMC 2013-2014 Dietetic Interns; interested DN graduate students; DN Faculty

Location: University of Kansas Medical Center (KUMC) SON B11 - W 8:30 AM – 11:45 AM, Aug 21, 2013

Workshop Instructors:
Diana Noland, MPH RD CCN LD
Leigh Wagner, MS RD LD
Randy Evans, MS RD LD
Emily Newbold
Katie George

Sponsor: Esperance Family Foundation Dietetics and Integrative Medicine Project Fund

---

PROGRAM SCHEDULE

8:30 AM — Introduction (Rachel Barkley)

8:40 AM — Pre Evaluation

8:55 AM — **WHAT** is Dietetics and Integrative Medicine?

9:15 AM — **WHY** Dietetics and Integrative Medicine?

9:25 AM — **HOW** does a dietitian apply Dietetics and Integrative Medicine in clinical practice?

- Ten Tenets of Dietetics and Integrative Medicine
- Methods:
    - Advanced Specialty Training
    - Functional Medicine Matrix
    - The Patient's Story
    - Inter-professional team participation
- Tools
    - Medical History/Diagnosis (universal)
    - Anthropometrics (universal)
    - MSQ (signs & symptoms) (complete handout)
    - Nutrition Physical Exam / BIA (Interactive session)
    - I-D-U Nutrition Status Assessment
    - Intervention / Monitoring and Evaluation:
        - Whole Low-Contaminated Food and water
        - Dietary Supplements
            - Ethics / Legal use of dietary supplements
            - Therapeutic intervention with dietary supplements
        - Team Referral Network

10:15 AM — ***BREAK*** 15 minutes: Water – Tea - Snack

10:30 AM — **Case Studies**: DIM Nutrition Care Process – Assessment, Diagnosis, Intervention, Monitoring and Evaluation (ADIME)

11:25 AM — Post Evaluation

11:30 AM — Closing – Q&A

Handouts: 1. *JADA* June 2011 SOP/SOPP DIFM 2. Ten Tenets of DIM 3. DIM KUMC Graduate Certificate 4. Changing Landscape in Nutrition and Dietetics: A Specialty Group in Integrative and Functional Medicine. Integrative Medicine (Apr/May 2012).

KUMC Dietetic Internship Dietetics and Integrative Medicine Orientation Workshop, Aug 21, 2013 — 1

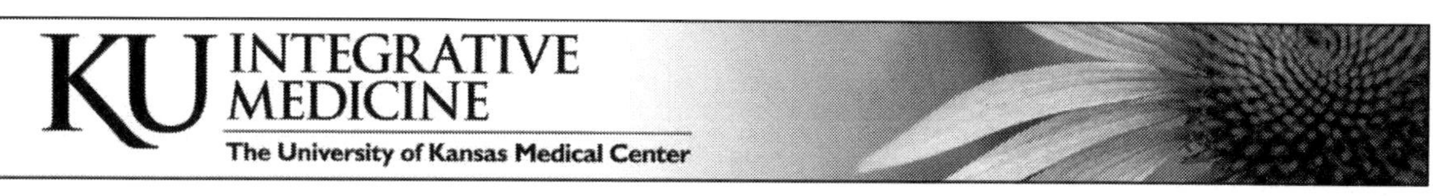

Dietetics & Nutrition Dietetic Internship Workshop

"Dietetics & Integrative Medicine (DIM) Nutrition Care Process Workshop"

Attendees: All KUMC Dietetic Interns; interested DN graduate students; DN Faculty
Location: University of Kansas Medical Center (KUMC) 1014 Orr Major
Date: Tuesday, January 21, 2014, 8:30 am – 3:30 pm
Workshop Instructors:
Diana Noland, MPH RD CCN LD, Leigh Wagner, MS RD LD, Randy Evans, MS RD LD
Sponsor: Esperance Family Foundation DIM Project Fund
Exhibitor: Xymogen

PROGRAM: ***"Dietetics & Integrative Medicine (DIM) Nutrition Care Process Workshop"***

Key Message: *"Individualized nutrition care improves chronic disease conditions."*

8:00 am	Sign-in / Exhibit / Pick up Workshop Materials
8:30 am	Introduction (Dr. Drisko, Dr. Sullivan, Adrienne Baxter)
8:45 am	Introduction / Pre- Evaluation / Review: DIM Dietetics' Role in Healthcare & NCP (Noland)
9:15 am	The Integrative application of the Nutrition Care Process for Heart Disease (Wagner/Evans)
9:45 am	***NCP: DIM Assessment*** (Noland/Wagner/Evans)
10:30 am	*BREAK / Medical Food, Exhibit, Functional Foods Snacks & Coffee / Tea*
10:55 am	Interactive Session Part I: Nutrition Physical Exam (Noland/Wagner/Evans)
12:00 Noon	***NCP: DIM Nutritional Diagnosis*** driven by assessment data (Noland/Wagner)
12:30 pm	*LUNCH BREAK (bring lunch to Workshop)*
1:00 pm	Tour of KU Integrative Medicine (Wagner/Evans)
1:30 pm	***NCP: DIM Intervention***- developing metabolic priorities / Considering Use of Dietary Supplements (Noland)
2:15 pm	***NCP: DIM Monitoring & Evaluation*** for successful outcomes / Post-Evaluation (Noland/Wagner/Evans)
2:30 pm	Meet Dietetics & Integrative Medicine (DIM) Practitioners with Q&A

- Leigh Wagner, MS RD LD (PhD Cand.)
- Randy Evans, MS RD LD
- Diana Noland, MPH RD CCN LD
- Outside-KC DIM Practitioner ________________TBD
- Outside-KC DIM Practitioner ________________TBD

3:30 pm	Closing remarks

KU Integrative Medicine | Mail Stop 1017 | 3901 Rainbow Blvd. | Kansas City, KS 66160 | (913) 588-6208 | Fax (913) 588-0012 | http://integrativemed.kumc.edu/

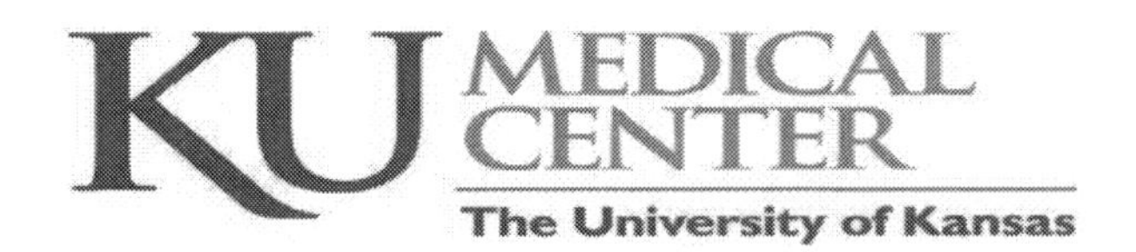

Business and Dietary Supplement Workshop 2014
Dietetic Internship | Dietetics & Integrative Medicine

Attendees: All KUMC Dietetic Interns; interested DN graduate students; DN Faculty

Location & Date:
University of Kansas Medical Center (KUMC)
Room - Orr Major 1014
Monday 2:00PM - 5:00PM, April 28, 2014

Workshop Instructors:
Diana Noland, MPH RD CCN LD
Leigh Wagner, MS RD LD
Randy Evans, MS RD LD

Sponsor: Esperance Family Foundation Dietetics & Integrative Medicine Project Fund

Guest Speakers: Kathy King, RD LD, Author of *The Entrepreneurial Nutritionist*; Mary Willis, MS RD LD, Amy Schleper, MS RD LD; Sally Berry, MS RD LD

1 WEEK BEFORE WORKSHOP – Survey Monkey Pre-evaluation (email)

HANDOUTS

Folders:

Program | Business Plan 101 | DSHEA Act of 1994 | Speaker Bios

Emailed:

Program | Metagenics Quality Brochure | "Dietitians Recommend Supplements" JADA 2012 | Code of Ethics | "Dietary Supplements" The IntegrativeRDN newsletter | "Preventative Medicine as a Viable Financial Model" (link) | Office of Dietary Supplements brochure

RESOURCES

www.integrativerd.org www.nutraingredients-usa.com www.lef.org

www.newhope360.com/nutrition-business-journal http://www.designsforhealth.com/

Business & Dietary Supplements Workshop | Program | April 28th 2014 1

PROGRAM

2:00 Introduction (Adrianne Baxter)

2:05 Entrepreneurial Principles (EP book cover/FNT first page) (Noland)

- Code of Ethics (Cover page photo)
- Income Range
- Negotiating a contract
- Malpractice Insurance

2:20 Business Practice Models

- Private Practice – Independent Contractor
  - Solo office (D Noland photo)
  - Group office: Julie Starkel, Ayleen Video
  - Internet Practice (Gay Riley photo or video)
  - Out-patient Consulting
  - Mentorship: Susan Allen Mentoring Program
  - Combining professions (RD-MD, RD-PT, RD-Pharm, RD-DC, RD-Atty)
- Employee
  - Medical Office Group (Leigh Wagner/Randy Evans-slide photo-talk 10-15 min)
  - Hospital Out-patient
  - LTC (LTC RD and facility photo)
- Self-employed entrepreneur – owner
  - -Sheila Dean video
- Self-employed entrepreneur – Farming
  - -Prairie Birthday Farm (Linda Hezel, PhD RN http://www.prairiebirthdayfarm.com/)

3:00 Dietary Supplements

- Ethics / Legal use of dietary supplements
- Therapeutic intervention with dietary supplements
  - Training
  - Quality
  - Legal
- Nutritional Pharmacy Management
  - In-office (SFM office photo, M Haskell office photo, Deb Ford photo)
  - Off-site (Metagenics, Xymogen, Thorne, Designs for Health, Emerson Ecologics)
  - Health Food Store Nutraceutical Pharmacies (health food store photo)
- Current trends in use of dietary supplements

3:20 Break

3:30 A Plan for Business (e-myth photo)

- Deciding if it's the right fit for you?
- E-myth (Business 101 Handout)

3:45 Meeting Practitioners in Dietetics & Integrative Medicine with Q&A

- Kathy King, RD LD – 15 min LIVE/Audio
- Mary Willis, MS RD LD – 15 min (onsite)
- Amy Schleper, MS RD LD – 15 min (onsite)
- Sally Berry, MS RD LD – 15 min (onsite)

4:50 Closing

Survey Monkey Post-evaluation – 2 days after workshop (email)

Business & Dietary Supplements Workshop | Program | April 28th 2014 2

KU Dietetics and Integrative Medicine

Real Food for *Really* Healthy Living

What is Dietetics and Integrative Medicine? DIM is a new type of nutrition therapy that focuses on the whole person, lifestyle, biochemical individuality and environmental influences. The United States is facing an epidemic of chronic diseases that are preventable by diet and lifestyle. An Integrative Dietitian assesses YOUR nutritional status and plans with YOU to meet YOUR health needs. Consider an Integrative assessment to improve any medical condition or for "early detection" of nutrient imbalances to keep YOUR body functioning in wellness.

KU Dietetics and Integrative Medicine: The KU Integrative Medicine is an emerging center for DIM. Nutrition services include personalized nutrition consultations with a nutrition physical exam, laboratory analyses, body composition testing, and personalized nutritional planning. In addition to one-on-one consultations, the Healing Foods Kitchen offers a place to learn to live a lifestyle rich in real foods. These classes are open to the Kansas City community as well as campus staff, students and patients.

Why whole foods? Eating a diet rich in "whole foods" is the use of *Food as Medicine*. *Whole, real, unprocessed* food is the most compatible fuel for our bodies. Foods grown in nutrient-rich soils produce nutrient-rich foods. An Integrative Dietitian can personalize a whole foods diet to assist YOUR body to function at its greatest potential.

Why specific nutritional supplement? When the Integrative Dietitian completes a full, individualized assessment, YOUR unique nutritional needs are identified. From that information, sometimes specific, *pharmaceutical-grade* nutritional supplements may be necessary to support YOUR body, speed healing, and reach YOUR optimal nutritional status.

The Healing Foods Kitchen: Seasonal classes are offered each month based on healthy, whole foods that nourish the mind-body-spirit. Classes are casual and conversational. Tasting, smelling and touching new and different foods are highly encouraged. Taste foods you've never heard of or those you've seen and always wanted to try. Class prices range from $15-25, depending on menu offerings.

Leigh Wagner, MS, RD
Medical Nutrition Therapy and Nutrition Education
KU Integrative Medicine
lwagner@kumc.edu
913-588-6208
Website: http://integrativemed.kumc.edu

Dietetics and Integrative Medicine

What is Dietetics and Integrative Medicine?

Dietetics and Integrative Medicine is the future of nutrition care for chronic disease. In general, it is the advanced practice of nutrition assessment, diagnosis, intervention, and monitoring at the molecular and cellular levels that focuses on the promotion of optimal health and the management and prevention of diet- and lifestyle-related diseases.

DIM is at the core of Integrative Medicine, as a foundational approach to health. The Consortium of Academic Health Centers for Integrative Medicine defines Integrative Medicine as *"the practice of medicine that reaffirms the importance of the relationship between practitioner and patient, focuses on the whole person, is informed by evidence, and makes use of all appropriate therapeutic approaches, healthcare professionals and disciplines to achieve optimal health and healing."* Nutrition is a key piece of the various therapeutic approaches that is evidence-based and allows for a deep therapeutic relationship between client and practitioner. Dietitians in Integrative Medicine take the necessary time to investigate the root cause of a client's health problems associated with nutritional imbalances, whether from inadequate intake, digestion or utilization.

Why Do We Need Dietetics and Integrative Medicine?

- The prevalence of complex, chronic diseases is escalating globally, from heart disease and diabetes to irritable bowel syndrome, chronic fatigue, fibromyalgia, mental illness, and rheumatoid arthritis and other autoimmune disorders.
- Chronic diseases are diet- and lifestyle-related diseases and require solutions in diet and lifestyle. A major strength of DIM is its focus on the molecular mechanisms that underlie disease, which provides the basis for targeted, innovative solutions that can restore health.
- The current healthcare system fails to account for the unique genetic makeup of each individual or the ability of foods, toxins, and other environmental factors to influence gene expression. The interaction between genes and environmental factors is a critical component in the development of chronic disease and plays a central role in the Dietetics and Integrative Medicine approach.
- Most nutrition professionals are not adequately trained in integrating nutrition assessment at the molecular and cellular levels with emerging research in nutrition and nutritional genomics. These advanced practice skills are essential for preventing and managing today's chronic disorders.

How is a Dietetics and Integrative Medicine Practitioner Different?

The Dietetics and Integrative Medicine (DIM) Practitioner represents an advanced level of nutrition professional. The DIM Practitioner functions as the physician's primary partner on the chronic care team and is the expert in using diet, nutrition and lifestyle approaches, including nutritional genomics, for preventing and managing chronic disease. The specialty knowledge and advanced skills of the DIM Practitioner includes more advanced knowledge in nutritional and functional testing of nutrients and nutritional imbalances. All of this makes a DIM practitioner unique within healthcare and able to participate within healthcare in ways never before possible.

University of Kansas Medical Center | **Integrative Medicine** 1

Ten Tenets of Dietetics and Integrative Medicine (DIM)

University of Kansas Medical Center
KU Integrative Medicine

"First, do no harm."

1. **Individualized Integrative Medical Nutrition Therapy (MNT) optimizes wellness.**
2. **Genomic uniqueness of an individual contributes to integrative MNT interventions in addition to practice and evidence base medicine.**
3. **Listening to the patient's story is the basis of the therapeutic relationships between providers and their clients to maximize health outcomes.**
4. ***"Food as epigenetic medicine"* – appropriate foods and targeted nutrients* for an individual can act as epigenetic messages to promote wellness.**
5. **Whole low-contaminated foods and targeted nutrients* specific for the individual provide the basis of integrative MNT.**
6. **Correct nutritional insufficiencies as well as deficiencies to optimize nutrient metabolism and lower risk of chronic disease.**
7. **Manage chronic disease inflammation through food and targeted nutrients.**
8. **Use of targeted nutrient* therapies can reduce toxin damage to metabolism.**
9. **Beliefs and community relationships influence nutritional health (mind-body).**
10. **Know when you are not the expert. Collaborate with other members of the integrative care team.**

The etiology of the current chronic disease epidemic is often due to a lifetime of poor diet and lifestyle choices as well as harmful environmental exposures.

targeted nutrients: therapeutic use of isolated or combined nutrients that can be administered as dietary supplements, medical foods, topical cutaneous, intramuscular or intravenous injections.

 1

IV. Dietetics and Integrative Medicine (DIM) Learning Objectives

Learning objectives include both didactic and self-motivated learning. The certificate and the MS degree program training are expected to result in competence in:

- The practice of dietetics and integrative medicine (DIM), either in a private practice, in an academic setting or an institutional setting.
- Conducting and/or assisting with basic research in DIM to advance and broaden the evidence base.
- The education, mentorship, and training of students and colleagues in the basic principles and practices of DIM.

There are a number of core areas where, upon satisfactory completion of the certificate and fellowship training programs, individuals are expected to show an in-depth understanding, both in theory and in practice and within a community, management, or clinical setting:

A. Foundational Concepts of DIM

1. Define and describe the role *systems physiology* plays in DIM. Consider the complex interaction between genetics, the environment and lifestyle overtime and resulting health. (Clinical, Community)
2. Describe the meaning of the phrase "Structure equals function" in relation to nutritional status and health. (Clinical, Community)
3. Give 2 examples of the health and nutritional influence of stress or beliefs (thoughts, feelings, culture, religion, spirituality, other) on a patient's/client's health. (Clinical, Community)

B. DIM, Nutrition Care Process: Assessment and Diagnosis

4. Identify three (3) textbook references for Dietitians and healthcare practitioners in Integrative Medicine (Clinical, Community)
5. Clearly state three (3) distinguishing aspects of a nutrition assessment from the perspective of Dietetics and Integrative Medicine Assessment compared to a typical nutrition assessment. Describe how they're similar and how they differ. (Clinical, Community)
6. List five (5) of the many signs of nutritional deficiency or insufficiency that can be noted upon administering a Nutrition-Focused Physical Exam. (Clinical)
7. List two (2) companies, which are commonly, used for outside nutritional testing or laboratory assessments. (Clinical)
8. Name three (3) conventional and three (3) functional nutritional laboratory assessments that are useful in designing a successful nutritional assessment within

the context of Dietetics and Integrative Medicine. Be able to discuss why and under what circumstances they might be most useful. (Clinical)

9. Using a Bioelectric Impedance Analysis (BIA) device, analyze body composition of a patient/client. Discuss the differences between BIA and other body composition tests, measurements and devices (BMI, Bod Pod, DEXA). Describe what is being measured by each assessment and the advantages or disadvantage for each. Be able to discuss why and under what circumstances they might be most useful. (Clinical)
10. Within the context of the patient's individual story, analyze a food diary for content and quality of (Clinical):
    a. Fat, Protein, Carbohydrate, Fiber, Liquid (water/other), Phytonutrients
    b. Sunlight exposure with emphasis on residence (location, latitude) and Vitamin D food intake
    c. Meal Timing and Snacking
    d. Supplements and Medications
    e. Toxin load
11. Assess patient lifestyle factors that contribute to nutritional status (sleep, physical activity/inactivity, beliefs, etc.). (Clinical, Community)
12. Regarding other aspects of lifestyle (in addition to dietary intake), describe the impact of the following lifestyle factors and how these may affect nutritional status (Clinical, Community):
    a. Sleep and sleep quality, circadian rhythm
    b. Community and family/friend support
    c. Food access, preparation or other limits on a healthy nutrition lifestyle
    d. Belief system regarding: healthy, religion/spirituality, cultural or other
13. Describe nutritional influences on the following principles of Dietetics and Integrative Medicine (Clinical, Community):
    a. Inflammation
    b. Immune regulation
    c. Long Latency Nutritional Insufficiencies (aka "Long Latency Deficiency Disease")
    d. Epigenetics/gene expression
    e. Body Composition
14. Using the Natural Medicines Comprehensive Database or Natural Standard database, check interactions or drug-induced nutrient depletions (DINDs) for medications, dietary supplements, herbal supplements, etc. (Clinical)
15. List at least two (2) common Nutrition Diagnostic Statements used to diagnose nutrition problems used often in DIM (E.g. Altered gastrointestinal function; altered nutrition-related laboratory values; altered nutrient utilization; etc.). (Clinical)

C. DIM, Nutrition Care Process: Intervention and Monitoring and Evaluation

16. Be able to describe, verbally or in written form, the decisions considered in recommending an elimination diet and the purpose of the timing and removal of a specific food or foods. (Clinical)
    a. List and describe three (3) different types of elimination diets (FODMAPs, comprehensive elimination, Histamine, Nightshades, Gluten, Casein, etc.)
    b. Describe how to plan and monitor the reintroduction, rotation, and/or challenge of eliminated foods.
17. Describe when nutritional supplementation is appropriate and outline key things to monitor for a patient or client (lab values). Explain instances when it would be inappropriate to recommend supplementation. (Clinical, Community)
18. Have the capability to effectively and efficiently search for scientific literature to support interventions for patients or clients. (Clinical, Community)
19. Discuss the physiological, biological and scientific basis of various "diets" (Consistent Carbohydrate, "Cardiac" Diet, Modified Elimination, Ketogenic, other). Discuss the appropriate application of each to populations versus individuals. (Clinical)
20. Discuss the importance of monitoring individualized nutrition interventions. Give 2-3 strategies (action steps) to monitor a patient. (Clinical)

D. Food Quality and Regulation

21. Describe the importance of soil quality, mineral/nutrient content, and its effect on nutritional recommendations. (Community)
22. Describe Endocrine-Disrupting Chemicals (EDCs) and list 2 common substances or groups of substances that would be considered EDCs. Name ways to avoid EDCs through food or lifestyle efforts. (Clinical, Community)
23. Describe instances when food quality would be higher or lower when produced: locally, organically, conventionally, in various growing conditions. State other reasons you might consider nutritional quality or content of endocrine-disrupting chemicals. (Clinical, Community)
24. Describe five (5) key aspects of a successful local food system. Describe the differences and similarities from hospital or other foodservice experience(s) you have had. (Community, Management)
25. Be able to independently plan, organize and prepare for a cooking demonstration. (Community, Management)
26. Be able to correctly write a recipe: correctly listing ingredients, describing instructions and altering ingredients to meet needs of those with food sensitivities/allergies, those avoiding excess sodium, and other specific dietary needs. (Community, Management)

E. Community Nutrition

27. List general nutrition recommendations that can be given in a group setting. (E.g. Whole foods and minimally-refined foods are optimal for most people; many people benefit from a primarily plant-based diet; Low-toxin food optimizes health; Dietitians in Integrative Medicine must do an individualized nutrition assessment to determine a patient's/client's nutrition status). (**Community**)
28. List or name various community-based organizations and/or websites that could help dietitians, healthcare practitioners or the lay public to access whole, real, minimally refined foods. (**Community, Clinical**)

F. Expected Competencies in Computer Technology

The student exhibits sufficient competence in computer technology to:

- Receive electronic mail communications from the course instructor.
- Open electronic mail attachments.
- Use research databases and explore internet web sites.
- Download computer software slide presentations provided for class session notes.
- Own, purchase and install, or be willing to access through the Instructional Technology Center at the University of Kansas Medical Center, Microsoft Power Point® and Microsoft Word® computer applications.

How to Think Like an Integrative RD

Biochemical individuality is a foundational tenet of Dietetics and Integrative Medicine (DIM); each person has a different lifestyle, family, culture, community, and genetic makeup. In effect, each person has a different nutritional status. DIM interventions are specific for each individual and are based on an individual nutrition assessment. The DIM dietetic internship will provide DIM experiences in the clinical, community and the food service rotations. Individualized care is accomplished easier in a **clinical setting**, working one on one with a client or patient. In the **community setting,** DIM is more challenging as the Integrative Dietitian is working with a population in which only part of the time a single intervention may be appropriate. Similarly, in **food service management**, an Integrative RD prioritizes the use of the highest quality of foods to promote healing, i.e., to use "food as medicine". Each Dietetic Internship rotation – clinical, community and food service – will emphasize and use varying degrees of the DIM tenets. Thus, the following will help you *think like an Integrative RD* throughout each of your dietetic internship rotations.

Integrative dietitians practice can be complex because it focuses on the individual and attempts to identify underlying causes for symptoms or conditions. Integrative RD patients are often in poor health and interventions require major changes in diet and lifestyle. These changes are necessary to allow for healing and to improve possible underlying metabolic causes of chronic health conditions or disease. While DIM practice can be complex, it focuses on a simple principle: the use of real, whole foods our bodies are designed to recognize and promote optimal health.

Community: Among a population, it's difficult to provide specific nutrition recommendations. Thus, addressing Biochemical Individuality will not always be possible, especially in a community setting. An individualized nutrition assessment is critical – though not always feasible – for an DIM Intervention to be successful. When you are asked specific nutrition questions by individuals during a presentation or in a group, you should remind the group that each person in the room has a different nutritional status and, thus, unique nutritional needs/recommendations.

Tenet: Food as medicine – Food acts as information to message our genes.
Beliefs and community influence health (Mind-Body).
Chronic disease is most often due to a lifetime of diet & lifestyle choices.

How to think like an Integrative RD: Community Perspective

Food is Medicine:

a. Whole Foods are Foundational
b. Food quality and minimization of toxins through food and food service/preparation

Lifestyle: In KU Integrative Medicine, we provide lifestyle education directly through cooking classes in the Healing Foods Kitchen. Other important Lifestyle categories include:

a. Mind-body-spirit c. culture e. nature / sunlight
b. Environment d. family f. community / laughter

Environmental Impact: Nourishing food comes from nourished soil, and therefore it is important for Integrative RDs to care for the land on which our food is grown.

KUMC | Integrative Medicine 1

Food Service Management: Through KU Integrative Medicine, the student's major experience with foodservice management is through KU Healing Foods Kitchen Cooking Classes. However, most of students' hours for food service (FS) management are spent outside of KU Integrative Medicine's Healing Foods Kitchen.

Tenet: Whole foods and targeted nutrients are the basis of medical nutrition therapy.
Toxins can alter nutrient metabolism.

How to think like an Integrative RD: FS Management Perspective

Food is Medicine:

a. Whole Foods are Foundational and meet biochemical needs
b. Food quality and minimization of toxins through food and food service/preparation

Lifestyle: In KU Integrative Medicine, we provide lifestyle education directly through cooking classes in the Healing Foods Kitchen. Other important Lifestyle categories include:

a. Mind-Body-Spirit
b. Environment
c. Culture
d. Family
e. Nature / Sunlight
f. Community / Laughter

Environmental Impact: Nourishing food comes from nourished soil, and therefore it is important for Integrative RDs to care for the land on which our food is grown.

Clinical: This is the biggest and most in-depth application DIM.

Tenet: Safe and individualized nutrition care optimizes wellness.
Biochemical individuality provides the evidence base of the individual.
Food and targeted nutrients are primary factors in chronic inflammation management.
Efficient nutrient metabolism supports optimal function.
The therapeutic relationship maximizes outcomes.

How to think like an Integrative RD: Clinical Perspective

You will do nutrition assessments during every rotation of your internship. What's most critical about thinking like an Integrative RD is to realize that NOT All NUTRITION INTERVENTIONS ARE APPROPRIATE FOR ALL PEOPLE/DIAGNOSES/ILLNESSES.

a. Biochemical Individuality is critical
b. Assess what the person is ingesting on a regular basis
c. Furthermore, think also about...
   1. How the individual is DIGESTING, ABSORBING AND UTILIZING the food, beverage, nutrients
   2. What environmental exposures may affect their ability to digest/absorb/utilize their nutritional intake

Future experiences & Reading: You will learn more as you spend more time in Integrative Medicine. In the meantime, you can refer to the foundational references, (see list).

a. IFMNT Radial
b. 7 Principles of DIM

Orientation to KU Integrative Medicine

Welcome to our clinic! KU Integrative Medicine (IM) was founded in 1998 with Jeanne Drisko, MD operating solely with another physician and an infusion nurse. They operated out of two small rooms at the end of the OBGYN hall at KU Medical Center. Since then, the clinic has grown to house 3 Medical Doctors,one Naturopathic Doctor (ND), one Advanced Practice Registered Nurse (APRN), two Registered Dietitians, two Neurofeedback Technicians, a Clinical Research Coordinator, and an amazing support staff!

Things to know about KU Integrative Medicine:

- **Days & Hours of Operation**: Monday-Friday, 8:30 am – 5:00 pm
- **Friday Chart Review**: Every Friday at noon in the KU IM Conference Room, the KU IM has a presentation or professional development activity followed by a meeting to review complex cases and discuss patients.
- **Dress**: Business attire. Practitioners do not wear white coats
- **How to Address Practitioners**: All practitioners in the clinic are referred to on a first-name basis between practitioners. This varies between patient and practitioner.
- **Healing Foods Kitchen and other Cooking Classes**:
    - Cooking classes are held at least once monthly, generally at the beginning of the month.
    - Classes in the HFK are held between 12:00-1:30 pm, with some variation depending on the menu.
    - You may keep your food in the refrigerator with exceptions for limits on space surrounding cooking class (Wednesday afternoon through Thursday afternoon)
    - Please refer to Orientation to KU Healing Foods Kitchen document (Week 4 documents).

- **Integrative Medicine Modalities: KU Integrative Medicine Services**
    - Integrative & Functional Medical Consultations
    - Naturopathic Medical Consultations
    - Nutrition Consultations
    - Cooking Demonstrations
    - Neurofeedback
    - IV and IM Nutritional Therapies

- **Integrative Medicine Modalities: Referral Services**
    - Acupuncture
    - Massage Therapy
    - Chiropractic
    - Physical Therapy
    - Medical Specialties
    - Energy healing
    - Attunement
    - Reike
    - Others, as needed

KU Integrative Medicine is based on 4 Pillars of the University of Kansas Medical Center:

- **Patient Care**: Individualized care for patients and clients is the main focus of KU IM.
- **Education**: Nutrition, nursing, and medical students and medical residents and fellows shadow each of the practitioners, including the registered dietitian nutritionist (RDN). Presentations are also periodically given to educate campus student organizations.
- **Service**: Campus and community presentations, cooking classes, group classes, and other community outreach is important to KU IM. Additionally, many staff members serve on local and national boards and committees within the Integrative Medicine community.
- **Research**: KU IM conducts translational research: from basic lab sciences to clinical research We also house a growing nutrition-focused evidence based library on Mendeley and EndNote.

Practitioners	**Specialty**
Jeanne Drisko, MD	Medical Director
Jody Krukowski, ND	Naturopathic Doctor
Ourania Stephopoulus, MD	Internist
Anna Esparham, MD	Pediatrician
Elizabeth Schrick, RN	Infusion Nurse
Leigh Wagner, MS, RDN	Registered Dietitian Nutritionist
Randy Evans, MS, RDN	Registered Dietitian Nutritionist & Operations Manager
Tiffany Burch	Neurofeedback Technician
Teri Mayo	Neurofeedback Technician
Emily Curran, APRN	Advanced Practice Registered Nurse
Staff	
Janet Ink	Executive Director
Nancy Lynn	Patient Service Representative
Crystal Lowe	Patient Service Representative
Research Team	
Jean Sunega	Clinical Research Coordinator
Qi Chen, PhD	Primary Investigator

KU DIM Assessment Process

Background

The initial nutrition assessment at KU Integrative Medicine (KU IM) is based on the Nutrition Care Process established by the Academy of Nutrition and Dietetics (The Academy), and is summarized, as follows:

Assessment
Diagnosis
Intervention
Monitoring
Evaluation

Chart Review and Preparation

The RDN reviews the paper and/or electronic medical record for information about the client's health history, nutrition history, anthropometrics, and any other information that could be helpful to begin to evaluate the person's nutritional status.

Papers or documents that can be helpful for nutrition consultations

- Nutrition intake forms submitted prior to nutrition consultation
- While reviewing the chart, complete the "Blank Nutrition Assessment & Consultation Summary Form"
- Blank "Progress Note" to write notes during appointment (lined paper with the client's name, Medical Record Number (MRN) and Date of Birth (DOB))
- Charge Sheet (varies by practice)
- Nutritional supplement list and company contact information packet (varies by practice)
- List of supplements available at KU Hospital Outpatient Pharmacy

KU Integrative Medicine – Leigh Wagner MS, RD, LD

Before Appointment

Prior to the actual consultation/appointment, the patient service representative (PSR) will need to take care of technical information, paperwork and other items:

- PSR: Confirm that patient has filled out all necessary forms & take photo (if approved and appropriate). If not, prepare forms that need to be completed and explain each one in detail, if necessary. Chart should be prepared ahead of time.
    - Notice of Privacy Practices (PSR)
    - HIPPA Authorization (PSR)
    - Diet Prescription or specific KU IM Referral form (pink or blue form)
    - Integrative Nutrition Intake Form (self or physician-referred)
    - Diet Diary (1 to 3-day history)
    - Fats and Oils Questionnaire
    - Medical Symptoms Questionnaire
- Photograph (taken by PSR): Take a photograph of the client to place in the chart. This will be used for ease of recognition and better recall of client story and team approach to care.
- Dietitian (RDN): Introduce yourself, welcome and ask how the person prefers to be addressed. Lead client to private, quiet consultation room. Invite the client to sit in designated chair in counseling area. If a family member or friend of the client wants to join the consultation and is 18 years or older, ask client for permission.
- When necessary, ask the client whether a dietetic intern can observe the appointment.

KU Integrative Medicine – Leigh Wagner MS, RD, LD

Nutrition Assessment Process

Background and explanation of assessment

- Explain to client, when necessary, the uniqueness of Dietetics and Integrative Medicine by providing the handout "What is DIM?"
- Ask client to state his or her most important goals to achieve during the session. Be sure to address these goals during the session and in the visit summary
- Briefly explain the nutrition assessment process, when necessary
  - In-office assessments: Bioelectric Impedance Analysis (BIA), weight, waist circumference, nutrition physical exam, others
  - Review of Nutrition Intake Forms, Medical Symptoms Questionnaire (MSQ), Fats & Oils Questionnaires, and any others
  - Ask client to sign MSQ
  - Review Diet Diary. If not completed, take a 24-hour dietary recall
  - Develop intervention of a nutrition action plan and supplement plan

In-office assessments and measurements

In-office assessments (not all of these tests are completed at every visit on every client)

- Nutrition Physical Exam
- Anthropometrics: Height, weight, waist circumference
- Bioelectric Impedance Analysis (BIA): Measurements taken on a massage or acupuncture table or other surface client can easily and comfortably lay supine
- 02 Sat (Respiratory issues)
- Hand Grip Strength Measurement
- Blood Pressure and Pulse
- Frame Size Assessment

Other assessments/measurements not currently used in KU IM

- Other circumferences (Pediatric: Head; Sports: bicep; Muscle injury: atrophy of specific muscle(s); Amputation)
- Zinc Tally
- Iodine Patch Test
- Urinary pH
- Urinary Ascorbic Acid

KU Integrative Medicine – Leigh Wagner MS, RD, LD

Review forms with client

- Nutrition Intake Forms (Initial Comprehensive or Brief Follow-Up Form)
    - Fill in blanks and ask questions in areas needing clarification or expansion
    - Ask additional questions, if necessary
- Diet Diary
- Review important findings in lab work / note labs needing to be monitored / retested and timeline
- Review BIA results and other measurements

Develop and discuss priorities, and create nutrition action plan

- Review most important nutrition/lifestyle changes to accomplish goals within anticipated time and client adherence to plan
- Review supplement recommendations for understanding, tolerance, manageability
- Discuss important lifestyle changes (exercise, sleep, stress management, food preparation, procurement)
- Discuss whether further laboratory testing is recommended
- Set measurable goals for next appointment
- Write and provide a copy to the client of the Nutrition Action Plan for the client to have record and reference to his/her nutritional goals and actions

Review other recommendations

- If recommended, explain any further nutritional laboratory testing recommended by you, the physician, or Advanced Practice Registered Nurse (APRN)
- Schedule follow-up, "Touch Base", phone call within a week for 10-15 minutes to answer questions and monitor progress of Nutrition Action Plan
- Plan time for follow-up visit: 1-6 months, depending on the complexity of the case and nutrition action plan

Documentation and Follow-up

- After appointment, organize the chart, notes and laboratory results.
- Ensure action items are followed-up and completed (email articles, "to-dos", recipes, laboratory requisition, testing kits, etc.)
- Document (write, type, dictate) the nutrition note and finalizing by signing and submitting to the referring doctor for review and/or signature.
- Write the nutrition and supplement plan, if necessary

KU Integrative Medicine – Leigh Wagner MS, RD, LD

- What should be done prior to the next visit, (Labs, diet diary, etc.)
- Document treatment goal(s) and plan for client
- Based on Nutrition Assessment, Develop nutrition diagnostic statements and intervention (plan) by following the Nutrition Care Process (NCP) form for Nutrition Diagnostic Statements, PES:
  - Problem
  - Etiology
  - Signs/Symptoms

Definition of Terms and Acronyms

KU IM: University of Kansas (KU) Integrative Medicine
AND or "The Academy": The Academy of Nutrition and Dietetics (formerly, American Dietetic Association or "ADA")
PSR: Patient Services Representative
MSQ: Medical Symptoms Questionnaire
EMR: Electronic Medical Record
AVS: After Visit Summary
NCP: Nutrition Care Process
PES: Problem Etiology Signs & Symptoms
HPI: History of Present Illness
PMH: Past Medical History

Appendix I
Tools of the Trade for Clinical Nutrition Assessment

The functional medicine practitioner uses a variety of methods for nutritional assessment in order to obtain a complete understanding of a patient's nutrition status. Through careful history taking, physical findings, anthropometric measurements, standard and functional blood chemistry analysis, dietary intake and lifestyle assessment, the practitioner is able to evaluate fundamental imbalances and apply effective interventions. In addition, environmental, genetic and psychological components are addressed to gain a more comprehensive approach to managing or restoring health. Each of these tools provide important information as to how key processes are affected and help the practitioner prioritize the treatment plan.

> The tools that are discussed in this section are provided on the IFM website www.functionalmedicine.org. These may be used as is, or they may be customized to meet the specific needs of the practitioner.

Medical Symptom Questionnaire

The Medical Symptom Questionnaire (MSQ) is a tool that quantifies the incidence of symptoms and their frequency. When this tool is administered at regular intervals during patient follow-ups, it provides a quick measure of improvement. This tool evaluates symptoms over the past 30 days and in certain cases it may be used to assess symptoms over the past 48 hours. The patient simply rates each symptom on a scale of zero to four, with zero indicative of "never or almost never" having the symptom to four, for more frequent and severe effects of a symptom. All of the individual scores are added and the total score is rated as follows:

Optimal	Less than 10
Mild (Toxicity)?	10 – 50
Moderate	50 – 100
Severe	Over 100

Nutrition Physical Exam

The nutrition physical exam is a key component of the patient assessment. While the physician can complete an extensive physical, there may be signs specific to nutrient status. It is important to understand the place for nutrition exam findings within the functional medicine matrix and in the continuum of health. Use the **Nutrition Physical Exam** tool to assist with the evaluation of the patient. The following table summarizes exam findings and their nutritional implications.

SYSTEM	SIGN	NUTRIENT or CONDITION
Mouth	Glossitis	Deficiencies of riboflavin, niacin, biotin, B6, B12, folate, iron, zinc
	Angular stomatitis, Cheliosis	Deficiencies of riboflavin, niacin, biotin, B6, iron, zinc
	Gingivitis, Gingival bleeding	Vitamin C deficiency
	Parotid hyperplasia, dental erosions	Bulimia nervosa

Eyes	Xerophthalmia, Night blindness, Photophobia, Xerosis, Bitot's spots, Corneal ulceration, Corneal scarring	Deficiency of Vitamin A
	Dilopia	Toxicity of Vitamin A
	Nystagmus, Lateral gaze deficit	Thiamin deficiency
	Optic nerve atrophy, Blindness	Vitamin B12 deficiency
	Retinitis Pigmentosa, Visual deficits	Vitamin E deficiency
	Kayser-Fleischer ring, Sunflower cataract	Copper toxicity
Skin	Seborrheic-like dermatitis	Deficiencies of vitamin B6, zinc
	Impaired wound healing	Deficiencies of vitamin C, zinc
	Erythematous or scaly rash at sun-exposed areas (e.g., extremeties and neck) (Casal's necklace)	Niacin deficiency
	Perifollicular petachiae, Ecchymosis (bruising)	Vitamin C deficiency
	Easy bruising	Vitamin K deficiency
	Dry flaky skin	Essential fatty acid deficiency
	Depigmentation	Protein-energy malnutrition
	Yellow or orange discoloration	Carotenoid excess
	Pallor	Anemia due to deficiencies of iron, vitamin B12, folate
Nails	Koilonychia (spoon-shaped nails)	Iron deficiency
	Discolored or thickened nails	Selenium toxicity
Hair	Swan-neck deformity	Vitamin C deficiency
	Discoloration, dullness, easy pluckability	Protein-energy malnutrition
Cardiovascular	High output congestive heart failure	Thiamin deficiency
	Cardiomyopathy and heart failure	Selenium deficiency
Gastrointestinal	Stomatitis, Procitis, Esophagitis	Niacin deficiency
	Hepatomegaly	Hepatic steatosis due to obesity, deficiency of choline, carnitine
Musculoskeletal	General or proximal weakness, bone tenderness, fracture	Vitamin D deficiency
	Weakness	PEM, hypophosphatemia, hypolkalemia, hypomagnesemia, vitamin D deficiency, iron deficiency
	Muscle wasting	PEM
	Carpopedal spasm	Hypocalcemia
Neurologic	Peripheral neuropathy	Deficiencies of B6, B12, E, thiamin; B6 toxicity
	Mental status changes	Deficiencies of thiamin, B6, B12, niacin, biotin
	Delerium	Hypophosphatemia, hypermagnesemia
	Dementia	Deficiencies of vitamin B12, thiamin, niacin

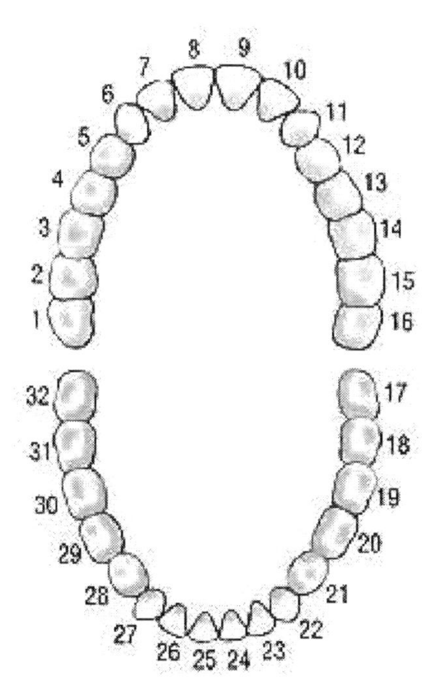

Dental Assessment

The dental assessment is an important part of the nutrition physical exam. The practitioner should evaluate overall dental health, number of amalgam fillings, root canals, extractions, as well as dental hygiene. The **Tooth Chart** enables the practitioner to make notations about the patient's dental history so that this information can later be studied in relationship to organ systems. On the tooth chart, simply circle teeth with amalgams, make an X over missing teeth, highlight root canals in one color and crowns in another color, and make notations if the patient has bridges.

KEY:

Silver Amalgam Fillings - Yellow Highlight (Note S for small, M for medium and L for large sized fillings)
Root Canals – Circle in RED pen
Crowns – Make a BLUE square around the tooth
Bridges – Circle the affected teeth and connect with GREEN pen
Missing Teeth – Black out with a **BLACK** marker

Anthropometric Measurements

Anthropometry, or the measurement of body size, weight and proportions, can be used to evaluate nutritional status. These physical measurements are useful for evaluating overnutrition as in obesity, or undernutrition, such as malnutrition and wasting due to disease or protein malnutrition. Common measurements include height, weight, skin-fold thicknesses, girth measurements and body composition and are most valuable to the practitioner when they are recorded accurately over a period of time. These tools help monitor the effects of nutritional interventions as well as to reflect a person's overall growth and development.

Body Mass Index (BMI) = body weight (kg) / height (m)^2

To determine body mass index, measure height to the nearest half inch and multiply by .0254 (to convert it to meters). Record weight to the nearest half pound and multiply by .454 (to convert it to kilograms).

SCORE	CATEGORY
Under 18.5	Underweight
18.5 – 24.9	Optimal weight
25 – 29.9	Overweight
30 or greater	Obesity

Height and Weight

The measurement of height and weight, calculated as Body Mass Index (BMI), can be used as a general measure of adiposity. While BMI is useful in large population studies, it does not accurately reflect the body composition or ratio of lean-to-fat tissue, of an individual. There are other clinical tools that can be used for this purpose, however; BMI is a simple, low cost, non-invasive method for assessing an individual's overall fatness.
Measure height using a stadiometer or

height rod rather than relying on a patient's note of his or her height. There are many inexpensive, wall-mount height scales that are appropriate for the clinical setting. Body weight should be measured using a standard physician's balance beam scale or a portable strain gauge digital scale. Strain gauge scales do not use springs and instead use a strain gauge transducer to measure weight and display it digitally. This type of scale is inexpensive, highly accurate and more reliable than a standard digital scale.

Waist Circumference

The measurement of waist circumference is an excellent clinical tool for assessing an individual's pattern of fat distribution. An excessive amount of visceral fat is associated with an increased risk for morbidity and mortality and is an independent risk factor for obesity, metabolic syndrome and type 2 diabetes.[1,2] An older method for determining central adiposity, waist-to-hip ratio, us used less often as a clinical tool. It should be noted that this measurement may not be as useful for those less than 60 inches tall or with a BMI of 35 or greater, however; the baseline measurement can still serve as a valuable tool for monitoring changes.

Measure the waist at the level of the top of the iliac crest (hip bone). This is generally the smallest area below the rib cage and above the umbilicus (belly button).	
WOMEN	**35** inches or lower is optimal
MEN	**40** inches or lower is optimal

Body Composition

Body fat distribution is and important concept in assessing nutritional status and the health implications of obesity. Estimating fat and lean (protein) tissue is an important component of body composition and is usually expressed as a percentage. Certain factors can affect the measurement of the fat-free or lean tissue such as age, degree of fitness and the body's state of hydration. There are several methods for assessing body composition that are common tools in the clinical setting. With all methods, strict adherence to the established protocols must be followed to obtain accurate results.

Skin-fold Measurements – Skin-fold measurements, the thickness of a double fold of skin and compressed subcutaneous adipose tissue, are a means of assessing percent body fat and are practical in the clinical setting. The validity depends on the accuracy of the measurement technique. Skin-fold calipers are used and a variety of measurements are taken from different sites on the body. Common sites for measurement include, triceps, biceps, subscapular, suprailiac, abdomen, upper thigh and calf. There are a number of different protocols utilizing these sites that yield an individual's estimate of body fat percent, however; the triceps skinfold is an easy site to access and very practical in a clinical setting. Though skin-fold measurements yield a percent body fat, the individual site measurements are also a good way to monitor patient progress. Thus, skin-fold measurements are a widely used method of indirectly estimating an individual's body composition.

Hydrostatic Weighing – A technique for determining whole body density is hydrostatic, or underwater, weighing. This method yields a more accurate estimation of body fat percentage and is considered the gold standard, but is impractical in a clinical setting. This technique also requires cooperation from the person being measured since he or she must be submerged and remain still long enough for an accurate measurement to taken. Hydrostatic weighing remains the standard laboratory technique to which most other methods for assessing body composition are often compared.

Air Displacement Plethysmography – The fundamental principle behind the air-displacement plethysmography method for measuring body composition uses the inverse relationship between pressure and volume to measure total body densitometry. One example of a commercially available product is the "Bod Pod." One advantage of this method is that it is more convenient and comfortable than underwater weighing. In general, the air-displacement plethysmography method shows agreement between two other criterion methods (hydrostatic weighing and dual-energy X-ray absorptiometry); however, some studies show significantly different estimates of body composition. Though this method is a promising technique for clinicians, further research is needed.

Bioelectrical Impedance Analysis (BIA) – The BIA is a useful tool for estimating body composition because it is non-invasive and has been shown to be as good or slightly better than skin-fold measurements when compared to underwater weighing. This technique is based on the principle that lean tissue has a higher electrical conductivity and lower impedance than fatty tissue due to its electrolyte content relative to water. In BIA analysis, the instrument generates an alternating electrical current, which is passed through the body by mean of electrodes. The body's resistance to this current what is measured. It is important that the individual is adequately hydrated since dehydration will result in an overestimation of body fat. Also, because BIA instruments rely on regression equations for their calculations, the method is good only if the appropriate equations are used. This is one of the weaknesses of BIA and the reason why some instruments are better than others. Thus, BIA is a convenient, non-invasive and safe method for estimating body composition and an ideal tool for the clinical nutritional assessment. Inexpensive, portable BIA scales are widely available and have been validated in research on older adults.[4]

Bioelectrical Impedance Analysis (BIA)

The BIA is also an important functional tool in evaluating the metabolic status of patient. The type of BIA referred to in this Guide is the "total body scan" positioning electrodes on hands and feet. It not only provides information about body composition (lean and fat mass), but also provides data about hydration, cell membrane fluidity and cell electrical potential. There are a variety of total body scan commercial products available: Biodynamics, ImpediMed and RJL machines. The BIA machine is non-invasive, portable and inexpensive, making it valuable for the functional medicine practitioner, as well as having been used in over 3000 research studies.

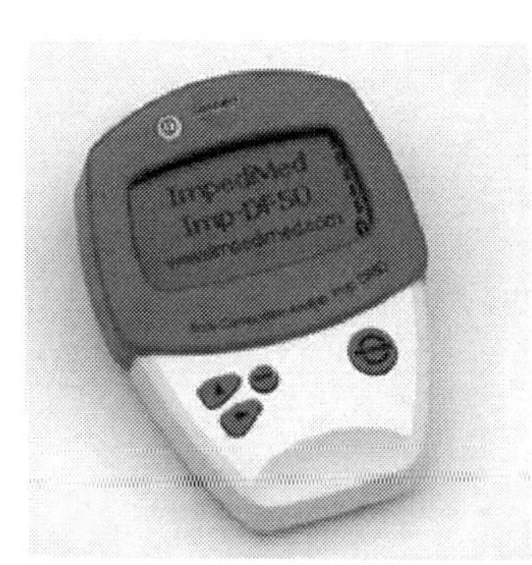

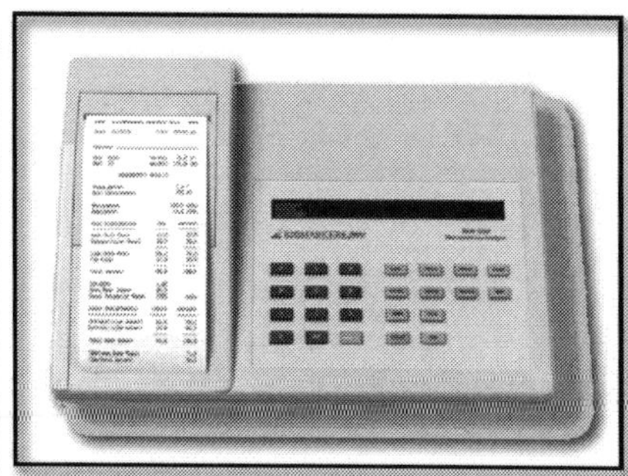

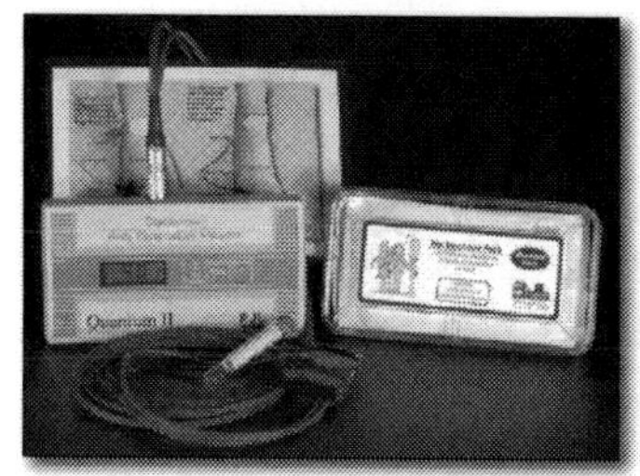

DF50 for Body Composition
www.impedimed.com

BIA 310 Bioimpedence Analyzer
www.biodyncorp.com

I BIA Analyzer
Lsystems.com

Once a patient is assessed, the practitioner can take the print-out from the machine, or downloaded to computer software, and tape it to a form which explains the results. A sample BIA form is provided in the tool kit and provides a concise way to keep record of the measurements and explain the results to the patient. Results may be compared over time to monitor progress and intervention methods. Normative data are provided in Table xxx at the end of this section.

Bioimpedance analysis (BIA) has become a widely accepted method in healthy and research study populations, for the determination of body composition due to its simplicity, speed (5-10 minutes) and noninvasive nature. BIA was first used over 30 years ago to measure the total water content of the body. The method involves passing an extremely low strength electrical current through the body and measuring the impedance to the flow of this current.

BIA is based on two key concepts:

1. The Fact That the Body Contains Water and Conducting Electrolytes.
   When a current is passed through the body, the water-containing fluids primarily conduct the electrical current. Water is found both inside the cells, intracellular fluid (ICF) and outside the cells, extracellular fluid (ECF). At low frequency, current passes through the ECF space and does not penetrate the cell membrane. (Figure 1).
2. That Impedance a Fixed Strength Current and Signal Frequency Can Measure Extracellular Fluids
   Based on these concepts a value for impedance can be calculated from a fixed strength current being passed through the body, which is inversely proportional to the amount of fluid. By appropriate choice of signal frequency, this can be made specific for extracellular fluid or for total fluid determinations.

Figure 1 [Ask Impedimed for a good copy of this picture and if we can use it]

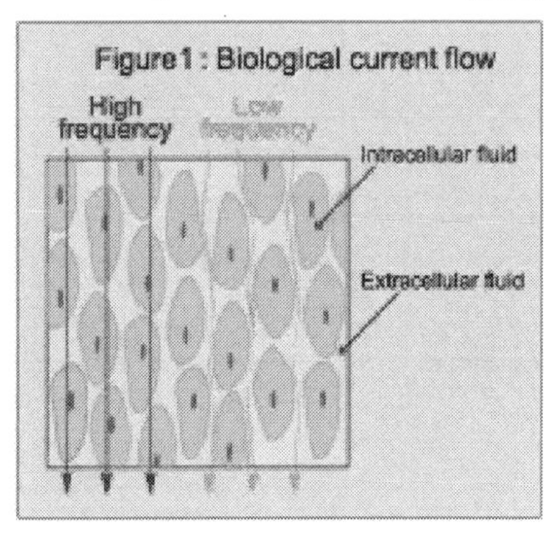

NOTE: The BIA test is reimbursable through most insurance companies and Medicare

Interpretation of BIA Results

Phase angle is a general indicator of cellular health and provides information about the cell membrane potential at the tissue level. It is a measurement of cell membrane fluidity. As the membrane becomes rigid, receptor function decreases. You can infer insulin resistance with lower phase angles. Intact healthy cells produce a higher phase angle; exercise and dietary liquid oils can increase phase angle. Damages oils decrease phase angle.

Body Capacitance is an indicator of the cell wall ionic potential (how strong is the batter charge?). All movement of energy and compounds require biochemical ionic charge. This value is primarily dependent on mineral electrolytes and pH. When capacitance it too low, you should check mineral status (serum electrolytes, calcium, magnesium and blood pressure). If they clinically support low mineral status, consider increasing dietary sea salt and magnesium and reducing calcium intake. If capacitance is high, check serum calcium, electrolytes, blood pressure and dietary intake of calcium. Oxidative stress, free radical damage also affects this result. Optimum numbers reflect a healthy cell (see chart). The body capacitance number can move up or down fairly rapidly. This is considered the oxidative stress number. Optimum capacitance for males is about 1300 and for females is about 900.

Total Body Water as a percentage of **fat-free mass** is a marker of hydration. If this result is <69% the patient should be put on hydration protocol and retested in 24-48 hours as values below this level indicate dehydration. This is an accurate indicator of hydration even when the person is significantly overweight.

Total Body Water (TBW/total weight) as a percentage of **total weight** can show dehydration but is also related to % body fat. If a person's weight falls in the overweight or obese categories, then consider the inverse relationship between total body fat and TBW (total body water may show lower values). This is due to lean body mass being approximately 70% water and body fat being around 10% water. This value can decline with age.

Basal Metabolic Rate (BMR) represents the estimated number of calories metabolized at rest during a 24-hour period. About 70% of a human's total daily energy expenditure is due to the basal life processes within the organs of the body. About 20% of one's energy expenditure comes from physical activity and another 10% from thermogenesis, BMR decreases with age and the loss of lean body mass and can increase as lean body mass increases, since lean mass is metabolically active. The BMR value is important for providing patients with estimated daily calorie intake plus caloric need adjustments for physical activity or energetic requirements (like infection).

Body Mass Index (BMI) is a useful measure to assess obesity as it correlates to overall fatness in both men and women, which can help identify health risks. Since this value is a relationship between height and weight, it may not be appropriate for some lean/muscular individuals. To calculate BMI:

$$\text{Body Mass Index} = \text{Weight in kilograms} / (\text{Height in meters})^2$$

Classifications from the National Heart, Lung and Blood Institute are as follows:

Body Mass Index	Classification
Less than 18.5	Underweight
18.5 to 24.9	Normal/Healthy
25 to 29.9	Overweight
30 to 34.9	Obese Class I

35 to 39.9	Obese Class II
40 or greater	Extremely Obese

Fat-free Mass (FFM) or lean body mass is the total non-fat parts of the body and includes all the body's water and metabolically active tissues. It includes both body cell mass and extracellular mass and is the source of all metabolic caloric expenditure.

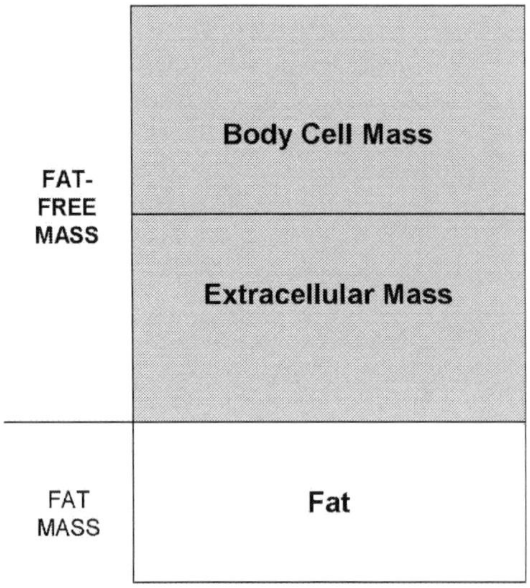

FAT-FREE MASS	**Body Cell Mass**
	Extracellular Mass
FAT MASS	**Fat**

Body Cell Mass (BCM) contains metabolically active components of the body such as muscle cells, organ cells, blood and immune cells. BCM also includes intracellular water and the active portion of fat cells, but not the stored fat lipids.

Extracellular Mass (ECM) contains the metabolically inactive parts of the body components including bone, minerals , blood plasma and extracellular water.

Fat Mass (FM) is the total amount of storage fat in the body and includes both subcutaneous and visceral fat. Subcutaneous fat is the body's main energy reserve and is stored beneath the skin and above muscle tissue. Visceral fat is located deeper within the body, also serves as an energy reserve and a cushion between organs. Fat mass is expressed as a percentage of your total body weight and reflects both essential fat and storage fat. It's important to remember that a certain amount of fat is *essential* to the normal functions of the body. Norms for percent body fat are presented below.

MALES		***FEMALES***	
Essential	2-4%	Essential	10-12%

Athlete	< 10%	Athlete	< 17%
Lean	10-15%	Lean	17-22%
Normal/Healthy	15-18%	Normal/Healthy	22-25%
Above Average	18-20%	Above Average	25-29%
Over-fat	20-25%	Over-fat	29-35%
Unhealthy/Obese	> 25%	Unhealthy/Obese	> 35%
***Sources**: Adapted from ACSM's Guidelines for Exercise Testing and Prescription, 6th Ed., 2000 and ACSM's Resource Manual for Guidelines for Exercise Testing and Prescription, 4th Ed., 2001*			

Intracellular and Extracelular Hydration Homeostasis

What does it mean electrolyte homeostasis? As we know, the electrolytes sodium, potassium, magnesium and calcium with their corresponding anions: chloride, phosphate and bicarbonate are represented within and without the cells at very different concentrations.

For those electrolytes a transcellular concentration difference exists with varying gradients between the intra- and extracellular space. Naturally, there is a tendency for concentration differences to go toward an equilibrium. It is a characteristic sign of life, however, that the cell shows a continuous effort against this tendency to maintain those given gradients with an expense of energy in the form of a dynamic electrolyte homeostasis. From the concentration gradients an electric voltage of the cell results, which we call the electric potential and which is calculable according to Nernst's equation:

$$\text{Nernst: } E = \frac{RT}{nF} \ln CE / CI$$

Cells that are shaped "round like grapes" show that the cells are well hydrated with Intracellular water (ICW) and Extracellular water (ECW) in balance with each other as controlled by the Sodium-Potassium Pump. When the ICW is lower than optimum, it indicates the cells are dehydrated, and is likely low in Potassium which is the primary mineral in ICW. One could visualize the cell will be shaped "more like a raisin." If the cell is over-hydrated, it will look like a water balloon that is too full and about "ready to pop". These are analogies a practitioner can use in explaining this to a patient. Therefore, ICW and ECW balance is needed for healthy cell functioning as well as cell wall integrity for proper function.

Sodium-Potassium Pump (Na+/K+ Pump or NAKA)

It is important to have a good understanding of the Sodium-Potassium Pump function, to more fully understand the use of the ICW and ECW measurements on the BIA testing. Active transport is responsible for the observation that cells contain relatively high concentrations of potassium ions but low concentrations of sodium ions. The mechanism responsible for this is the sodium-potassium pump that moves these two ions in opposite directions across the plasma membrane. The ionic transport conducted by sodium pumps creates both an electrical and chemical gradient across the plasma membrane

Some key examples include:

- The cell's resting membrane potential is a manifestation of the electrical gradient, and the gradient is the basis for excitability in nerve and muscle cells.
- Export of sodium from the cell provides the driving force for several facilitated transporters, which import glucose, amino acids and other nutrients into the cell.

- Translocation of sodium from one side of an epithelium to the other side creates an osmostic gradient that drives absorption of water. Important instances of this phenomenon can be found in the absorption of water from the lumen of the small intestine and in the kidney. (Wikipedia http://en.wikipedia.org/wiki/NaKATPase)

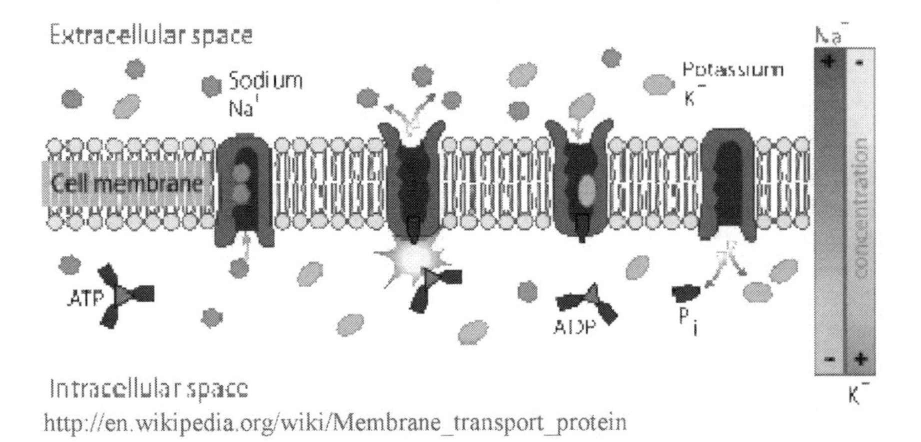

http://en.wikipedia.org/wiki/Membrane_transport_protein

Controlling cell volume

One of the important functions of Na+-K+ pump is to maintain the volume of the cell. Inside the cell there are a large number of proteins and other organic compounds that cannot escape from the cell. Most, being negatively charged, collect around them a large number of positive ions. All these substances tend to cause the osmosis of water into the cell that, unless checked, can cause the cell to swell up (high ICW). The Na+-K+ pump is a mechanism to prevent this. The pump transports 3 Na+ ions out of the cell and in exchange takes 2 K+ ions into the cell. As the membrane is far less permeable to Na+ ions than K+ ions the sodium ions have a tendency to stay there. This represents a continual net loss of ions out of the cell. The opposing osmotic tendency that results operates to drive the water molecules out of the cells. Furthermore, when the cell begins to swell, this automatically activates the Na+-K+ pump, which moves still more ions to the exterior.

The N+/K+ Pump can also function as signal transducer as discovered within the last decade, many independent labs have demonstrated that in addition to the classical ion transporting described above, this membrane protein can also relay extracellular binding signals into the cell. Medications can effect the functioning of the pump and cause alterations in its ability to balance ICW and ECW.

To remain viable, all cells are required to maintain a low intracellular concentration of sodium. In polarized epithelial cells like enterocytes, low intracellular sodium is maintained by a large number of Na+/K+ ATPases - so-called sodium pumps - embedded in the basolateral membrane. These pumps export 3 sodium ions from the cell in exchange for 2 potassium ions, thus establishing a gradient of both charge and sodium concentration across the basolateral membrane.

Depending on cell type, there are between 800,000 and 30 million pumps on the surface of cells. They may be distributed fairly evenly, or clustered in certain membrane domains. An example of clustering is in the basolateral membranes of polarized epithelial cells in the kidney and intestine. (website: http://en.wikipedia.org/wiki/NaKATPase#Controlling_cell_volume)

For instance in the intestine, virtually all nutrients from the diet are absorbed into blood across the mucosa of the small intestine. In addition, the intestine absorbs water and electrolytes, thus playing a critical role in maintenance of body water and acid-base balance.

It's probably fair to say that the single most important process that takes place in the small gut to make such absorption possible is establishment of an electrochemical gradient of sodium across the epithelial cell boundary of the lumen. This is a critical concept and actually quite interesting. Also, as we will see, understanding this process has undeniably resulted in the saving of millions of lives.

In rats, as a model of all mammals, there are about 150,000 sodium pumps per small intestinal enterocyte which collectively allow each cell to transport about 4.5 billion sodium ions out of each cell per minute (J Membr Biol 53:119-128, 1980). This flow and accumulation of sodium is ultimately responsible for absorption of water, amino acids and carbohydrates. Also, dietary sources of protein, carbohydrate and fat must all undergo the final stages of chemical digestion just prior to absorption of, for example, amino acids, glucose and fatty acids.

Abnormalities in the functioning of the Na+/K+ Pump are thought to be involved in several pathologic states, particular heart disease and hypertension. Well-studied examples of this linkage include:

- Several types of heart failure are associated with significant reductions in myocardial concentration of Na+-K+-ATPase that drives the control of the pump.
- Excessive renal reabsorption of sodium due to oversecretion of aldosterone has been associated with hypertension in humans. This is important to consider for patients with significant adrenal stress.

Regulation of Sodium Pump Expression and Activity

It is important to consider cellular insufficiencies in any of these key nutrients involved in the Na+/K+ Pump function: Sodium, Potassium and Magnesium. Magnesium and potassium especially have a close relationship in this process. J Physiol Vol 315 pp 421-446 The magnesium dependence of sodium-pump-mediated sodium—potassium and sodium—sodium exchange in intact human red cells, Peter W. Flatman* and Virgilio L. Lew. Key nutrients effect sodium pump activity. Each of these key nutrients can become a rate-limiting cofactor in the function of the pump. This does not preclude that Chloride and Calcium to not have a part to play, but less so that than the primary three noted. Disorders of electrolyte homeostasis are known at many diseases and clinical situations. They have serious consequences for the cell. The function of the Sodium-Potassium Pump has a large part to play in this homeostasis. For instance Mg-deficiency is followed by a K-deficiency, which cannot be equalized by K alone: a refractory hypokalemia always needs additional Mg supply for its restitution. Potassium and magnesium have been shown to be synergist, and when replacing one, it is beneficial to replace the other. Dorup I, and Clausen T, Correlation between magnesium and potassium contents in muscle: role of Na(+)-K+ pump, Am J Physiol Cell Physiol 264: C457-C463, 1993.Magnesium especially is known as a facilitator of the pump by increasing the ATPase activity and is necessary for the function of the sodium/potassium pump. Conversely, a magnesium deficiency promotes pumping sodium out of the cell, and pumping potassium into the cell may be impaired by decreasing the activity of the pump. It is suggested that this leads to an increase in intracellular Na+, resulting in a change in the membrane potential, and may contribute to the arrhythmias associated with magnesium deficiency. Effects of Dietary Magnesium on Sodium-Potassium Pump Action in the Heart of Rats, Publication No. 252 of the Bureau of Nutritional Sciences, Manuscript received 7 April 1987. Revision accepted 24 August 1987. Peter W. F. Fischer and Alexandre Giroux Prescription diuretics tend to deplete magnesium and potassium. In this situation, magnesium foods or supplementation intake can normalize both magnesium and potassium levels in the muscle and other tissues. P. Wester. "Magnesium," Am J Clin Nutr 45 suppl (1987): 1305-1312

(Dyckner T., Wester, P.O. (1979): Ventricular extrasystoles and intracellular electrolytes before and after potassium and magnesium infusions in patients on diuretic treatment Am. Heart J. 97, 12. From K and Mg-deficiency a Na/Ca-overload of the cell with aggravating consequences will follow: impaired activity and vitality with electric instability. Low Mg, which is responsible for development of a Ca-overload is also able to restore electrolyte homeostasis by sufficient supply competitively. The pathophysiologic relations for development of a cellular imbalance and its restitution concern the Na/K-pump, the Ca-pump and the Na/Ca-exchange. The clinical applications of Mg therefore are manifold: recovery under diuretic treatment, coronary heart disease, arrhythmias, perioperative electrolyte therapy, transcellular shifts, coronary dilatation and so on. Wang, R., Flink, E.B., Dyckner, T. et al. (1985): Magnesium depletion as a cause of refractory potassium repletion Arch. Intern. Med. 145, 1686.

Did you know? Among US adults, 68% consumed less than the recommended daily allowance (RDA) of magnesium, and 19% consumed less than 50% of the RDA. Just (National Health and Nutrition Examination Survey 1999–2000 [NHANES])

Major hormonal controls also exist over pump activity can be summarized as follows:

- Thyroid hormones appear to be a major player in maintaining steady-state concentrations of pumps in most tissues. ICW/ECW ratios should trigger consideration of thyroid function.
- Aldosterone is a steroid hormone with major effects on sodium homeostasis. It stimulates both rapid and sustained increases in pump numbers within several tissues. ICW/ECW ratios should trigger consideration of adrenal/HPA function.
- Insulin is a major regulator of potassium homeostasis and has multiple effects on sodium pump activity. Within minutes of elevated insulin secretion, pumps have increased affinity for sodium and increased turnover rate. Sustained elevations in insulin causes upregulation of the pump. In skeletal muscle, insulin may also recruit pumps stored in the cytoplasm or activate latent pumps already present in the membrane.
- Catecholamines have varied effects, depending on the specific hormone and tissue.

Ewart HS, Klip A: Hormonal regulation of the Na(+)-K(+)-ATPase: mechanisms underlying rapid and sustained changes in pump activity. Am J Physiol 269:C295, 1995.

Geering K: Na, K-ATPase. Curr Opin Nephrology Hypertension 6:434, 1994.

Jorgensen PL, Hakansson KO, Karlish SJD: Structure and mechanism of Na,K-ATPase: Functional sites and their interactions. Annu Rev Physiol 65:817-849, 2003.

Lingrel JB, Kuntzweiler T: Na+, K+-ATPase. J Biol Chem 269:19659, 1994.

Drug-Nutrient Interactions

Medications, such digitalis and ouabain, can cause binding of these widely-used drugs to sodium pumps and will specifically inhibits the pump's activity. Drug-nutrient interactions should be considered when an ICW/ECW is imbalanced.

Intracellular water (ICW) can change with age and reflects the cells ability to retain optimum fluid compartment inside and outside the cell. Balance is needed in order to maintain cellular integrity. High numbers can indicate toxicity; a need for detoxification or a need for EFAs, magnesium, or sodium. Low numbers show a need for potassium, and possibly magnesium. Control of ICW is dependent on the function of the sodium-potassium pump. Potassium is the dominant mineral intracellularly and sodium the dominant extracellular mineral. Magnesium is the primary cofactor to drive the Na-K pump.

Extracellular water (ECW) is the volume outside the cell mass. Higher values may be related to fluid retention and symptoms of edema. Ideally, the ratio of ICW to ECW should be about 55:45 which would may indicate a lower level of toxicity in the body.

Standard Blood Chemistry

Laboratory testing is essential for the assessment of both clinical and sub-clinical nutrient deficiencies and provides the most objective and quantitative data on nutritional status. For many practitioners blood chemistry and CBC analysis compares a test result with the conventional laboratory reference range. Unfortunately these ranges are designed to identify disease states and pathology. Thus if a person falls within the "normal" range they are deemed healthy, but still may have markers for sub-clinical nutrient deficiencies. Functional medicine practitioners look at laboratory results in a much more comprehensive manner in an attempt to detect problems with optimum function of bodily systems long before a disease manifests. As such, the functional medicine practitioner focuses on physiologic function and will look for areas of imbalance as a marker of health rather than simply the presence of pathology as a marker of disease. This provides the practitioner with the opportunity to intervene and optimize function. The **Blood Chemistry Functional Analysis** tool can assist the practitioner with providing comprehensive view of results with both the conventional and functional reference ranges.

Three reasons for high serum potassium
1) dehydration
2) significant catabolism
3) compromised renal function.

Recommended Labs
For those clinicians who are not licensed to order blood chemistry testing, the Recommended Nutritional Labs form can be a useful tool. For example, a dietician or clinical nutritionist can provide the patient with this form that the patient takes to the doctor, in order to have certain labs completed for the nutritional assessment.

<note for functional/optimum ranges in the table below, black is from Sam Queen, Blue is from Michael Wald and Red is from Dicken Weatherby>

Blood Chemistry Functional Analysis

Serum Marker		***Nutritional Considerations***
Glucose, Fasting Ref. Range 60 – 115 (mg/dl) Optimum 75 – 90 Pre-diabetes 98-115 Diabetes >126	*High*	Glucose control dysfunction, Insuline Resistance, Hi GI meal prior evening, "Dawn Phenomenon" nocturnal glycogen secretion, toxicity interfering with Insulin Sensitivity, Dehydration
	Low	Hypoglycemia, low mineral status (Mg, Cr, Zn, V), toxicity, adrenal imbalance, thyroid dysfunction, pre-diabetes
Hemoglobin A1C Ref. Range 5.0-7.0 Optimum 5.0-6.0	*High*	2-3 months prior poor glucose management
	Low	Good glucose management or hyperinsulinemia with Insulin Resistance

 13

Insulin, fasting	*High*	Insulin Resistance, primary pancreatic dysfunction
Ref. Range 0 – 17 (uU/mL) Optimum 0 - 10	*Low*	
Blood Urea Nitrogen (BUN)	*High*	
Ref. Range 10 – 20 (mg/dl) Optimum 10 – 12 / 10 - 16	*Low*	
Creatinine	*High*	
Ref. Range .6 – 2.0 (mg/dl) Optimum .6 – 1.0	*Low*	
Glomular Filtration Rate (GFR)	*High*	
	Low	
Uric Acid	*High*	
Ref. Range 2.5 – 8.5 (mg/dl) Optimum 3.5 – 5.5	*Low*	
Sodium	*High*	
Ref. Range 135 – 145 (mEq/L) Optimum 138 - 142	*Low*	
Potassium	*High*	
Ref. Range 3.6 – 5.0 (mEq/L) Optimum 4.4 – 4.7	*Low*	
Chloride	*High*	
Ref. Range 98 – 109 (mEq/L) Optimum 101 – 107 / 100 - 104	*Low*	
Carbon Dioxide (C02)	*High*	
Ref. Range 20 – 30 (mEq/L) Optimum 23 – 27 / 25 - 30	*Low*	
Total Protein	*High*	
Ref. Range 6.0 – 8.5 (gm/dl) Optimum 7.0 – 7.4	*Low*	
Albumin	*High*	
Ref. Range 3.5 – 5.0 (g/dl) Optimum 4.3 – 4.8	*Low*	
Globulin	*High*	
Ref. Range 1.2 – 3.0 (gm/dl) Optimum 2.2 – 2.4	*Low*	
A/G Ratio	*High*	
Ref. Range 1.2 – 2.2 Optimum 1.8 – 2.2 / 1.4 – 2.0	*Low*	

 14

AST (SGOT) Ref. Range 8 – 40 (U/L) Optimum 15 – 30 / 10 - 20	*High*	
	Low	
ALT (SGPT) Ref. Range 0 – 45 (U/L) Optimum 12 – 30 / 10 - 25	*High*	
	Low	
Gamma Glutamyltransferase (GGT) Ref. Range 0 – 65 (U/L) Optimum 15 – 30 / 10 - 35	*High*	
	Low	
Alkaline Phosphatase Ref. Range 20 – 140 (U/L) Optimum 50 – 75 / 70 - 100	*High*	
	Low	
Bilirubin, total Ref. Range .2 – 1.5 (mg/dl) Optimum .5 - .8 / 0 - .2	*High*	
	Low	
Calcium Ref. Range 8.5 – 10.5 (mg/dl) Optimum 9.4 – 9.8	*High*	
	Low	
Magnesium Ref. Range 1 – 4 (mmol/L) Optimum 3 - 6	*High*	
	Low	
Phosphorus Ref. Range 2.5 – 4.5 (mg/dl) Optimum 3.6 – 4.2 / 3.2 – 4.0	*High*	
	Low	
Gliadin AB IGA Ref. Range 0 – 20 (units) Optimum 0 - 15	*High*	
	Low	
Gliadin AB IGG Ref. Range 0 – 20 (units) Optmum 0 – 15 F / 0 – 10 M	*High*	
	Low	
Serum Iron Ref. Range 40 – 190 (ug/dl) Optimum 80 - 99	*High*	
	Low	
Ferritin Ref. Range 20 – 350 (mcg/L) Optimum 20 - 120	*High*	
	Low	
White Blood Cell Count (WBC) Ref. Range 4500 – 9000 /mm3 Optimum 5000 - 7500	*High*	
	Low	

Red Blood Cell Count (RBC) Ref. Range 4.2 – 6.0 (mil/mm3) Optimum 4.8 – 5.0	*High*	
	Low	
Hematocrit (HCT) Ref. Range 36 – 48% Optimum 41 – 45%	*High*	
	Low	
Hemoglobin (HGB) Ref. Range 12 – 16 (gm/dl) Optimum 13.5 - 15	*High*	
	Low	
Mean Corpuscular Volume (MCV) Ref. Range 83 – 99 units Optimum 83-99 / 83 – 93.45	*High*	
	Low	
Mean Corpuscular Hemoglobin (MCH) Ref. Range 28 – 32 (pg) Optimum 28 – 32 / 27 – 31.45	*High*	
	Low	
Mean Corpuscular Hemoglobin Concentration (MCHC) Ref. Range 32 – 36 (g/dl) Optimum 32 – 36 / 31.5 – 34.45	*High*	
	Low	
Red Cell Distribution Width (RDW) Ref. Range 10 – 16.9 % Optimum 10 – 12 %	*High*	
	Low	
Neutrophils Ref. Range 40 – 75 % Optimum 60 – 65 %	*High*	
	Low	
Lymphocytes Ref. Range 25 – 45 % Optimum 30 – 40 %	*High*	
	Low	
Monocytes Ref. Range 2 – 8 % Optimum 4 – 5 %	*High*	
	Low	
Basophils Ref. Range 1 – 3 % of WBC Optimum < 1 %	*High*	
	Low	
Eosinophils Ref. Range 0 – 4 % Optimum 0 – 2 %	*High*	
	Low	
Platelet Count Ref. Range 150 – 400 (100c/ml) Optimum 200 - 250	*High*	
	Low	

 16

Total Cholesterol Ref. Range 150 – 240 (mg/dl) Optimum 180 – 219 / 160 - 180	*High*	
	Low	
High Density Lipoprotein (HDL) Ref. Range ≥ 45 (mg/dl) Optimum ≥ 50	*High*	
	Low	
Low Density Lipoprotein (LDL) Ref. Range ≤ 130 mg/dl Optimum ≤ 100	*High*	
	Low	
TC/HDL Ratio Ref. Range ≤ 4.0 Optimum ≤ 3.4	*High*	
	Low	
Triglycerides Ref. Range 40 – 149 (mg/dl) Optimum 50 – 85 / 75-100	*High*	
	Low	
Lipoprotein(a)	*High*	
	Low	
Homocysteine Ref. Range 0 – 11.4 (MICROmol/L) Optimum 0 - 6	*High*	
	Low	
C-Reactive Protein, ultra sensitive Ref. Range 0 – 4 (mg/dl) Optimum 0 - 2	*High*	
	Low	
Erythrocyte Sedimentation Rate (ESR) Ref. Range 0 – 25 (mm/hr) Optimum 0 – 10 / 0 - 8	*High*	
	Low	
Fibrinogen Ref. Range 175 – 400 (mg/dl) Optimum 175 - 350	*High*	
	Low	
Thyroid Stimulating Hormone (TSH) Ref. Range .35 – 6.0 (uU/ml) Optimum 1.3 – 6.0??	*High*	
	Low	
Free T4	*High*	
	Low	
Free T3	*High*	
	Low	

 17

Thyroid Peroxidase Antibodies (TPO)	*High*	
Ref. Range 0 – 20 (iu/ml) Optimum 0 - 2	*Low*	
Estrone (E1)	*High*	
	Low	
Estradiol (E2)	*High*	
Ref. Range 0 – 50 (pg/mL) Optimum 0 - 40	*Low*	
Estriol (E3)	*High*	
	Low	
Progesterone	*High*	
	Low	
Testosterone	*High*	
	Low	
Dehydroepiandostrerone (DHEA)	*High*	
Ref. Range M=180-1250/F=130-980 mg/dl Optimum 250 - 1500	*Low*	
Vitamin B12	*High*	
	Low	
Folate	*High*	
	Low	
Vitamin D (25-hydroxy, D3)	*High*	
Ref. Range > 30 ng/dl Optimum > 60	*Low*	
H. Pylori Antibodies	*High*	
	Low	
Antigliadin	*High*	
	Low	
Food Allergies (IgE/IgG)	*High*	
	Low	

 18

Medical History and Diagnosis

Generally, a patient's medical history will be obtained through the initial intake questionnaire. Accurately assessing all of the factors and comprehensively managing them is the best way to identify underlying causes of illness and also helps the practitioner formulate a treatment plan. For an Initial Assessment prior to seeing a patient, the **Nutritional/Medical Intake Questionnaire** is one tool that collects all medical information and history of diagnosis. This form may be customized to collect a variety of diet and health-related information. This is usually not repeated more often than annually, depending on patient outcomes and condition.

Family History and Genotype
The collection of details relating to family history of illness can provide important clues to a patient's current health challenges and may also provide information about genotype. As part of the intake form, it is important to include a section or a separate page (if detailed information is desired) relating to family history.

Diet and Nutrient Data
Measurement of nutrient intake is an important and widely used indicator of nutrition status. There are a variety of tools available that can be used to assess the eating and supplementation habits of an individual, which can be used individually or collectively.

Food logs are a frequently used tool and usually range from 1 to 7 days. With this method of reporting food intake, the individual keeps a record of all foods eaten including, portion sizes, time consumed and beverages. Some clinicians ask for additional information such as where the meal was eaten, the mood of the individual, water intake, sleep habits, activity levels, and a description of daily bowel movements. The 3-day Diet Diary is a popular tool since it is generally easy enough for the patient and contains sufficient information for the practitioner. More recent research has shown the 7 day food log to be more accurate than the 3 day, but each practitioner can use this tool as fits his or her assessment styles.

If the patient provides a detailed food diary, the practitioner may also use **computerized analysis** to get a general idea of nutrient intake. There are many programs available that provide client reports and recommendations, however; these programs are often time-consuming for the practitioner. If this type of analysis motivates a patient, there are many online sources where individual's can keep detailed records of their food intake. This may be extremely valuable for the person who has a healthy diet but does not believe he or she needs vitamin/mineral supplementation, since many of these programs show the levels of micronutrients.

The practitioner can also administer a **24-hour diet recall**, especially if the patient has difficulty completing a food log. In the 24-our recall, the practitioner asks the patient to recall in detail all the food and beverages consumed during the last 24 hours or the previous day. This is a quick way for the practitioner to obtain some detailed information on the types of foods consumed. Though there are some limitations to this method, such as poor memory and over or under reporting of food intake, it remains a useful tool in the clinical setting.

Food frequency questionnaires assess food and nutrient intake by determining how frequently a person consumes certain types of foods. The more common questionnaires used in nutritional epidemiology are the Harvard University Dietary Assessment and the National Cancer Institute Quick Food Scan. Other questionnaires have been developed based on the information desired by the practitioner.

The **Fats and Oils Worksheet** is another great tool for the assessment of balanced intake of beneficial and essential fatty acids, as well as assessment of intake of damaged fats. When used in conjunction with BIA, it can provide important information about cell membrane health. This is a good screening if you do not have an RBC Fatty Acid Test to refer. The worksheet is divided into 5 sections:

- Omega 9 Fats
- Omega 6 Fats
- Omega 3 Fats
- Beneficial Saturated
- Damaged Fats

The patient is asked to fill out this worksheet, writing the number of times per week they ingest the listed foods. Any essential fatty acid supplements should also be noted. For overall balance of fatty acids, about 50% of their fat calories should come from Omega 9 fats, 30% from Omega 6 fats of the low heat processed or food sources, 10% from Omega 3, and 10% from beneficial saturated fats, and 0-2% of daily fat calories from damaged oils. From this overall picture of the patient's fat intake, the practitioner can easily spot imbalances in the various categories and make appropriate dietary recommendations. Most of the body fat composition is determined by dietary intake. The absorption of the fats is mostly determined by adequate bile and pancreatic lipase levels, so this survey information can be a good beginning in evaluating a person's Oil/Fatty Acid nutrition status. Note if a patient has had their gallbladder removed or a gastric bypass, both alter availability of bile for fat and fat-soluble vitamin emulsification in the gut and then absorption.

History of Dieting

A person's **history of dieting** or following specific diet programs will also provide information useful to the clinician. Ask questions such as:

- Have you followed any popular diet programs that you feel have worked well for you?
- Do you notice that you feel better or worse when eating certain types of foods? If so, which foods?
- Have you ever tried a vegetarian diet? Macrobiotic diet? Low carbohydrate diet? Blood Type Diet? Others?
- Do you currently follow and specific eating guidelines?
- What foods of your ancestral heritage do you eat regularly?

You may even choose to ask some questions about the person's relationship to food. For example, is the patient an "emotional" eater? Is there a history or current pattern of disordered eating? A careful list of well-thought-out questions can offer important clues about the individual's nutritional lifestyle.

There are other factors to consider in taking a dietary history that the practitioner can include as part of the patient intake form, many of which can have an impact on nutrition status.

- Weight changes
- Unusual meal pattern
- Appetite
- Satiety
- Discomfort after eating
- Chewing/swallowing ability

- Food likes/dislikes
- Taste changes/aversions
- Allergies (if known)
- Nausea/vomiting
- Bowel habits
- Living conditions
- Ability to purchase & prepare foods
- Snack consumption
- Alcohol/drug use
- Access to health care
- Ability to pay for food

Supplement and Medication Intake
Lastly, be sure to obtain a detailed list of nutritional supplements the person is currently taking. It is important to note the brand names, dosages and consistency with taking supplements. In many cases, the practitioner will ask the client to bring in the bottles. The functional medicine practitioner ensures that the supplements are appropriate for the individual and free from toxic ingredients.

Environmental and Occupational Exposure

As part of the patient's history-taking, it is important for the practitioner to know if there are any environmental exposure issues that may be contributing to an illness or poor health. Asking questions about work and home exposure of potential environmental toxins can provide valuable information for completing a comprehensive nutritional assessment.

There are many occupations that expose a person to various toxins:

OCCUPATIONS	ENVIRONMENTAL EXPOSURE
Information technology (computers, laptops), flight attendants, electricians, jobs with heavy cell phone use,	Electromagnetic radiation
Painters, construction, hairdressers, nail salon workers, exterminators, maids	Chemical toxins, heavy metals
Firefighters, police, toll booth collectors, machinists	Heavy metals, air pollutants, chemicals
Landscapers, gardeners, agricultural workers, farm workers, city workers (parks)	Pesticides, herbacides

In addition the practitioner should ask about daily exposure to household chemicals and cleaners. Cleaning supplies, bug sprays, cosmetics, toiletries, detergents can all pose a toxic risk. Use of the **Environmental Sensitivity Questionnaire** is a valuable tool for this purpose. It may be included as part of the Nutrition/Medical Intake questionnaire or as a separate document.

Other environmental disruptors of metabolism include
- inhalants
- food toxins
- cosmetic toxins
- dental toxins
- household
- water
- Energetic toxins
- Emotional toxins

- Iatrogenic pharmaceutical reactions
- Occupational environment (heavy metals and petrochemicals)

Lifestyle Data

As part of comprehensive history-taking, it important to obtain information about the person's overall lifestyle. These are included in the Nutrition Medical Intake provided with this Guide. The following are sample questions that can be incorporated in a patient intake form:

- Please describe your **physical activity** habits?
- Do you smoke? Drink alcohol?
- What do you do for daily relaxation?
- Do you eat "on the run" or while doing something else (driving, working, etc.)?
- Do you take vacations? If so, how often and where to you go?
- How much sleep do you get on weeknights? Weekends? Do you feel rested upon waking?
- Do you prepare your own meals?
- Do you eat out frequently or visit fast food establishments?
- Do you travel for work? If so how much?
- What do you do for fun?
- What are your religious/spiritual beliefs? Do you believe your life has meaning?
- Describe your "self-care" habits.
- Evaluate your relationships with others and your community.

If a patient's main concern strongly relates to a lifestyle habit, the practitioner may use a questionnaire that is more specific to that habit. For example, the **Sleep Questionnaire** will provide detailed information that can assist with an appropriate intervention.

References Books Used for this Section

Mahan, LK and Escott-Stump, S. Krause's Food, Nutrition and Diet Therapy (11th Edition), Philadelphia 2004, Saunders

Lee, RD and Nieman, D. Nutritional Assessment (Fourth Edition), New York 2007, McGraw-Hill

Queen, HL (Sam). The Basic 100 (Third Review Edition)

Wald, Michael. Blood Lab Test Descriptions and Cancer Markers, Mt. Kisco 2007, Blood Logic

Lord, R and Bralley, JA. Laboratory Evaluations for Integrative and Functional Medicine (2nd Edition), , 2008

Websites

Zinc Tally - Metagenics -- http://www.metagenics.com/products/detail.asp?pid=26
Bioimpedance Analysis – www.biodyncorp.com; http://rjlbia.com; www.impedimed.com
Air Displacement Plethysmography – www.bodpod.com
Genova Diagnostics – www.gdx.net (Education PPT Resources)
Metametrix Laboratory – www.metametrix.com (Education PPT Resources)
Doctor's Data
Spectracell
Neuroscience

Recommended Reading/Office Resources

Biodynamics Corporation, *Clinician Desk Reference for BIA Testing,* 2003-2005.

Bralley, Lord, *Laboratory Evaluations for Integrative and Functional Medicine (2nd Edition)*, 2008

Gibson RS, *Principles of Nutritional Assessment*, Second Edition, Oxford Universtiy Press, 2005.

Katz DL, *Nutrition in Clinical Practice, Second Edition*, Lippincott Williams & Wilkins, 2001, 2008.

Mahan K, et. al. Krause's Diet Therapy, 2008

Lombardo GT, *Sleep to Save Your Life:The Complete Guide to Living Longer and Healthier Through Restorative Sleep, 2006.*

Queen HLS, *The Basic 100, Third Review Edition,* Institute for Health Realities, 2001.

References for Endnote

BMR reference for % - Template:Exercise Physiology. McArdle, William D. 2nd edition. 1986. Lea & Febigier, Philadelphia.

Integrative & Functional Medical Nutrition Therapy (IFMNT) Radial

Lifestyle
•Food
•Culture
•Environment
•Movement
•Nature
•Relationships
•Sleep
•Stress
•Spirituality
•Sunlight
•Supplements
•Traditions

Negative thoughts & beliefs

Systems Signs & Symptoms
Nutrition Physical
•Circulatory
•Digestive
•Endocrine
•Immune
•Integumentary
•Lymph
•Musculoskeletal
•Nervous
•Reproductive
•Respiratory
•Skeletal
•Urinary

Environmental Exposures

Biomarkers
• Anthropometrics
• Digestion/Absorption
• Genomics/SNPs
• Immune/Inflammatory
• Metabolic/Energy
• Macronutrients
• Micronutrients
• Organic Acids
• Toxins

Metabolic Pathways/ Networks
•Anabolic / Catabolic
•Nutrient Cofactors
•Cellular Respiration
•Eicosanoid Series
•Biotransformation
•Steroidogenic Pathway
•Urea Cycle

Pathogens

Core Imbalances
•Cellular Integrity
•Digestion
•Detoxification
•Energy Metabolism
•Inflammation/Oxidative stress
•Neuro-Endocrine-Immune
•Nutritional Status

Allergens & Intolerances

Personalized Nutrition Care
Assessment
Diagnosis
Intervention
Monitoring
Evaluation

FUNCTIONAL MEDICINE MATRIX

Retelling the Patient's Story

Antecedents

Triggering Events

Mediators/Perpetuators

Physiology and Function: Organizing the Patient's Clinical Imbalances

Assimilation

Defense & Repair

Structural Integrity

Mental

Emotional

Spiritual

Energy

Communication

Biotransformation & Elimination

Transport

Modifiable Personal Lifestyle Factors

Sleep & Relaxation	Exercise & Movement	Nutrition	Stress	Relationships

Name:__________ Date:__________ CC:__________

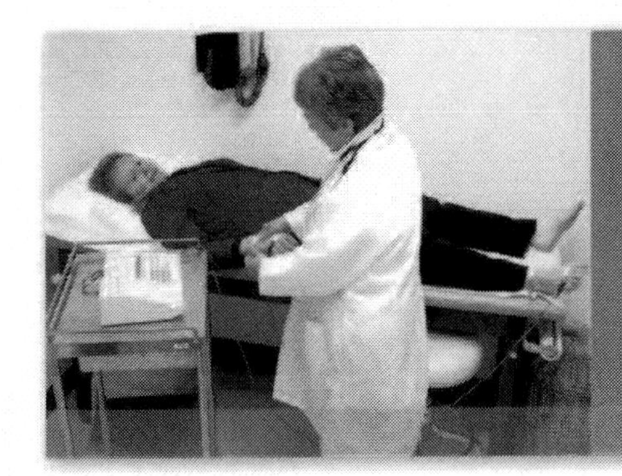

What Is a BIA?
(And why do you need one?)

Bioelectrical Impedance Analysis or Bioimpedance Analysis (BIA) is a method of assessing your "body composition"—the measurement of body fat in relation to lean body mass. It is an integral part of a health and nutrition assessment.

Why Is Body Composition Important to My Health?

Research has shown that body composition is directly related to health. A normal balance of body fat is associated with good health and longevity. Excess fat in relation to lean body mass, known as altered body composition, can greatly increase your risks to cardiovascular disease, diabetes, and more. BIA fosters early detection of an improper balance in your body composition, which allows for earlier intervention and prevention. BIA provides a measurement of fluid and body mass that can be a critical assessment tool for your current state of health.

BIA also measures your progress as you improve your health. Improving your BIA measurement, or maintaining a healthy BIA measurement, can help keep your body functioning properly for healthy aging. Your BIA results can help guide us in creating a personalized dietary plan, including nutritional supplements when appropriate, and exercise to help you maintain optimal health and well-being for a lifetime.

How Does a BIA Work?

BIA is much more sophisticated than your bathroom scale, but just as simple—and almost as quick. BIA is performed in our office with the help of a sophisticated, computerized analysis.

This analyzer "calculates" and estimates your tissue and fluid compartments—using an imperceptible electrical current passed through pads placed on your hand and foot as you lie comfortably clothed on an exam table. In just minutes, we'll have detailed measurements to help create an effective, personalized program for you.

Follow-up Tests

We can conduct a series of follow-up BIA tests to monitor your health and measure your progress.

Guidelines for Assessment

For the most accurate results, the following guidelines should be followed:

1. **Do not eat for 4 hours prior to testing.**
2. **Do not exercise for 12 hours prior to testing.**
3. **Do not consume alcohol for 24 hours prior to testing.**
4. **Drink at least 1 quart of water one hour before your test.**
5. **Do not drink caffeine the day of your test.**
6. **Do not wear pantyhose.**
7. **Do not put lotion on your hands and feet.**

Follow-up Appointment:

FirstLineTherapy®

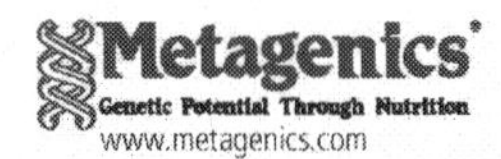

www.metagenics.com

MET1323 6/5/08

Nutritional Supplementation: Assessment of Need

Who

Patient/Client: person being evaluated for assessment of nutritional status and needs recommendations by a nutritionist/RD to functional optimally (heal or prevent)
Nutritionist/RD: healthcare practitioner capable of employing the Nutrition Care Process and is armed/prepared with safeguards to ensure a patient or client will meet optimal needs and avoid toxic levels of a nutrient that could alter other micronutrient status or metabolic status/function. Nutritionist it's aware and assessing structure and function and assessing the patient/client from a "systems biology" lens and approach.

What

Targeted nutrients or "nutrient groups" (minerals/electrolytes, b-vitamins, fat-soluble vitamins, etc.)
Identify a reason that a patient/client may or may not be able to meet optimal health/wellness, at least in the short term, taking a nutritional/dietary supplement. This is determined by either blood or other lab values or by dietary intake review and matched with skill in the nutrition-focused physical exam, medical and surgical histories, and any other health history or lifestyle factors that would contribute to the patient being able or unable to meet his or her needs.
Route: Oral/IV/IM/topical
Third party tested, cGMPs, USP certified
No fillers, gluten, etc.

How

IDU is an assessment tool used to determine a persons nutritional status via Intake, Digestion and Utilization review and assessment

When

When the RD/Nutritionist determines that a patient/client needs a nutrient or group of nutrients beyond the intake,digestion, utilization of the patient currently through typical dietary intake.
When blood/lab values indicate that there is nutritional insufficiency, excess, imbalance
Blood, urine, stool testing, functional and otherwise

Where

Supplements may be available:
In stores: Whole Foods, Natural Grocers, other high integrity store or outlet
Online: supplement companies that require the reference to or advisement of a healthcare practitioner (MD, RD, RN, DO, ND, PharmD, etc.) to dispense (Emerson, Xymogen, Natura, Metagenics)

Healthcare clinics: Some IM and general internal medicine practices, chiropractors, others, sell nutritional/dietary supplements out of their clinics
Outpatient pharmacies: E.g. KUH outpatient pharmacy sells many nutritional supplements out of the outpatient pharmacy (account with Emerson, Xymogen)

Regulatory/Advisory Organizations

FDA: what it DOES and DOES NOT mandate/regulate
Codex Alimentarius (Latin: "Book of Food"): Goal: protect health of consumers. Collaboration between the WHO and FAO (UN) and established in 1961 by FAO, WHO joined in 1962

Nutrition in the context of the BIG PICTURE

Does the patient/client eat an overall healthy diet with wide variety of nutritional intake of food groups, etc.?
If so, and imbalances exist, then nutritional or dietary supplements may be appropriate (taking into account the nuances of the individual and potential medication interactions, etc.)
Supplements may not make a difference in general/overall outcomes of patient health
Monitoring is absolutely necessary and "stop dates" must be given: either stop completely or stop and re-evaluate to adjust dosage
Nutrients work in groups
Target nutrients as much as possible to avoid unintended confounding/interactions
Minimize financial burden without sacrificing the patient's health and need for high quality nutritional supplements, when appropriate.

Supplements for obesity-related pain

(Robert A Bonakdar - Director of pain management at Scripps)
Turmeric
Resveratrol
Omega 3s
Vitamin D3
L carnotite
CoQ 10
Probiotics
Tea
Flavonoid-rich foods

Dietetics and Integrative Medicine Practicum Overview

Year 1	**All-Student Activities**	**Practicum Activity**	**Coursework**
Fall Term	**Early Fall (August)** Workshop: Introduction to Dietetics and Integrative Medicine	Clinical Rotation with KU Hospital	General Dietetics and Nutrition Curriculum
Spring Term	**Early Spring (January)** Workshop: Evidence in practice for Dietetics and Integrative Medicine, practice applications, Nutrition Physical Exam, Case Studies, Clinical Scenarios	**8-weeks (248 hours)**: Community Rotation (KU Integrative Medicine) **8-weeks (248 hours)**: Management Rotation (various sites/locations)	General Dietetics and Nutrition Curriculum
Spring Term	**Late Spring (April)** Entrepreneurship in Nutrition Business aspects of Nutritional Supplements	Students switch after each 8 week rotation (Community and Management rotations)	General Dietetics and Nutrition Curriculum
Summer Term	**None**	**8-weeks (248 hours)**: • Area of Interest Rotation (KU Integrative Medicine) • Center for Mind-Body Medicine "Food as Medicine"	DN 880 Dietary and Herbal Supplements (2-3 credits) May start writing literature review for thesis to begin fall semester
Year 2	**Graduate Assistanceship**	**Research Activities**	**Coursework**
Fall Term	16-20 hours weekly: work as a Graduate Research Assistant (GRA) or Graduate Teaching Assistant (GTA) with DN Faculty on relevant work or teaching.	**Masters' Thesis**: With an advisor from Dietetics and Nutrition Department, work on research project through the lens of Dietetics and Integrative Medicine	General Dietetics and Nutrition Curriculum DN 881 Introduction to Dietetics and Integrative Medicine (3 credits)
Spring Term	16-20 hours weekly: work as a Graduate Research Assistant (GRA) or Graduate Teaching Assistant (GTA) with DN Faculty on relevant work or teaching.	**Masters' Thesis:** With an advisor from DN Department, work on research project through the lens of Dietetics and Integrative Medicine	DN 882 A Nutrition Approach to Inflammation and Immune Regulation
Summer Term		**Masters' Thesis:** Complete research, write thesis and defend thesis with oral defense.	DN 980 Nutrigenomics and Nutrigenetics in Health and Disease (3 credits)

The University of Kansas Medical Center | KU Integrative Nutrition | Leigh Wagner, MS, RD, LD | Integrative Nutritionist | http://integrativemed.kumc.edu
3901 Rainbow Blvd, MS 1017 | Kansas City, KS 66160 | (913) 588-6208 | Fax (913) 588-0012 | E-mail: integrativemedicine@kumc.edu 06282012

Outline of Nutrition Practicum: Community Rotation

General Practicum Reference Documents

0.1 Dietetics and Integrative Medicine – Practicum Guidelines
0.2 Outline of Community Practicum (8-week format and Required/Optional format)
0.3 Learning Objectives for Practicum
0.4 10 Tenets of Dietetics and Integrative Medicine
0.5 Dietetics and Integrative Medicine: Why, What and How?
0.6 Intern Check List
0.7 How to Think Like a Dietitian in Integrative Medicine
0.8 Dietetics and Integrative Medicine from the Intern Perspective
0.9 Time Sheet

Weeks 1-2: General Orientation to KU Integrative Medicine & Intro to Dietetics and Integrative Medicine

Activities and Documents: Weeks 1-2
1.1 Orientation to KU IM Clinic
1.2 Orientation to KU Integrative Medicine, Nutrition Care Process
1.3 Orientation to Nutrition Care Process, Tools of the Trade, and general assessment tools
1.4 Ten Tenets of Dietetics and Integrative Medicine
1.5 Radial Conceptual Diagram and application
1.6 Pre- and Post-Evaluation for Dietetics and Integrative Medicine Practicum Experience

Other Activities

- Lecture on Introduction to Dietetics and Integrative Medicine
- Case Studies
- Clinical Practice and Assessment
- Video: The Blood Sugar Solution (Dr. Mark Hyman)

Week 3: Orientation to Integrative Medicine Modalities

Activities

- Rotate with Infusion Nurse and Nurse Practitioner in the Infusion Clinic
- Rotate with Medical Doctors (MDs) and Fellows in the clinic
- Rotate with the Naturopath (ND)
- Rotate with Neurofeedback technicians
- Rotate with other IM practitioners outside KU IM: Acupuncturist, massage therapist, etc.

Week 4: Whole food preparation & Targeted Nutrients
KU Healing Foods Kitchen and Outpatient nutrition pharmacy

Activities

- Assist with acquisition of food products, grocery shopping list, communication between food delivery service and whole foods
- Rotate 1-2 days with Lisa Markley, MS, RD – Culinary Nutritionist and Registered Dietitian at Whole Foods Market
- Prepare for and assist with Healing Foods Kitchen Demonstration in the KU Integrative Medicine Healing Foods Kitchen
- Rotate with Seth Williams, PharmD at KU Outpatient Pharmacy

Week 4 Documents

4.1 Orientation to KU HFK and Student Responsibilities.docx
4.2 Cooking class outline intern orientation.docx
4.3 OUTLINE - TEMPLATE cooking class.doc
4.4 Kitchen Checklist V1.docx
4.5 Recipe Format & Instructions.docx
4.6 Example Recipe Format - Chicken & Coconut Milk.docx
4.7 Grocery List Template.docx

Week 5-6: Clinical Nutrition Practice

Activities

- Observe and work with the Dietitian
- Participate with the Dietitian to complete the Nutrition Care Process: ADIME
- Observe and assist with:
  - Nutrition Physical Exam
  - Bioelectric Impedance Analysis (BIA) for Body Composition
  - Reviewing Nutrition Intake Forms
  - Assessing the diet history
  - Documenting and assessing the influences of the "patient story" (history) on the patient's nutritional health status

Weeks 5-6 Documents

1.3 Tools of the Trade for Clinical Nutrition Assessment
5.0 KU Integrative Medicine, Nutrition Care Process
5.1 Motivational Interviewing
5.2 Consultation Guidelines
5.3 Daily, Weekly and Monthly Procedural Checklists
5.4 Integrative Medicine Paper Chart Orientation
5.5 Nutrition Physical Exam
5.6 Bioelectric Impedance Analysis (BIA) Reference (Metagenics handout)

5.7 References for Dietetics and Integrative Medicine (Text & Electronic)
5.8 IFM Matrix
5.9 Timeline of Health History (blank)

6.0 KU Integrative Medicine, Nutrition Intake Forms and Medical Symptoms Questionnaire (MSQ)
6.1 KU Integrative Medicine Fats & Oils Questionnaire
6.2 KU Integrative Medicine Dental Form
6.3 Diet Diary Form & Instructions
6.4 Plate and [A] Protein, [B] Carbohydrates, [C] Fats & Oils Patient/Client Handouts
6.5 IDU – Ingestion, Digestion, Utilization
6.6 Table of Specialized Diets
6.7 GI Tract Assessment Table
6.8 GI Nutrient Absorption Sites
6.9 Dietary Withdrawal Guidelines

7.0 Nutritional Supplementation Needs Assessment
7.1 How to Prepare to Observe a Nutrition Consultation
7.2 Blank Nutrition Assessment & Consultation Summary Form
7.3 Reading Assignment Reflections Form

Week 7: Research in Nutrition

Activities

- Review the Nutrition Evidence Based Library on Mendeley
- Rotate with the clinical research coordinator to observe and assist with research activities and processes
- Rotate with or interview basic sciences team (PhDs and/or students) to learn about laboratory-based research (in vivo and in vitro)

Week 7 Documents

7.0 Criteria for Student Research projects for Dietetics and Integrative Medicine
7.1 Research Projects for Interns

Week 8: Community Nutrition

Activities

- Rotate with Healthy Eating Specialist at Whole Foods Market: Healthy Foods Shopping Tours, Healthy Foods Shopping Tour, Healthy Cooking Classes
- Rotate at a sustainable, local, organic (low-toxin) farming operation (If you are not already connected to a local grower: www.localharvest.org can help you find one nearby)
- Rotate with a local restaurant that serves locally-sourced foods (as described in previous bullet)

- Prepare and assist with campus and/or community presentations, activities, and classes:
  - Food is Medicine (KUMC campus organization)
    - Community Supported Agriculture (CSA)
    - Campus presentations
    - Campus organic garden
  - KU Hospital Mid-America Cardiology group (Cardiac Rehabilitation), Collaboration with White Heart Learning Center: Three-class series of nutrition information and cooking demonstration
  - Turning Point: the Center for Hope and Healing: Presentations
  - Greater KC Psychological Association: Nutrition and Mental Health presentation
  - Midwest Cancer Alliance: Kitchen Therapy monthly classes: "Cooking up Comfort" classes for cancer survivors and their caregivers

Reference Document

8.0 Community Nutrition Resources and Websites

The University of Kansas
School of Allied Health and KU Integrative Medicine
Department of Dietetics and Nutrition
Graduate Certificate Dietetic Internship Program

DN 827 Practicum
Dietetics and Integrative Medicine (DIM)
Community Nutrition Supervised Practice Guidelines
Fall 20 and Spring 20****

Total Hours	**At least 248 hours over 8 weeks**
DI Program Director	**Rachel Barkley, MS, RD, LD**
Contact information	**Phone: 913-588-7683 Email: rbarkley@kumc.edu**
Preceptor:	**See assignment list for preceptor and contact information**

Intern Responsibilities for the DIM Community Nutrition Supervised Practice Experience

Interns assume responsibility for assigned clients, projects, areas, employees, and events. Routine activities may include, but are not limited to the following:

1. Meet daily with the preceptor or assigned supervisor to discuss performance, plan daily activities, review completed work, submit reports, discuss problems and justify decisions.
2. Complete all orientation activities, review orientation materials to identify themes related to DIM practice and become familiar with the policies and procedures of the organization.
3. Determine the rationale for any changes made in reports, projects, and other work by preceptor and make or implement the recommended revisions.
4. Record and report pertinent information as requested by the preceptor and other personnel.
5. Communicate effectively with clients, family members, clinician's and other staff.
6. Assess priorities so work is completely in an effective and efficient manner.
7. Assess performance based on ability to successfully accomplish assigned competencies and activities.
8. Review the competencies, suggested activities listed for the rotation, and maintain a record of those completed along with examples of work accomplished to fulfill the competencies. Present this record to the preceptor for approval and signature periodically throughout the experience.
9. When unfamiliar with a condition or service, research the condition or service, and nutrition/health/social/economic/political implications of the condition or service.
10. Be familiar with diet therapies and nutrition recommendations utilized in DIM, common therapeutic diets and the rationale for their use, e.g., elimination diets, sugar/cancer.
11. Collect and interpret information from the medical records and other sources for assigned clients or groups. Use available recommended internet & textbook resources.
12. Assess nutritional risks/status of assigned clients or groups.
13. Identify nutritional problems and goals for assigned clients or groups while understanding and communicating Integrative approaches are based on individual assessments.
14. Strive to improve nutritional status and care of assigned clients or groups.
15. Design and implement appropriate nutrition care plans or interventions for assigned clients or groups.
16. Determine the rationale for any changes made in the plans of care by preceptor or other staff and implement the revised plan.
17. Evaluate the educational and counseling needs of clients and other groups and effectively meet those needs by consultation or referral to other services.
18. Calculate nutrient content of recipes or foods consumed.

19. Arrange for other services/referrals for assigned clients or groups as needed.
20. Record pertinent information about client needs and care plans in medical and other health/social record systems as required and as approved by preceptor.
21. Provide chart notes and/or other required documentation of client care to the preceptors for review and approval.
22. Communicate in a timely and appropriate manner about client care and other assigned tasks with the health care team and other personnel.
23. Attend pertinent departmental and other meetings as assigned by preceptor.
24. Read and study appropriate references in order to be able to satisfactorily complete competencies and activities for the rotation.
25. Complete the weekly time sheet and submit to preceptor for signing.
26. Complete written self-evaluation of performance midway and at the end of the rotation. This can be done more often if desired by the preceptor.
27. Request that the preceptor(s) complete evaluations of intern midway (or more often if desired by preceptor) and at the end of the food and nutrition services management rotation.
28. Ensure that the preceptor(s) has the correct forms in time to complete the evaluations.
29. Set up a meeting with the preceptor(s) to review the written performance evaluation of intern performance at the end of each evaluation period.
30. Plan and complete assigned projects, counseling, and presentations.
31. Provide preceptor with evaluation forms to use in rating the quality of the projects, counseling, and presentations.
32. Submit the completed checklist and work to Graduate Teaching Assistant by the due date.
33. Meet with the Dietetic Internship Program Director as requested to review progress.

Preceptor Responsibilities for the Community Nutrition Supervised Practice Experience

The preceptors:

1. Ensure that the intern is adequately oriented to the facility, services and programs offered.
2. Provide intern with direction and pertinent information needed during the workday.
3. Assign the intern an appropriate workload. At the beginning of the rotation the preceptor will assign the intern simpler work assignments and progressively increase the difficulty of the work assignments as the intern's skills develop.
4. Tell the interns with whom to check in and out with each workday.
5. Verify and sign the weekly time sheet that is submitted by the intern.
6. Meet daily with the intern to discuss activities and problems encountered during the workday.
7. Evaluate the intern's performance and provide verbal feedback throughout the experience.
8. Provide intern with guidance throughout the experience by reviewing and approving worked assigned to intern.
9. Verify that the intern completed required activities by reviewing competencies, suggested activities and assignments.
10. Present the intern with his/her philosophy about concerning community health, social, and nutrition services.
11. Makes any changes he/she deems necessary in an intern's plan of action for assigned work.
12. Report concerns about intern performance to the Dietetic Internship Program Director as soon as possible so that they are addressed in a timely manner.
13. Complete the written evaluation of the intern's performance mid-way (or more often if desired by preceptor) and at the end of the rotation. Meet with the intern at the end of each evaluation period to discuss the written performance evaluations (usually every 4 weeks or more often).
14. Provide the intern with direction in the completion of the assignments (project and in-service or class).

15. Evaluate the assignments (project, counseling, and in-service or class) completed by the intern using the forms provided.
16. Evaluate the intern while counseling a client.
17. Complete the "Preceptor Evaluation of Supervised Practice Experiences" form at the end of the rotation.

Objectives for Community Nutrition Supervised Practice Experience

The intern provides nutrition care in the community setting under the supervision of a public health nutritionist or registered dietitian or other qualified professional.
The intern:

1. Screens clients or communities for nutritional, health, and social risks while communicating Integrative approaches are based on in-depth individual assessments.
2. Collects and assesses nutrition, health, and other data from at risk individuals or communities.
3. Develops nutrition plans and interventions for individuals or communities.
4. Implements nutrition plans and interventions for individuals or communities.
5. Provides needed referrals for high-risk individuals or communities.
6. Documents care provided in medical and/or program records.
7. Assists in the evaluation of nutrition, health, and other services provided to individuals or communities by the community health program.
8. Reviews the quality improvement program in place at the assigned clinical education facility.
9. Provides individual and/or group nutrition counseling/education to meet needs of clients and groups served by the community health program or agency based on the ten tenets of Dietetics and Integrative Medicine (DIM).
10. Participates in the completion of projects and other assigned activities necessary to provide quality nutrition and health care to clients and groups served by the community health program or agency.
11. Interacts with health professionals, administrators, legislators, and others to learn more about health, nutrition, and social services in the community served.
12. Performs in accordance with the values of the Academy of Nutrition & Dietetics as stated in the "Code of Ethics for the Dietetic Profession".
13. Conducts an on-going evaluation of knowledge and skills in the clinical setting based on feedback from preceptors and self; and modifies performance as indicated by the evaluation process.
14. Participates in activities as assigned by the dietetic internship program director, graduate faculty and preceptors.
15. Assists preceptor with any responsibilities assigned by community/group education and/or cooking classes.

Experiences for DIM Community Nutrition

The intern and preceptor use this list to aid in planning activities for the experience to meet competencies. The intern is not required to complete all of the suggested activities on the list as these serve as a general guide to plan the experience.

- ✓ Interact with patients, clients, health professionals, staff, students and others to develop oral and written communication and interpersonal skills.
- ✓ Interview different professionals working with the agency or program to learn what roles they fulfill and what key health concerns they see in the community.
- ✓ Attend and participate in inter- and intradepartmental or agency meetings.
- ✓ Review the organizational chart, policies and procedures for the agency or program employee manual, and job descriptions.
- ✓ Conduct and supervise health and nutrition screenings of individuals or groups to identify those at risk.
- ✓ Conduct and supervise health and nutrition assessments of individuals or groups at risk and identify health and nutrition care plans/interventions recommended.
- ✓ Provide health and nutrition care interventions to at risk individuals and groups.
- ✓ Conduct and participate in community based health promotion programs.
- ✓ Investigate a health and nutrition problem in the community and develop, or revise an intervention addressing the problem.
- ✓ Review or compile a list of food, nutrition, and social service resources in the area.
- ✓ Observe a variety of community nutrition and health programs in the area. Examples: organic local farm, Good Natured Family Farms (farms with an integrative approach.
- ✓ Identify reference books, publications, and journals used by community health professionals.
- ✓ Read chapters or articles from the difference references at the facility on topics related to community health, nutrition or social issues.
- ✓ Discuss the readings with the preceptor.
- ✓ Participate in the use of mass media for community education or the promotion of community health and nutrition initiatives or services.
- ✓ Revise or develop educational materials for use by clients or professionals served by the community nutrition agency or program.
- ✓ Plan, develop, market, conduct, and evaluate at least one in-service training session for employees and/or nutrition classes for clients.
- ✓ Plan, develop, market, coordinate, and participate in a community health screening, health fair, intervention, or other community health project.
- ✓ Identify computer resources and applications specific to integrative community health and nutrition services.
- ✓ Review local, state, and federal regulations that affect the community health and nutrition services provided by the agency/program.
- ✓ Communicate with the appropriate local, state, and/or federal legislators and administrative staff regarding community health, nutrition, and social legislation and policies.
- ✓ Review the budget for the community health and nutrition agency/program with the preceptor.
- ✓ Discuss community health, nutrition, economic and social needs of the clients or groups served by the agency or program with the preceptor.
- ✓ Identify interventions to address the needs identified for the clients or groups served and discuss your recommendations with the preceptor.

Community Nutrition Project

The intern completes many projects during the experience. The intern and preceptor select a project that is evaluated as part of the final course grade. In some cases, it may be one large project. In other cases, it is several smaller projects that are evaluated as a whole.

Guidelines for the project encompass the following criteria. These form the basis by which the project is evaluated by the preceptor.

1. The project meets an existing identified need of the facility. (see list of potential community projects)
2. The project should be of serious value to the facility and constitute something that is utilized after the intern leaves.
3. The project allows the intern to fulfill one or more competencies for the rotation.
4. The completed project is professional in content and quality.
5. A written one-page description of the project is submitted to the preceptor for review and approval during the first four weeks of the rotation and before the intern begins work on the project.
6. The intern describes the project on Angel course web site weekly blog after approval by the preceptor.
7. It is the intern's responsibility to complete the project. In order to produce a quality project this will involve time spent outside of scheduled rotation hours.
8. The preceptor(s) and Dietetic Internship Program Director receive a written report describing the completed project or an actual copy of the project.
9. The preceptor uses the "Evaluation of Project" form to grade the project. It is the intern's responsibility to ensure the appropriate forms are available to the preceptor(s) for evaluating the project.
10. The completed evaluation(s) of the project is submitted to the Dietetic Internship Program Director upon completion of the experience.
11. A passing score is earned on the graded project. If the intern fails to earn a passing score on the first attempt, the preceptor suggests improvements and they are made by the intern to reach a passing score. In some cases, a totally new project may be assigned.

Project ideas – See lists of DIM community projects. These are suggestions only; the preceptor probably has many ideas for projects.

1. Create audiovisual or printed materials (e.g., cooking class vignettes, handouts, tapes, web site, posters, etc.) on some aspect of education and training for personnel or clients, use the new materials with personnel, and evaluate the effectiveness of the new materials.
2. Develop a new education and training program or complete a major revision of an existing education and training program for personnel or clients, teach the new or revised program to personnel, and evaluate the effectiveness of the program.
3. Conduct studies to determine need for services or the quality and effectiveness of services, present findings of studies, and implement plans to address problems identified.
4. Participate in the collection and analysis of market research related to integrative community health and nutrition services, (i.e., Food Is Medicine (FIM), Greater Kansas City Food Policy Coalition (GKCFPC), KC Food Circle, KC Community Gardens, Cultivate KC).
5. Plan, organize, direct, and/or evaluate one of the following: health fair, health screening, health intervention program, legislative event, etc.
6. Implement portion of a computer application related to community health and nutrition services and report on the impact of the new application.
7. Write and revise policies and procedures for the facility or community health agency.
8. Develop, implement, and evaluate protocols or standards of care for clients.

9. Develop, prepare, evaluate, standardize, and/or analyze nutrient content of recipes for clients.

In-Service Training for Personnel AND/OR Nutrition and Health Education Program for Clients

The intern plans and conducts one or more in-service training or education programs presented to staff, clients or others groups during the experience. The training or education programs may be for employees or clients served by the agency or program or for other organizations or groups. The preceptor determines the topic for the training or education programs that the intern is leading.

The intern is responsible for preparing and collecting materials needed to effectively lead the training or education program (e.g. audiovisual aids, handouts, equipment, etc.). The preceptor or other designated staff attending the training or education program evaluates the presentation by the intern. The intern is responsible for ensuring that the preceptor or other staff has the evaluation form to rate the performance of the intern leading the training session.

The intern is responsible for submitting the completed evaluation forms and samples of materials used during the in-service training or education programs to the Dietetic Internship Program Director at the end of the experience. A passing score is earned on the evaluation of the presentation. If the intern fails to earn a passing score on the first attempt, another training or education program is conducted by the intern and evaluated by the preceptor or other staff.

Nutrition Counseling Evaluation

The preceptor observes the intern counseling clients and evaluates her/his performance using the form provided. A passing score is earned for the evaluation of a counseling session. If the intern fails to earn a passing score, another consult is completed by the intern, observed and evaluated by the preceptor. If individual client counseling is not possible at the community nutrition site, the intern completes counseling during the clinical nutrition and practice area of interest rotations.

7

DN 827 Practicum: Check List of Items to Submit for Community Nutrition

- ✓ The following items are submitted to the GTA when the experience is finished or by the end of final exam week.
- ✓ A check list and materials are submitted upon completion of the supervised practice experience.
- ✓ The items are placed in the same order as on the check list.
- ✓ The check list and items are submitted in a manila file folder labeled with the intern's name, rotation, semester, and year.
- ✓ After review of materials by the GTA the folders are passed to the DI Program Director for final review and assignment of course grades.
- ✓ When all items are completed satisfactorily assign grade of S (satisfactory) is assigned.
- ✓ A grade of I (incomplete) is assigned if work is incomplete.
- ✓ A grade of U (unsatisfactory) is assigned if the work quality does not meet standards.

Intern Name ____

Facility or Site ____

Submission Date __________________________

Semester ___**Fall 20**** OR ___**Spring 20****

___ Copy of project or description of project
___ Completed project evaluation by preceptor
___ Four week performance evaluation completed by preceptor (1 or more)
___ Four week performance evaluation completed by intern (1 or more)
___ Final performance evaluation completed by preceptor
___ Final performance evaluation completed by intern
___ In-service or class evaluation form and samples of materials used for class
___ Nutrition counseling evaluation
___ Competencies completed with examples and preceptor signature
___ Preceptor evaluation of experience
___ Intern evaluation of experience
___ Weekly blogs (5)
___ Time sheets signed by preceptor

- At least 248 hours for Community Nutrition

___ Proof of attendance at two professional meetings during each semester

- Provide title, date, location, and competencies completed

Comments:

DN 827 Community Nutrition 20**-20**

Competencies for Supervised Practice Experiences

The Commission on Accreditation of Dietetic Education Programs developed competencies for Accredited Dietetic Internship Programs.

For each semester of the dietetic internship the intern fulfills competencies and provides a written example of work that fulfills the competencies. If all competencies are not completed by the end of the program, the intern documents class work or other supervised practice or work experiences to show how the intern accomplished the competencies.

The intern is responsible for maintaining this document of the competencies achieved. The preceptor reviews it with the intern and verifies the competencies met by the intern during the supervised practice experience. The intern copies and pastes this list of competencies and types examples of work accomplished for the competencies. The preceptor signs the list verifying work accomplished. If competencies are accomplished through graduate course work, the intern asks the faculty to verify the competencies fulfilled and sign instead of the preceptor. The intern submits the updated competencies list to the Dietetic Internship Program Director at the end of each semester.

Intern name ____

Scientific and Evidence Base of Practice: integration of scientific information and research into practice

DI 1.1 Select appropriate indicators and measure achievement of clinical, programmatic, quality productivity, economic or other outcomes, ex., elimination diets, general principles of IN approach, (10 Tenets).

Example:

Preceptor signature and date:

DI 1.2 Apply evidence-based guidelines, systematic reviews and scientific literature in the nutrition care process and model and other areas of dietetic practice. Review the types of evidence and quality or evidence for nutrition research: compare randomized controlled trials between nutritional and pharmaceutical studies.

Example:

Preceptor signature and date:

DI 1.3 Justify programs, products, services and care using appropriate evidence or practice. Review the literature for various individualized nutrition interventions.

Example:

Preceptor signature and date:

DI 1.4 Evaluate emerging research for application in dietetics practice.

Example:

Preceptor signature and date:

DI 1.5 Conduct research projects using appropriate research methods, ethical procedures, and statistical analysis.

Example:

Preceptor signature and date:

Professional Practice Expectations: beliefs, values, attitudes and behaviors for the professional dietitian level practice

DI 2.1 Practice in compliance with current federal regulations and state statutes and rules, as applicable and in accordance with accreditation standards and the ADA Scope of Dietetics Practice Framework, Standards of Professional Performance and Code of Ethics for the Profession of Dietetics.

Example:

Preceptor signature and date:

DI 2.2 Demonstrate professional writing skills in preparing professional communications (e.g., research manuscripts, project proposals, education materials, policies and procedures)

Example:

Preceptor signature and date:

DI 2.3 Design, implement, and evaluate presentations considering life experiences, cultural diversity, and educational background of the target audience.

Example:

Preceptor signature and date:

DI 2.4 Use effective education and counseling skills to facilitate behavior change.

Example:

Preceptor signature and date:

DI 2.5 Demonstrate active participation, teamwork and contributions in group settings.

Example:

Preceptor signature and date:

DI 2.6 Assign appropriate patient care activities to DTRs and/or support personnel considering the needs of the patient/client or situation, the ability of support personnel, jurisdictional law, practice guidelines, and policies within the facility.

Example:

Preceptor signature and date:

DI 2.7 Refer clients and patients to other professionals and services when needs are beyond individual scope of practice.

Example:

Preceptor signature and date:

DI 2.8 Demonstrate initiative by proactively developing solutions to problems.

Example:

Preceptor signature and date:

DI 2.9 Apply leadership principles effectively to achieve desired outcomes.

Example:

Preceptor signature and date:

DI 2.10 Serve in professional and community organizations.

Example:

Preceptor signature and date:

DI 2.11 Establish collaborative relationships with internal and external stakeholders, including patients, clients, care givers, physicians, nurses, and other health professionals, administrative and support personnel to facilitate individual and organizational goals.

Example:

Preceptor signature and date:

DI 2.12 Demonstrate professional attributes such as advocacy, customer focus, risk taking, critical thinking, flexibility, time management, work prioritization, and work ethic within various organizational cultures.

Example:

Preceptor signature and date:

DI 2.13 Perform self-assessment, develop goals and objectives and prepare a draft portfolio for professional development as defined by the Commission on Dietetics Registration. (Note: This is completed in the spring semester for the Practice Area of Interest experience that takes place in the summer semester.)

Example:

Preceptor signature and date:

DI 2.14 Demonstrate assertiveness and negotiation skills while respecting life experiences, cultural diversity and educational background.

Example:

Preceptor signature and date:

Clinical and Customer Services: development and delivery of information, products, and services to individuals, groups, and populations.

DI 3.1 Perform the Nutrition Care Process and use standardized nutrition language for individuals, groups and populations of differing ages and health status, in a variety of settings.

Example:

Preceptor signature and date:

DI 3.1a Assess the nutritional status of individuals, groups, and populations in a variety of settings where nutrition care is or can be delivered.

Example:

Preceptor signature and date:

DI 3.1b Diagnose nutrition problems and create problem, etiology, signs and symptoms (PES) statements.

Example:

Preceptor signature and date:

DI 3.1c Plan and implement nutrition interventions to include prioritizing the nutrition diagnosis, formulating a nutrition prescription, establishing goals and selecting and managing intervention.

Example:

Preceptor signature and date:

DI 3.1d Monitor and evaluate problems, etiologies, signs, symptoms, and the impact of interventions on the nutrition diagnosis.

Example:

Preceptor signature and date:

DI 3.2 Develop and demonstrate effective communication skills using oral, print, visual, electronic and mass media methods for maximizing client education, employee training and marketing.

Example:

Preceptor signature and date:

DI 3.3 Demonstrate and promote responsible use of resources including employees, money, time, water, energy, food and disposable goods.

Example:

Preceptor signature and date:

DI 3.4 Develop and deliver products, programs or services that promote consumer health, wellness and lifestyle management merging consumer desire for taste, convenience and economy with nutrition, food safety and health messages and interventions.

Example:

Preceptor signature and date:

DI 3.5 Deliver respectful, science-based answers to consumer questions concerning emerging trends.

Example:

Preceptor signature and date:

DI 3.6 Coordinate procurement, production, distribution, and service of goods and services.

Example:

Preceptor signature and date:

DI 3.7 Develop and evaluate recipes, formulas, and menus for acceptability and affordability that accommodate the cultural diversity and health needs of various populations, groups and individuals.

Example:

Preceptor signature and date:

Practice Management and Use of Resources: strategic application of principles of management and systems in the provision of services to individuals and groups

DI 4.1 Use organizational processes and tools to manage human resources.

Example:

Preceptor signature and date:

DI 4.2 Perform management functions related to safety, security, and sanitation that affect employees, customers, patients, facilities, and food.

Example:

Preceptor signature and date:

DI 4.3 Apply systems theory and a process approach to make decisions and maximize outcomes.

Example:

Preceptor signature and date:

DI 4.4 Participate in public policy activities, including both legislative and regulatory initiatives.
Example:

Preceptor signature and date:

DI 4.5 Conduct clinical and customer service quality management activities.

Example:

Preceptor signature and date:

DI 4.6 Use current informatics technology to develop, store, retrieve and disseminate information and data.

Example:

Preceptor signature and date:

DI 4.7 Prepare and analyze quality, financial, or productivity data and develops a plan for intervention.

Example:

Preceptor signature and date:

DI 4.8 Conduct feasibility studies for products, programs or services with consideration of costs and benefits.

Example:

Preceptor signature and date:

DI 4.9 Obtain and analyze financial data to assess budget controls and maximize fiscal outcomes.

Example:

Preceptor signature and date:

DI 4.10 Develop a business plan for a product, program or service inducing development of a budget, staffing needs, facility requirements, equipment and supplies.

Example:

Preceptor signature and date:

DI 4.11 Complete documentation that follows professional guidelines, guidelines required by health care systems and guidelines required by practice setting.

Example:

Preceptor signature and date:

DI 4.12 Participate in coding and billing of dietetics/nutrition services to obtain reimbursement for services from public or private insurers.

Example:

Preceptor signature and date:

KU Integrative Medicine
and
School of Human Sciences – Department of Dietetics and Nutrition
KU Integrative Nutrition Project

Nutrition Evidence-Based Library (NEBL)
Time Sheets

Students complete and submit time sheets weekly or bi-weekly to the advisor. The advisor and student sign the time sheet each week or every other week. The intern submits the signed time sheet to the advisor (lwagner@kumc.edu). The student keeps a copy of the time sheets for his/her own records. Submit time sheets monthly and at end of the experience.

Student Name ______________________________

Supervised Practice Experience______________________________

Site: ______KU Integrative Medicine______________________

Week ending 30/30/2012

Day of week	Clock In	Clock Out	Hours worked	Excused hours
Monday				
Tuesday				
Wednesday				
Thursday				
Friday				
Saturday				
Sunday				
Total hours worked	XXXXXXXXXXX	XXXXXXXXX		

I certify that the hours recorded above represent my supervised practice experience hours this week.

____
Student's signature and date

I certify that the hours recorded by the student are correct.

____
Advisor's signature and date

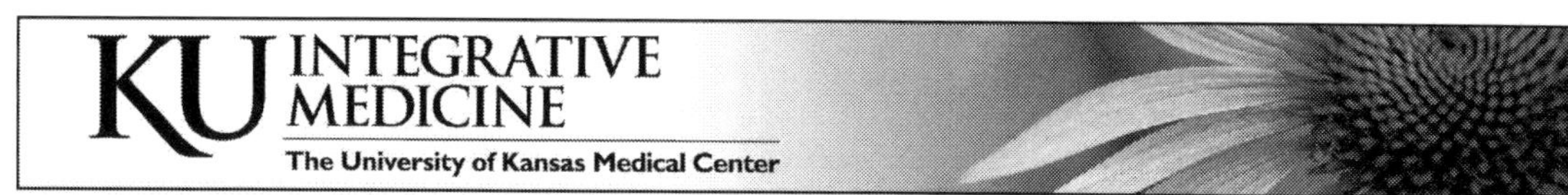

Pre-Post Evaluation for DIM Internship

Name ______________________________ Date__________________________

1. What is an Elimination Diet?

2. What is the purpose of an Elimination Diet?

3. Name 5 of the 10 top food sensitivities/allergens?

4. What does it mean to have a leaky/permeable gut?

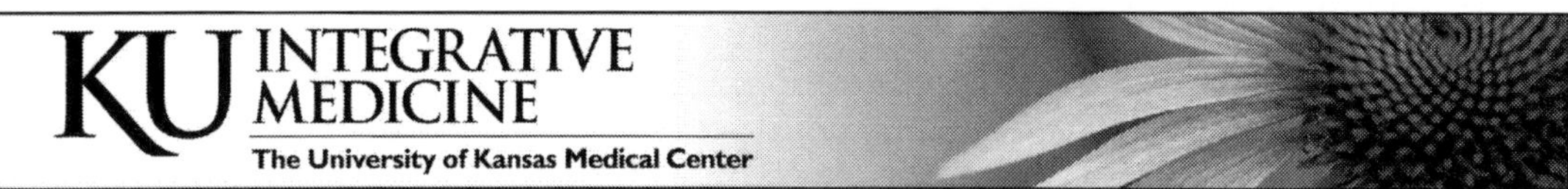

5. What does "IDU" stand for on the "IDU worksheet"?

6. What is the function of the "IDU" (Ingestion, Digestion, and Utilization) Nutrition Assessment Tool?

7. What does MAPDOM stand for?

8. List as many possible ways you can think of to cook/prepare vegetables.

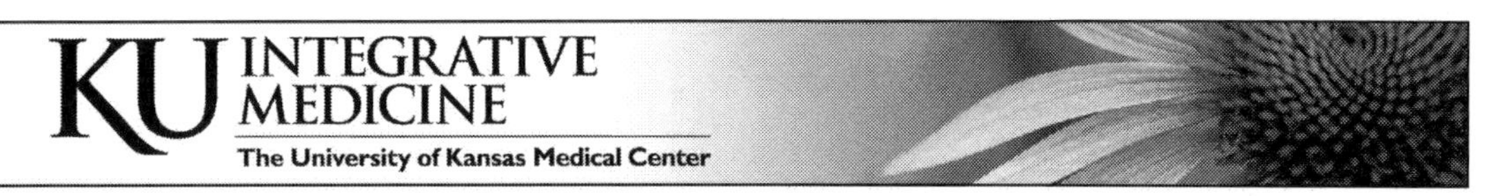

9. Although DIM really emphasizes the Individual Nutrition Assessment, what are some general dietary recommendations that would be appropriate for all people?

10. Please list and describe the Ten (or however many) Tenets of DIM.

11. Name two ways genetics affect nutrition recommendations or health

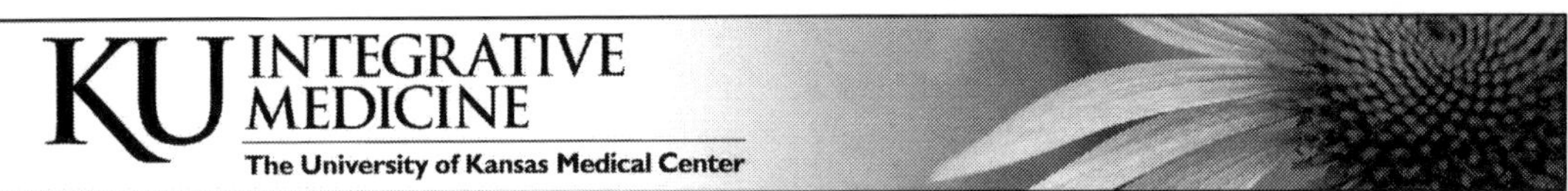

12. Name two ways the methylation cycle impacts health

13. What is the most common underlying cause for most chronic health conditions?

14. Briefly describe the difference between conventional nutrition therapy and integrative nutrition therapy

Dietetics and Integrative Medicine (DIM) Intern Checklist

Pre-practicum and orientation checklist (Module 1 Documents)

- ☐ DiSC, Meyer's Briggs or other workplace personality assessment
- ☐ Orientation to Dietetic Internship
- ☐ Lunch or other orientation to KU Dietetics and Integrative Medicine (DIM) program
- ☐ Orientation to KU Integrative Medicine, Nutrition Care Process
- ☐ Complete Pre-Practicum Evaluation

Clinical experiences checklist (Module 3 Documents)

- ☐ Read KU DIM Nutrition Care & Assessment Process
- ☐ Read Motivational Interviewing (MI) Document and watch web videos on MI basics
- ☐ Read Nutrition Consultation Guidelines
- ☐ Review KUMC Physical Exam Checklist
- ☐ Review IDU – Ingestion, Digestion, Utilization Document
- ☐ Review Table of Specialized Diets
- ☐ Review GI Tract Assessment Table
- ☐ Refer to GI Nutrient Absorption Sites
- ☐ Observe 12 total patients (minimum)
- ☐ Choose 1 patient/client to turn into "Case Report" and present at weekly team meeting
- ☐ Shadow each of the KU Integrative Medicine team members
    - Medical Doctor (MD)
    - Infusion Nurse (RN)
    - Naturopathic Doctor (ND)
    - Neurofeedback Technician
    - Research Coordinator
    - Advanced Practice Registered Nurse (APRN)
    - Clinical Psychologist (PhD)
- ☐ Rotate with other Integrative Medicine practitioners
    - Reiki or Attunement
    - Acupuncture
    - Massage Therapy
    - Physical Therapy
    - Biological Dentistry
    - Others...
- ☐ Bioelectric Impedance Analysis (BIA)
    - Observe BIA Analysis
    - Complete client BIA Analysis under supervision of RDN

- Complete client BIA Analysis alone & enter data into computer for patient printout

- ☐ Observe nutrition physical exam & take notes of your and RDN's observations
- ☐ Take notes in addition to RDN's clinic notes to assist with input on Nutrition Assessment
- ☐ Assist with nutrition supplement plan & recommended supplements for patients. Note dosage, frequency and time to re-evaluate
- ☐ Use Natural Medicines Comprehensive Database to check potential drug-nutrient interactions
- ☐ Research a supplement you are unfamiliar with in the Natural Medicines Comprehensive Database to learn about: Effectiveness, Dosage, Adverse E
- ☐ Utilize Dietitians in Integrative and Functional Medicine website for Natural Medicine Comprehensive Database, archived webinars, locating Integrative RDs nationwide, etc.
- ☐ Observe examples of patients exhibiting metabolic disturbances related to:
  - Cancer
  - Gastrointestinal dysregulation
  - Inflammation
  - Immune Dysfunction
  - Energy imbalance (overweight, underweight, mitochondrial disruption)
  - Autoimmune disorder
  - Endocrine disruption (Hypothyroidism, Diabetes, Metabolic Syndrome
- ☐ Watch archived webinars from Dietetics in Integrative and Functional Medicine (DIFM) web archives (www.integrativerd.org)

Community and/or Management-related experiences checklist (Module 2 and 5 Documents)

Healing Foods: Food as Medicine

- ☐ Prepare for and help organize cooking classes
- ☐ Assemble and/or prepare recipes, assess kitchen inventory, prepare grocery list and shop for food or submit to grocery delivery service
- ☐ Work at Sustainable Farm, Garden and/or foodservice operation to learn the importance of soil quality and health and sourcing foods to local businesses and working with consumers.
- ☐ Review all documents from Modules 2 and 5

Targeted Nutritional Supplements

- ☐ Shadow a nutritional pharmacist (PharmD) that manages a nutritional supplement formulary
- ☐ Review the Comprehensive Natural Medicines Database for supplement information

List of DIM Resources

Text Books/eBooks

- Bland, JS., Levin, B., Costarella, L., Liska, D., (2004) Clinical Nutrition, a Functional Approach. *2nd ed.,* IFM.
  - **ISBN-13: 978-0962485916**
  - **ASIN: B000CD1PWM**
- Erdman, J., MacDonald, IA., Zeisel, SH. (2012) Present Knowledge in Nutrition, *10th ed.*, Wiley-Blackwell.
  - **ISBN-13: 9781455746286**
  - **eBook: ISBN-13: 9780470963104**
  - ASIN: **B008MQ9AGO**
- Escott-Stump. S., (2011). *Nutrition & Diagnosis Related Care,*
  - **ISBN-13: 978-1608310173**
  - **eISBN-13: 9781451160758**
  - **ASIN: B0093CP9H0**
- Gaby, A.R., (2011). *Nutritional Medicine*, Fritz-Perlberg
  - **ISBN-13: 978-0982885000**
  - **ASIN: B005ERQLS4**
- Jones, D.S., *(ed)* (2010). Textbook of Functional Medicine, *3rd ed.* IFM
  - **ISBN-13: 978-0977371372**
  - **eBook: ASIN: B0083X7G6C**
- Lanham-New, S.A., Macdonald, I.A., Roche, H.M., (*eds*) (2010). *Nutrition and Metabolism*: 2nd *Ed.*
  - **ISBN-13: 978-1405168083**
  - **e ISBN-13: 9781444347692**
- Long-Roth, S., Nahikian-Nelms, (2013) Medical Nutrition Therapy: A Case Study Approach, *4th ed*
  - **ISBN-13: 978-1133593157**

- **eBook: ASIN: B00CIIHF2S**

- Lutz, CA., Przytuski, KR., (2011) Nutrition and Diet Therapy. *5th ed.*,FA Davis.
  - **ISBN-13: 978-0-8036-2202-9**
- Mahan, K., (2011). *Krause's Food and the Nutrition Care Process,13th ed.* Saunders
  - **ISBN-13: 978-1437722338**
  - **eBook: ASIN: B00EDS9JKC**
- Mataljan, G. (2006) The World's Healthiest Foods, Essential Guide for the Healthiest way of Eating. GMF Pub.
  - **ISBN-13: 978-0976918547**
  - **eBook: ASIN: B004XIZM7Q**
- Niculescu, M.D., Haggarty, P. *(eds) (*2011). *Nutrition in Epigenetics*, Wiley-Blackwell
  - **ISBN-13: 978-0813816050**
  - **eBook: ASIN: B004V4FH4A**
- Pizzorno, J., Katzinger, J., (2012) *Clinical Pathophysiology -A Functional Perspective with Companion Guide*
  - **ISBN-13: 978-1927017043**
- Pizzorno, JE., (2012) Textbook of Natural Medicine, *4th ed.* Churchill-Livingstone.
  - **ISBN-13: 9781437723335**
  - **eBook: ASIN: B00989QEQS**
- Rakel, D. (2012) Integrative Medicine, *3rd ed.*, Elsevier.
  - **ISBN-13: 9781437717938**
  - **eBook: ASIN: B008151Z9G**
- Stipanuk, M. (2012) Biochemical, Physiological and Molecular Aspects of Human Nutrition, *3rd ed.* Elsevier.
  - **ISBN-13: 9781455746286**
  - **eBook: ASIN: B00EEJUH2E**
- Weatherby, D., Ferguson, S. Blood Chemistry and CBC Analysis, (2004) Bear Mountain.

- **ISBN-13: 9780976136712**

Other references:

- *Advanced Nutrition and Human Metabolism: 5th Edition* (2012), Gropper, Smith
-
- *AAPI'S Nutrition Guide to Optimal Health: Using Principles of Functional Medicine and Nutritional Genomics* (2012), Kanumaury, Batheja
- *Biochemical, Physiological and Molecular Aspects of Human Nutrition (2013)*, Stipanuk, Caudill
- *Krause's Food, Nutrition and Diet Therapy* (2004), Mahan, Escott-Stump
- *Krause's Food and the Nutrition Care Process* (2012), Mahan, Escott-Stump
-
- *Integrative Gastroenterology* (2011), Mullin
-
- Integrative Medicine: Principles for Practice (2004), Kligler, Lee
-
- Integrative Medicine: 3rd Edition (2012), Rakel
-
- *Laboratory Evaluations for Integrative and Functional Medicine: 2nd Edition, Lord, Bralley*
-
- *Molecular Basis of Health and Disease* (2011), Undurti,
- *Nutrition and Diagnosis-Related Care (2012)*, Escott-Stump
- *Nutrition and Immunology (2000)*, Gershwin, German, Keen
- Nutrition in Epigenetics 2011,
- *Nutritional Medicine* (2011), Gaby
- *Nutrition and Metabolism: 2ndEdition* (2011), Lanham, MacDonald, Roche
- Pathophysiology by the Nutrition Society (England),
- Present Knowledge in Nutrition by Zeisel, etc.
- *Text Book of Biochemistry with Clinical Correlations*: 7th edition (2011), Devlin (editor)
- *Text Book of Functional Medicine (2010)*, Jones (editor)
- *The world's healthiest foods* (2007), Mateljan

Web Resources

- EBSCO databases
  - http://www.ebscohost.com/biomedical-libraries/AMED-The-Allied-and-Complementary-Medicine-Database
  - http://www.ebscohost.com/biomedical-libraries/medline-complete
  - http://www.ebscohost.com/academic/cinahl-plus-with-full-text
- Dieticians in Integrative and Functional Medicine (DIFM) website:
  - http://integrativerd.org/
- Natural Medicines Comprehensive Database

    - http://naturaldatabase.therapeuticresearch.com/home.aspx?cs=&s=ND
- Natural Standard Database
    - http://naturalstandard.com/databases/
- NCCAM
    - http://nccam.nih.gov/
- NIH/Office of Dietary Supplements
    - http://ods.od.nih.gov/Research/CARDS_Database.aspx
- Herbal Databases:
    - http://botanical.com/
    - http://www.herbmed.org/
- Basic Laboratory Reference Information for practitioners and/or patients
    - Lab Tests Online
        - http://labtestsonline.org/
    - Metametrix
        - http://www.metametrix.com/
    - HealthCheck
        - http://www.healthcheckusa.com/Nutrition-Profile/46898/
    - WellnessFX
        - http://www.wellnessfx.com/product
- Testing for food sensitivities and intolerances
    - http://www.alcat.com/landing/food-intolerance-testing.html
    - http://meridianvalleylab.com/food-allergy-testing/basic-foods-e-panel/

Journal Article References: Core Resources

1. American Dietetic Association Revised 2008 Standards Of Practice For Registered Dietitians In Nutrition Care; Standards Of Professional Performance For Registered Dietitians; Standards Of Practice For Dietetic Technicians, Registered, In Nutrition Care; And Standards Of Professional Performance For Dietetic Technicians, Registered." *Journal Of The American Dietetic Association* 108.9 (2008): 1538-1542.
2. Jones DS, Hofmann L, Quinn S. 21st Century Medicine: A New Model for Medical Education and Practice. Gig Harbor: Institute for Functional Medicine; 2009.
3. Triage Theory
    a. McCann J, Ames B. Vitamin K, an example of triage theory: is micronutrient inadequacy linked to diseases of aging? *American Journal Of Clinical Nutrition* [serial online]. October 2009;90(4):889-907.
    b. Ames B. Prevention of mutation, cancer, and other age-associated diseases by optimizing micronutrient intake. *Journal Of Nucleic Acids* [serial online]. September 22, 2010;2010
    c. McCann J, Ames B. Adaptive dysfunction of selenoproteins from the perspective of the triage theory: why modest selenium deficiency may

increase risk of diseases of aging. *FASEB Journal: Official Publication Of The Federation Of American Societies For Experimental Biology* [serial online]. June 2011;25(6):1793-1814.

d. Ames B. Optimal micronutrients delay mitochondrial decay and age-associated diseases. *Mechanisms Of Ageing And Development* [serial online]. July 2010;131(7-8):473-479.

4. Heaney R. Long-latency deficiency disease: insights from calcium and vitamin D. *American Journal Of Clinical Nutrition* [serial online]. November 2003;78(5):912-919.
5. Heaney R. The nutrient problem. *Nutrition Reviews* [serial online]. March 2012;70(3):165-169.
6. Diamanti-Kandarakis E. Endocrine-Disrupting Chemicals: An Endocrine Society Scientific Statement. Endocrine Reviews. 2009;**30**(4):293.

Reading Assignment Summary and Reflections Form

Name____________________________________ Date__________

Title of Book/Article/Chapter ____

Author____________________ Year ____________

Please give a 1-2 paragraph summary of the article's main ideas. You may only need one paragraph if it was a short excerpt or book chapter. This may mean summarizing the intent of a study, its main methods, results and a brief discussion of the conclusions. Please also give your own opinion of the results and conclusions drawn – be critical/skeptical of the findings.

Initial Reflections/Thoughts

One or 2 new facts/ideas you learned from the article

1.

2.

Take-home message of article/book/excerpt

What will you take from this reading that you can apply to your future as a nutritionist/dietitian?

What questions do you have after reading?

Orientation to KU Healing Foods Kitchen

Healing Foods Kitchen Guide

KU Integrative Medicine is fortunate to house a Healing Foods Kitchen within the clinic to teach patients, staff, students and the public how to cook the healthy, whole foods that we recommend: teaching people how to use Food as Medicine. This document outlines the student's role in the kitchen after the preceptor has determined the content of the cooking class. However, it is possible to delegate to the student the task of formulating or deciding on class recipes and content. The following assumes the preceptor has determined class content and recipes.

Students' Role in the Kitchen

The week prior to the cooking class:

- **Recipes:** At least a week or more before class, the preceptor or student(s) should choose appropriate recipes for the cooking class. When determined, the recipes can be formatted appropriately. Please see "Recipe Format & Instructions" Document, "Example Recipe Format – Chicken Breast with Tomato and Coconut" document for Recipe-writing instructions and guidance.
- **Ingredient Inventory**: Based on the recipes, a shopping list is developed. Upon completing the shopping list, check the current kitchen inventory to determine which ingredients are available and which are needed for the cooking class. Record amounts needed or mark/check-off the items already in stock. Check with a faculty advisor for possible substitutions. Please see the "Grocery Shopping Template" for guidance.
- **Grocery List**: Based on the Recipes, Ingredient Inventory and local, whole and organic food availability, create a shopping list to submit to take with you to the grocery store or to send to the grocery delivery service.
- **Grocery Shopping**: If you are tasked with doing the grocery shopping, take reusable bags and try to envision how the groceries can be organized based on recipes for ease of assembly and preparation. Complete grocery shopping at least by the morning or early afternoon of the day before class.
- **Grocery Delivery Service**: If there is a grocery delivery service available in your area, it may be economical to have an outside service shop for and deliver the groceries for cooking classes. If so, contact them with the grocery list and specifics to the email address provided for their services about a week before the cooking class. Groceries should be delivered by 1 pm the day before class to give ample preparation time and to identify any last-minute or missing items.

Week of the class / Evening before or morning before cooking demonstration:

- **Food Acquisition:** Food can be acquired a variety of ways: CSA pickup, farmer drop-off and/or grocery shopping or grocery delivery service. When the groceries place the groceries in the proper storage area, (refrigerator, freezer, cabinet). By 1 pm the day before cooking class, all ingredients should be accounted for. Any missing ingredients will need to be purchased for class.

Orientation to KU Healing Foods Kitchen

- **Food Preparation:** The day prior and the morning of cooking class, most foods should be cleaned, cut, measured, prepared for the cooking class. Leave some of the produce items to be "demonstrated" for the cooking class. Each recipe should be measured and assembled separately and either stored in the refrigerator or on the counter. Please use baking sheets, plates, bags or other equipment to keep all ingredients for a single recipe together.
- **Read recipes ahead of time:** It will be important to understand the flow of the cooking to supply the teacher the ingredients for upcoming recipes, as needed.

✓ Keep a portion of the foods (produce, herbs, spices, etc.) to demonstrated, and used as examples for students to observe. This is the purpose of the class!

✓ Using recipes note foods to be prepared during class. Most foods and ingredients are precut and measured but often-small portions are reserved for demonstration in class.

✓ Keep a compost bag sitting (in a bowl) for waste when prepping foods

✓ Items can be placed in the bowls covered with cellophane and labeled

✓ When portioning items for each recipe on a separate cooking tray to keep them together

✓ Note on each recipe foods which are prepped and ready for the class

✓ If portioning foods the day before the class – process only the foods that can keep overnight

Morning of Cooking Demonstration:

- **Class Preparation:** Finish preparing remaining foods and ingredients. Clean the kitchen floor and counter for the class.
- **Class Food Organization:** Ingredients should be labeled with name and amount of ingredient, as the recipes will be assembled or completed in the order of the class. As much as possible, organize the class recipes from left to right (or right to left), so that we can move as systematically as possible. Place the ingredients for each recipe in the order they will be used starting with the first ingredients used closest to where the teacher will stand. Note: Some recipes will need to remain on trays in the refrigerator or to the side because space is limited.
- **Place Settings:** The Patient Service Representatives have a "final attendance" list at the front desk of KU Integrative Medicine. Place table settings for the number of attendees enrolled for the class. Left side of plate is for forks, right side of plate is knife with blade facing plate and spoon on the outside. Glasses are filled with water on the top right side of the place setting. Recipes and note pages should be printed and placed under the place mats on the right side of the place setting. Pens should be provided for notes.

Cooking Class:

Orientation to KU Healing Foods Kitchen

- **Equipment:** Please prepare for use of blender, immersion blender, food processor, or other kitchen gadgets and equipment. Because space is limited, you may only need to be aware of the time these need to be ready for use during the class. Turn on the light in the exhaust hood (over the range top). Also, if the oven will be used in class, please turn it on to the correct temperature at the beginning of class.
- **Classes**: Classes move pretty quickly and can be a little hectic if there are a lot of questions from the audience.
- As the assistant, it is important to focus on what the teacher is doing to anticipate things she may need or help with cooking (listen for questions) as she works on many recipes at one time. The RDN will teach nutrition while cooking, so it will be helpful to assist her while somewhat limiting interaction with the audience to avoid confusion, as time is limited.
    - ✓ As recipes are started help with removing the covers from the ingredients and remove empty containers as they are used to clear the cooking space
    - ✓ Smaller items can be set in the sink while larger items can be loaded on the dish washer trays
    - ✓ The preceptor may ask you to help by cleaning appliances or other cooking utensils (like the food processor) if they are to be used for more than one recipe
    - ✓ As items are prepared you will serve them to the audience

After Class

- **Clean up**: You can run most of the cooking equipment and dishes through the washer. As one load is washing you can load the second rack to be washed and continue rotating. When dishes come out of the washer they can be put away, if they are still wet they should be dried with a towel then put away. Clean the counters and run the disposal (check for small measuring spoons in the disposal) and finish by sweeping the floor.

Orientation for Interns - Cooking Class Outline

The week prior to the cooking class:

Assemble recipes for the upcoming class
Using the recipes develop a shopping list (template)
Compare the completed shopping list with current kitchen inventory
You may need to check with Leigh to see if products (like spices or herbs we have can be substituted)
Once approved place/email the grocery order for delivery one full day before the class

Week of the class:

When the grocery order arrives compare it with the shopping list
Place the groceries in the proper storage area, (ie. Frig, freezer, cabinet)
Note anything missing or items still needed for the class

Evening before or morning before cooking demonstration:

It may be possible to cut, portion or chop some ingredients ahead of time, check with Leigh
Prep vegetables by washing, remove damage
Keep a compost bag sitting (in a bowl) for waste when prepping foods
Many items can be placed in the small bowls covered with cellophane and labeled
If portioning many items is may be helpful to put items for each recipe on a separate cooking tray to keep them together
Note on each recipe foods which are prepped and ready for the class
If portioning foods the day before the class – do only the foods that will keep overnight
Keep some produce, herbs and spices to be used as examples/prepared during the demonstration

Morning of Cooking Demonstration:

Finish prepping remaining foods and ingredients
Clean the kitchen floor and counter for the class
Recipes should be laid out according to the order of the cooking for the class (check with Leigh)
Group ingredients together on the counter around the range top
Layout the ingredients for each recipe in the order they will be used starting with the first ingredients used closest to where Leigh will stand
Once the recipes are laid out set the place mats, dishes and glasses for the attendees
Fill the water glasses and the water pitcher (try to keep glasses filled during class)
Place the recipes and handouts under the place mats/place a pen with the silverware

Some recipes will need to remain on trays in the refrigerator or to the side because space is limited
It will be important to understand the flow of the cooking to supply Leigh the ingredients for upcoming recipes as needed

Cooking Class:

Turn on the light in the exhaust hood (over the range top)
Classes move pretty quickly and can be a little hectic if there are a lot of questions from the audience
As the assistant it is important to focus on what Leigh is doing to anticipate things she may need or help with cooking (listen for ques) as she works on many recipes at one time

 1

Orientation for Interns - Cooking Class Outline

Leigh does education while cooking so it will be helpful to help her while staying out of the way and limiting interaction with the audience to avoid confusion with limited time
As recipes are started help with removing the covers from the ingredients and remove empty containers as they are used to clear the cooking space
Smaller items can be set in the sink while larger items can be loaded on the dish washer trays
Leigh may have you clean appliances or other cooking utensils (like the food processor) if they are to be used for more than one recipe
As items are prepared you will serve them to the audience

After the class

You can run most of the cooking equipment and dishes through the washer
As one load is washing you can load the second rack to be washed and continue rotating
When dishes come out of the washer they can be put away, if they are still wet they should be dried with a towel then put away
Clean the counters and run the disposal (check for small measuring spoons in the disposal)
Sweep the floor

 2

Class Outline

Before class

- Turn on dishwasher
- Fill water pitcher and place in refrigerator
- Set place settings
- Prepare handouts:
    - Print handouts: Recipes, Why Whole Foods, Stocking your Whole Foods Pantry, etc.
    - Print Evaluations (if there are none in the kitchen)
    - Place handouts at each place setting
- Fill water glasses (and teacups during fall/winter) at each place
- Place books at the corner of the counter for students to peruse

Today's Recipes:

1. Cool Sweet Potato Salad
2. Patriotic Quinoa Salad
3. Broccoli-Cauliflower Salad
4. Patriotic Parfait

Food Prep Before class (Teaching Topics/Points to Cover):

1. **Sweet Potato Salad (anti-ox rich potatoes orange = protection)**
   Boil/Cook Sweet potatoes
   Slice into ¼ inch thick pieces
   Slice onion and bell pepper
   Measure ingredients
   Mise en place

2. **Quinoa (protein-rich grain, fiber in beans)**
   Boil quinoa
   Chop veggies & measure
   Measure dressing ingredients
   Mise en place

3. **Broccoli-Cauliflower Salad – Teaching (detoxifying, especially with grilled meats - article)**
   Chop broccoli, cauliflower, onion
   Prep turkey bacon to cook during class
   Measure nuts, dried fruit, dressing ingredients
   Mise en place

4. **Parfait (Coconut MCFAs, antioxidants in blue/strawberries)**
   Wash fruit
   Measure Ingredients
   Mise en place

Class

Introduction:

1. **Instructor**: My name is Leigh Wagner – Nutrition Educator/Counselor most of my time and teach cooking classes for the other part of my time. I grew up in a food and health-focused home, and I love to help motivate people to make lifestyle changes and feel and live the benefits of **whole foods** lifestyle.

2. **Whole foods diet is not a fad**. It will not come in and go out of 'style'. Based on **our biochemistry**, eating a whole foods diet with organic, local, minimally-processed food is our **best fuel** for human life. Certain cells in our bodies require specific carbohydrates, fats, fibers, vitamins, minerals, etc. to function properly, and these are only completely provided by whole foods.

3. **Today's menu and Order of Operations: 1.** Sweet Potato Salad, 2. Patriotic Quinoa 3. Broccoli-Cauliflower Salad, 4. Parfait
   - **Recipe 2**: Quinoa should be cooking on stove
   - **Recipe 1**: Slice 1 potato and assemble ingredients, pour dressing over and marinate in fridge until later in class
   - **Recipe 2**: While potatoes marinating, take quinoa from stove and let cool (open and fluff), finish chopping (perhaps 1 pepper), assemble ingredients, pour dressing over top. Marinate in fridge until later.
   - **Recipe 3:** Cook turkey bacon (discuss alternatives), assemble salad ingredients, discuss alternatives to dried fruit and sunflower seeds. Nutritional content of sunflower seeds and the dried fruit. Crumble turkey bacon, assemble salad, pour dressing and mix.
   - **Recipes 1-3**: Serve
   - **Recipe 4**: While students enjoying salads, food-process the blueberries + coconut yogurt. Layer yogurt + fruit + almonds. Serve

4. **I am casual**, and I may not always explain every step that I take in the kitchen (sautéing, chopping, mincing broiling, boiling, etc.). **If you didn't catch something** that I added or did, please stop me and **ask** me to explain.

5. **No question is a stupid question:** Don't feel guilty about anything you eat or feel dumb about any questions you might have. We will talk about the foods we regularly eat, the places we shop, the questions we have, and the only progress that can be made is if we are as open and honest as possible. The bottom line is that we are all probably eating things we wish we didn't or want to learn more about the foods we aren't eating, so that we can make better choices to feel better. So, let's all share and question and wonder together!

6. **Taste, taste, TASTE**! If I am chopping something or you are wondering about a flavor I have mentioned, or we are preparing a food that you have never tasted: ask and TASTE!
7. **Class introductions:**
   - Go around and introduce ourselves
   - Why you are here/what interested you in the class
   - What level of cooking knowledge/experience (1-10... 1=none, 10=expert)
   - What level of nutrition knowledge (1-10)
   - What is a typical dinner meal for you? (fast, convenient, sit-down, restaurant...)

8. **Learning Objectives:**
   - Students will be able to cook/prep/choose...
   - Students will be able to name the benefits of...

Kitchen Checklist for Cooking Class

The week prior to the cooking class:

- Assemble recipes for the upcoming class
- Using the recipes develop a shopping list (template)
- Compare the completed shopping list with current kitchen inventory
- You may need to check with Leigh to see if products (like spices or herbs we have can be substituted)
- Once approved place/email the grocery order to KA Norris for delivery one full day (min) before the class

Note: during the growing season we will receive a CSA order each Tuesday. We will need to pickup and include these items in the kitchen inventory and may substitute products we expect or have on hand. We will also order locally grown products from Fair Share Farms and Birthday Prairie Farms

Week of the class:

- The grocery order should arrive on Tuesday or before 12:00pm on Wednesday prior to class.
- When the grocery order arrives compare it with the shopping list
- Place the groceries in the proper storage area, (ie. Frig, freezer, cabinet)
- **Note anything missing or items still needed for the class.** Missing or additional items will need to be picked up Wednesday evening

Evening before or morning before cooking demonstration:

- Food preparation: you will clean, wash, portion/chop most ingredients ahead of time. (Check with Leigh for specific items to be used for demonstration before portioning)
- Prep vegetables by washing, remove damage
- Keep a compost bag sitting (in a bowl) for waste when prepping foods
- Many items can be placed in the small bowls covered with cellophane and labeled
- If portioning many items is may be helpful to put items for each recipe on a separate cooking tray, plate, or bag to keep them together
- Note on each recipe foods which are prepped and ready for the class
- If portioning foods the day before the class – do only the foods that will keep overnight
- **Keep some produce, herbs and spices to be used as examples/prepared during the demonstration

Morning of Cooking Demonstration:

- Finish prepping remaining foods and ingredients
- Clean the kitchen floor and counter for the class
- Print recipes/handouts on colored paper for each student
- Recipes should be laid out according to the order of the cooking for the class (check with Leigh)
- Group ingredients together on the counter around the range top
- Layout the ingredients for each recipe in the order they will be used starting with the first ingredients used closest to where Leigh will stand
- Sticky notes/Labels for ingredients are placed next to each ingredient
- Once the recipes are laid out check with the front desk to get the count for the class, then set the place mats, dishes and glasses for the attendees
- Fill the water glasses and the water pitcher (try to keep glasses filled during class)
- Place the recipes and handouts under the place mats/place a pen with the silverware

Kitchen Checklist for Cooking Class

Cooking Class:

- Turn on the light in the exhaust hood (over the range top)
- Prepare equipment, appliances, cutting board and cooking utensils for each recipe
- As recipes are started help with removing the covers from the ingredients, remove empty containers and labels as they are used to clear the cooking space
- Smaller items can be set in the sink while larger items can be loaded on the dish washer trays
- Leigh may have you clean appliances or other cooking utensils (like the food processor) if they are to be used for more than one recipe
- You may need to assist with cooking as often many recipes are being prepared at one time
- As items are prepared you will serve them to the students

After the class

- Turn on the dish washer, put in the drain plug
- You can run *most* of the cooking equipment and dishes through the washer
- As one load is washing you can load the second rack to be washed and continue rotating
- When dishes come out of the washer they can be put away, if they are still wet they should be dried with a towel then put away
- Clean the counters and run the disposal (check for small measuring spoons in the disposal)
- Sweep the floor
- Remove the dishwasher drain plug and drain the dish washer

[Recipe Font: Franklin Gothic Book]

Recipe Title
[Centered, Bolded & 20 pt Font]

Recipe description
[Short, italicized description of the recipe]
[Centered, Normal, 12-point Font]

Ingredients [Bolded, 11 or 12 point Font, Left Justification]

List of ingredients
[Indent ¼ inch]
[11 or 12 point Font]
[Normal font (not bolded or italicized)]
[Use numbers (1, 2, 3, etc.)]
[Fully spell measurements: NO abbreviations, like"Tbsp" for 'tablespoon' or "c" for 'cup']

Directions [Bolded, 11 or 12 point Font, Left Justification]

1. [List ingredients in normal font using numbers and specific, systematic instructions for how to prepare the given recipe]
2. [Estimate times, additions, tips and tricks, rationale, etc.]
3. [Include time, temperature, and spell out Fahrenheit and/or Celsius. Be consistent with measurements used.]

[Reference should be given to any recipe used from a book, website or other resource that was not created by the author. If you adapt a recipe, please indicate this while citing the original recipe.]

[Insert KU Integrative Medicine Footer onto the document]

Curry Chicken Breast with Tomato and Coconut Milk

This savory and slightly sweet dish is a great introduction to Indian cuisine

Ingredients

2 tablespoons non-GMO canola oil or extra virgin olive oil
1 small red onion, cut in half lengthwise and thinly sliced
4 medium cloves garlic, minced
2 lengthwise slices fresh ginger (each 2 ½ inches long, 1 inch wide, and 1/8 inch thick), cut into matchstick strips (julienne)
1 ½ pound boneless, skinless chicken breasts, cut into 1-inch pieces
2 teaspoons Madras Curry Powder (store bought, contains coriander, cumin, mustard seeds, cloves, fenugreek, black peppercorns, red Thai or cayenne chiles, turmeric)
1 ½ teaspoons coarse sea salt
¼ cup unsweetened, light or regular coconut milk
1 large tomato, cored and finely chopped
2 tablespoons finely chopped fresh cilantro leaves and tender stems

Directions

1. Preheat a wok, stainless steel skillet or well-seasoned cast-iron skillet over medium-high heat. Drizzle oil down its sides. Add onion, garlic, ginger, and stir-fry until the vegetables are lightly browned (3-5 minutes).

2. Add chicken pieces and the curry powder, and cook until the meat is seared all over, about 5 minutes.

3. Sprinkle the salt over the chicken and pour in the coconut milk, which will immediately come to a boil. Cover, lower the heat to medium, and simmer, stirring occasionally, until the chicken is fork-tender and no longer pink inside (5-7 minutes). Remove the chicken pieces from the thin yellow sauce and place them in a serving bowl.

4. Raise the heat to medium-high heat and boil the sauce, uncovered, stirring occasionally, until it thickens, 3-5 minutes. Stir in the tomato and cilantro. Pour the sauce over the chicken and toss to bathe it with the curry. Serve immediately.

Recipe from 660 Curries by Raghavan Iyer, 2008: Workman Publishing; New York, NY.

The University of Kansas Medical Center | KU Integrative Nutrition | Leigh Wagner, MS, RD, LD | Integrative Nutritionist | http://integrativemed.kumc.edu

3901 Rainbow Blvd, MS 1017 | Kansas City, KS 66160 | (913) 588-6208 | Fax (913) 588-0012 | E-mail: integrativemedicine@kumc.edu

Grocery List for KA Norris Grocery Delivery Service

Please purchase groceries from _(Fill in name of Grocery Store or Market)_

Order to be delivered by

MM/DD/YY at/before __:__ am/pm

Email orders to: wnorris@kanorris.com

Item	#	Size	Brand	Other specifics
Produce				
Kale	*3*	*Bunches*		*Organic*
Pink Lady Apples	*3*	*Medium*		*Organic*
Carrots	*4*	*Medium*		*Organic*
Parsley	*1*	*Bunch*		*Organic*
Grocery				
70-80% dark chocolate chips	*1*	*~10-12 oz bag*	*Whole Foods*	*Prefer 80% cocoa*
Garbanzo beans	*2*	*16 oz cans*	*Eden Organics*	
Lemon Juice	*1 bottle*	*10 oz*		*Organic*
Bulk				
Raw Cashews		*2 cups*		
Raw almonds		*2 cups*		
Raisins and/or currants		*1 cup*		
Dried apple slices		*1 cup*		
Quinoa		*2 cups*		
Meat/Seafood				
Frozen Foods				

**** KA NORRIS, YOU MUST PROVIDE COPY OF GROCERY RECEIPT TO CUSTOMER****

Delivery Contact

Name

Phone #

Email

Delivery Address

KA Norris

Email orders to: wnorris@kanorris.com

P.O Box 2027, Kansas City, Kansas 66110
Office:913-262-6327 Fax: 913-828-4545

Whole Foods

7401 West 91st St
Overland Park, KS 66212 USA
map, directions & nearby stores

Phone 913.652.9633
Store contact form

Store hours:
7:30 a.m. to 10:00 p.m. seven days a week.

KU DIM Initial Assessment Process

Background

The initial nutrition assessment at KU Integrative Medicine (KU IM) is based on the Nutrition Care Process established by the Academy of Nutrition and Dietetics (The Academy), and is summarized, as follows:

Assessment
Diagnosis
Intervention
Monitoring
Evaluation

Chart Review and Preparation

The RDN reviews the paper and/or electronic medical record for information about the client's health history, nutrition history, anthropometrics, and any other information that could be helpful to begin to evaluate the person's nutritional status.

Papers or documents that can be helpful for nutrition consultations

- Nutrition intake forms submitted prior to nutrition consultation
- While reviewing the chart, complete the "Blank Nutrition Assessment & Consultation Summary Form"
- Blank "Progress Note" to write notes during appointment (lined paper with the client's name, Medical Record Number (MRN) and Date of Birth (DOB))
- Charge Sheet (varies by practice)
- Nutritional supplement list and company contact information packet (varies by practice)
- List of supplements available at KU Hospital Outpatient Pharmacy

Before Appointment

Prior to the actual consultation/appointment, the patient service representative (PSR) will need to take care of technical information, paperwork and other items:

- PSR: Confirm that patient has filled out all necessary forms & take photo (if approved and appropriate). If not, prepare forms that need to be completed and explain each one in detail, if necessary. Chart should be prepared ahead of time.
    - Notice of Privacy Practices (PSR)
    - HIPPA Authorization (PSR)
    - Diet Prescription or specific KU IM Referral form (pink or blue form)
    - Integrative Nutrition Intake Form (self or physician-referred)
    - Diet Diary (1 to 3-day history)
    - Fats and Oils Questionnaire
    - Medical Symptoms Questionnaire
- Photograph (taken by PSR): Take a photograph of the client to place in the chart. This will be used for ease of recognition and better recall of client story and team approach to care.
- Dietitian (RDN): Introduce yourself, welcome and ask how the person prefers to be addressed. Lead client to private, quiet consultation room. Invite the client to sit in designated chair in counseling area. If a family member or friend of the client wants to join the consultation and is 18 years or older, ask client for permission.
- When necessary, ask the client whether a dietetic intern can observe the appointment.

Nutrition Assessment Process

Background and explanation of assessment

- Explain to client, when necessary, the uniqueness of Dietetics and Integrative Medicine by providing the handout "0.8 What is DIM?"
- Ask client to state his or her most important goals to achieve during the session. Be sure to address these goals during the session and in the visit summary
- Briefly explain the nutrition assessment process, when necessary
    - In-office assessments: Bioelectric Impedance Analysis (BIA), weight, waist circumference, nutrition physical exam, others
    - Review of Nutrition Intake Forms, Medical Symptoms Questionnaire (MSQ), Fats & Oils Questionnaires, and any others
    - Ask client to sign MSQ
    - Review Diet Diary. If not completed, take a 24-hour dietary recall
    - Develop intervention of a nutrition action plan and supplement plan

In-office assessments and measurements

In-office assessments (not all of these tests are completed at every visit on every client)

- Nutrition Physical Exam
- Anthropometrics: Height, weight, waist circumference
- Bioelectric Impedance Analysis (BIA): Measurements taken on a massage or acupuncture table or other surface client can easily and comfortably lay supine
- 02 Sat (Respiratory issues)
- Hand Grip Strength Measurement
- Blood Pressure and Pulse
- Frame Size Assessment

Other assessments/measurements not currently used in KU IM

- Other circumferences (Pediatric: Head; Sports: bicep; Muscle injury: atrophy of specific muscle(s); Amputation)
- Zinc Tally
- Iodine Patch Test
- Urinary pH
- Urinary Ascorbic Acid

KU Integrative Medicine – Leigh Wagner MS, RD, LD

Review forms with client

- Nutrition Intake Forms (Initial Comprehensive or Brief Follow-Up Form)
  - Fill in blanks and ask questions in areas needing clarification or expansion
  - Ask additional questions, if necessary
- Diet Diary
- Review important findings in lab work / note labs needing to be monitored / retested and timeline
- Review BIA results and other measurements

Develop and discuss priorities, and create nutrition action plan

- Review most important nutrition/lifestyle changes to accomplish goals within anticipated time and client adherence to plan
- Review supplement recommendations for understanding, tolerance, manageability
- Discuss important lifestyle changes (exercise, sleep, stress management, food preparation, procurement)
- Discuss whether further laboratory testing is recommended
- Set measurable goals for next appointment
- Write and provide a copy to the client of the Nutrition Action Plan for the client to have record and reference to his/her nutritional goals and actions

Review other recommendations

- If recommended, explain any further nutritional laboratory testing recommended by you, the physician, or Advanced Practice Registered Nurse (APRN)
- Schedule follow-up, "Touch Base", phone call within a week for 10-15 minutes to answer questions and monitor progress of Nutrition Action Plan
- Plan time for follow-up visit: 1-6 months, depending on the complexity of the case and nutrition action plan

Documentation and Follow-up

- After appointment, organize the chart, notes and laboratory results.
- Ensure action items are followed-up and completed (email articles, "to-dos", recipes, laboratory requisition, testing kits, etc.)
- Document (write, type, dictate) the nutrition note and finalizing by signing and submitting to the referring doctor for review and/or signature.
- Write the nutrition and supplement plan, if necessary

KU Integrative Medicine – Leigh Wagner MS, RD, LD

- What should be done prior to the next visit, (Labs, diet diary, etc.)
- Document treatment goal(s) and plan for client
- Based on Nutrition Assessment, Develop nutrition diagnostic statements and intervention (plan) by following the Nutrition Care Process (NCP) form for Nutrition Diagnostic Statements, PES:
    - Problem
    - Etiology
    - Signs/Symptoms

Definition of Terms and Acronyms

KU IM: University of Kansas (KU) Integrative Medicine
AND or "The Academy": The Academy of Nutrition and Dietetics (formerly, American Dietetic Association or "ADA")
PSR: Patient Services Representative
MSQ: Medical Symptoms Questionnaire
EMR: Electronic Medical Record
AVS: After Visit Summary
NCP: Nutrition Care Process
PES: Problem Etiology Signs & Symptoms
HPI: History of Present Illness
PMH: Past Medical History

Motivational Interviewing (MI)
DIM Practicum

Motivational Interviewing

Motivational Interviewing (MI) is "a collaborative person-centered form of guiding to elicit and strengthen a person's motivation for change." It is a counseling technique that is a client-centered and goal-oriented. Dietetics and Integrative Medicine (DIM) practitioners and other practitioners use MI mainly in the clinical setting when working with behavior change one-on-one with clients. The following document summarizes some of the key principles of MI based on a 5 Part Series on MI from the Australian Heart Association (February 2012). When observing clinical nutrition consults, look for MI in action. Page 2 has questions to help identify whether the practitioner is using MI.

4 Principles of MI

1. **Expressing empathy**: Reflective Listening
2. **Developing discrepancies**: How do client behaviors fit with who the client wants to be?
3. **Rolling with Resistance**: ↑ resistance, ↓ likely change; validate
4. **Supporting self-efficacy**: Build confidence and hope

Working with clients with chronic diseases means often practitioners are working toward behavior change. In MI, ***ambivalence*** is a foundational challenge. In MI, ambivalence refers to both the desire to change and the desire to maintain the status quo.

MI Spirit

Collaborative: Client and Practitioner working together to set goals & formulate solutions
Evocation: The practitioner inspires or elicits motivation from the client
Respect: The practitioner respects the client's choices, resources, ability to follow-through to change, and decision *not* to change, if that is a result of the session.

As you watch the video and as you shadow other healthcare practitioners, refer to page 2 for reflections while observing the practitioner and patient. Start by asking these questions:

1. Who is making the argument for change? Patient? Practitioner? Parent? Child? Spouse? Other?
2. Is the encounter patient-centered?
3. Is the encounter goal-directed?

O.A.R.S. SKILLS of MI

Open Questions: To elicit evocative spirit and avoid yes/no questions
Affirmations: Affirm the client's strengths and efforts. Sincerity is important.
Reflections: Reflections of what the client wants, needs or feels
Summary: Summarize what the patient believes. Repeat a summary of a compilation of what the patient needs or wants in terms of behavior change or non-change.

Motivational Interviewing (MI)
DIM Practicum

OBSERVING THE PRACTIONER (HEALTHCARE PROVIDER)

Does the practitioner...

- Use Open questions?
- Practice Reflective Listening?
- Show the "Righting Reflex"?
- Fall into the "expert trap"?

OBSERVING THE CLIENT

Does the patient demonstrate ambivalence (the desire to change with the desire to remain the same)?

Do you notice the client using "change talk"?

Change Talk:

1. **Desire for change**: What are the patient's desires, preferences and wishes for change?
2. **Ability to change**: If the patient were to change, what strategies would he or she use to achieve change? How would the patient change?
3. **Reasons for change**: Most predictive of an actual change made by patient/client.
   E.g. Get in shape, reduce risk of disease, for kids, etc.
4. **Need for change:** Visceral/emotional reasons for change. Values-based.

Do you notice the client using:

A) "Commitment language"?
   - Client's statements of commitment to actual change

   OR,

B) "Sustain talk"?
   - Clients' own arguments or reasons against change or desire for status quo, inability for change

KU Integrative Medicine

Nutrition Consultation Guidelines

Background

The main reason for these guidelines is to ensure that the Nutritionist (RDN) can build and maintain rapport with each client. It is also important to understand Integrative Medicine consultations:

- ✓ Patients are often very sick and in many cases making difficult nutrition and lifestyle changes at a time when they do not feel well.
- ✓ Patients often have a good understanding of basic nutrition principles.
- ✓ The RDN's style of nutrition therapy changes with each person and evolves during the consultation based on each person's knowledge, understanding, willingness-to-change, and specific health issues.

Prior to Consultation

1. Before the appointment try to become familiar with the patient's chart (electronic and/or paper). If it is not given to you, please ask the RDN how to and when is best to access the chart.

2. Be prepared for the consultation by understanding how the consult is conducted for new patients and returning patients. (See *KU Integrative Medicine Care Process* document).

During the Consultation

3. Allow the RDN to introduce you to the patient. Keep introduction brief to allow more time for the RDN and the patient.

4. Do not speak unless the RDN asks you to (or patient asks, but do not encourage). Be ready during the consult to assist the RDN when he or she asks. Limit your interaction with the patient so the RDN can efficiently conduct the consult; it is important the RDN can:
   a. Ask questions to build and maintain rapport.
   b. Use feedback to make appropriate nutrition recommendations based on answers, new labs, symptoms and concerns, etc.

5. If necessary, assist the RDN with: finding papers, labs, handouts, and make copies at the front desk.

6. During the consultation, remain silent, or "like a fly on the wall". Stay engaged in the practitioner/client conversation, as the RDN may request that you help research information, assist with making copies or help with other activities.

7. At the end of the consult, remember to thank the patient, assist them in checking out, gathering paperwork, remaining handouts, Bioelectric Impedance Analysis (BIA), etc.

8. Over time, you will be trained in conducting the BIA assessment.

9. The flow of each consultation is different with each patient. So, although it is preferable to do the BIA right away, it is often important to sit down and build trust/rapport with the patient to move smoothly to the next step in the Nutrition Assessment process.

10. It may be beneficial to take notes and follow the RDN's consultation to anticipate questions/responses. This will help you in the future to answer client questions.

The University of Kansas Medical Center | KU Integrative Nutrition | Leigh Wagner, MS, RD, LD | Integrative Nutritionist | http://integrativemed.kumc.edu
3901 Rainbow Blvd, MS 1017 | Kansas City, KS 66160 | (913) 588-6208 | Fax (913) 588-0012 | E-mail: integrativemedicine@kumc.edu

07242012

Name: ______________________ Date: __________

NUTRITION STATUS ASSESSMENT *I-D-U* WORKSHEET

Anthropometrics: Height _______ Weight _______ BMI _______ Body Fat % _______

BP ______/______ Pulse _______ Waist Circ. _______

Assessment	History/Physical	Labs/Procedures	Nutrition Diagnosis	Nutrition Intervention
Ingestion - Variations in food preparation, processing, packaging, organic vs. nonorganic, freshness, fortification, etc.				
Food – Nutrient Intake Relative Potency Toxin Intake Hydration				
Digestion - Adequacy of HCL and digestive enzymes, bioavailability, medications				
Digestion of Nutrients Enzyme deficiency Absorption of Nutrients Endotoxins Microbiome				
Utilization - MAPDOM - Intestinal competence, food allergies, mal-absorption, medications, microbial overgrowth				
Cellular & Molecular metabolism Hydration/fluid status				
MAPDOM Nutrient Requirements - affected by Disease states, stress, environmental factors, age, drugs, genetic differences				
Mineral Status Fiber				
Antioxidants Water Soluble Vitamin C / Phytonutrients				
Protein Status				
D / Vitamin D, A, K				
Oils/Lipid/Fatty Acids Status Vitamin E				
Methylation				
Sum total of previous factors influence assessment - Nutritional Status				

Noland 2012 Practitioner______________________ Date________

How to Prepare to Observe a Nutrition Consult

Look for clues pointing to the person's nutritional status from the "Body, Mind and Belief" perspective. You can summarize these "clues" and "evidence" from the patient's chart, verbal comments and nutrition intake forms on the "Blank Nutrition Assessment & Consultation Summary Form".

First, always remember the 7 principles of nutrition from an integrative perspective:

1. Biochemical Individuality
2. Inflammation
3. Immune Regulation
4. Long-Latency Nutrient Insufficiencies
5. Nutritional Toxicology & Epigenetics
6. Energy Metabolism – Cell to Body Composition
7. Lifestyle

Body Clues

- **Medical Diagnoses:** These provide clues to you, as medical diagnoses are identification of disease through symptoms. Often, these are clusters of symptoms that are standardized ways to help determine how to treat a patient from a medical perspective. These same symptoms can be clues about a person's nutritional status and/or his/her physiological malfunction.
- **Anthropometrics and Body Composition:** Weight, height, waist circumference, percent of ideal body weight, Phase Angle, or other measurements taken.
- **Nutrition Physical Exam:** Please refer to the "Nutrition Physical Exam" document to refer to the standard check list of physical clues to a person's nutrition status. This includes dental history.
- **Laboratory Values:** Conventional and functional labs showing high/low or high-normal and low-normal levels are clues to nutritional imbalances. When recording these, list the reference ranges. Labs from previous doctors in the past 2 or more years help tell the patient's "story". Looking at nutrient levels, refer to text book references like Escott-Stump's *Nutrition and Diagnosis-Related Care*, Stipanuk's *Biochemical, Physiological, and Molecular Aspects of Human Nutrition*, Gaby's *Nutritional Medicine* or Krause's *Food and Nutrition Care Process*. Learn about the signs and symptoms of deficiencies/insufficiencies or toxic levels of certain nutrients.
- **Environmental Exposures:** Asking about how a person grew up will give insight into exposures to toxins that could disrupt one's metabolism. Some of these exposures are called "endocrine-disrupting chemicals" (EDCs). For example, growing up on a farm near crop-spraying, working as a hair dresser with dyes, sprays and other chemicals, growing up in a city near high-traffic areas with smog, etc.
- **Histories:** A person's Family History, Past Medical History, Surgical History, Social History, and anything else that tells the patient's "story" will help piece together where his or her main imbalances lie.

- **Lifestyle:** Physical activity, sleep quality, income, stress (work, family, health, other), employment, family life, community support are all lifestyle factors that contribute to one's health.

Mind Clues

- **Nutrition Knowledge:** Has this person ever received nutrition education in the past? Was it a group session? Was it one-on-one counseling? What might be the biases of previous education and/or biases from the patient/client about you and your goals/motivations working with him or her? Ask the patient or client what of nutrition information he or she has received in the past. Do they research online, read books or magazines, have another practitioner who talks about nutrition, watch television, or have any other source of nutritional information?
- **Nutrition Literacy:** To what degree does this person understand "serving sizes", standard household measuring (cups, teaspoons, Tablespoons, etc.), label reading, what is a carbohydrate, fat, protein, calorie, vitamin or mineral?

Belief or "Spirit" Clues

- **Emotional Health and Wellbeing:** Does
- **Beliefs:** Beliefs about one's culture, what will make a person well or ill, religion, spirituality, agnosticism or atheism will all contribute to a person's motivation and decision-making.
- **Lifestyle:** One's stress is a lifestyle factor that can affect one's beliefs about health and wellness and/or one's motivation to make certain healthy or unhealthy decisions.

Pattern Recognition

Combine the above "clues" or "evidence" and notice patterns that emerge. Use the *Medical Symptom's Questionnaire (MSQ)* to notice these physical patterns, the patient intake form to notice all patterns. You are ready to see a patient and start evaluating the physical clues and evidence

KU Integrative Medicine Intake Form – New Patient

General Information

Date:

Name			
Preferred Name			
Date of Birth	Age:	Gender: ☐ M ☐ F	Height __'__" Weight_____
Genetic Background	☐ African American ☐ Native American ☐ Mediterranean	☐ Hispanic ☐ Caucasian ☐ Northern European	☐ Asian ☐ Other *(please note)*
Family Status	Marital Status: M S	Do you have children: Y N	Children Ages:
ABO Blood Type	*(circle one)* **O A B AB**	Have you ever had a blood transfusion? **Y N**	
Address			
Home Phone			
Cell Phone			
Work Phone		Occupation:	
Fax			
Email			
Best Way to Reach?			
Primary Physician	*Name:*		
	City:	*Phone:*	
Secondary Physician	*Name:*		
	City:	*Phone:*	
Referred by			

The University of Kansas Medical Center | KU Integrative Nutrition | Leigh Wagner, MS, RD, LD | Integrative Nutritionist | http://integrativemed.kumc.edu
3901 Rainbow Blvd, MS 1017 | Kansas City, KS 66160 | (913) 588-6208 | Fax (913) 588-0012 | E-mail: integrativemedicine@kumc.edu
12082012

1

Complaints/Concerns

What do you hope to achieve in your visit?

If you had a magic wand and could erase three problems, what would they be?
(list you three main **health** concerns)

1	
2	
3	

If you had a magic wand and could erase three problems, what would they be?
(list you three main **nutrition** concerns)

1	
2	
3	

When was the last time you felt well?	

Did something trigger your change in health?

The biggest Challenge (s) to reaching my nutrition goals is/are?

In the past, I have tried the following techniques, diets, behaviors, etc. to reach my nutrition goals...

What makes you feel better?	
What makes you feel worse?	
What is the lowest body weight that you have been comfortably able to maintain for at least 2 years in your adult life, since around age 30?	

The University of Kansas Medical Center | KU Integrative Nutrition | Leigh Wagner, MS, RD, LD | Integrative Nutritionist | http://integrativemed.kumc.edu
3901 Rainbow Blvd, MS 1017 | Kansas City, KS 66160 | (913) 588-6208 | Fax (913) 588-0012 | E-mail: integrativemedicine@kumc.edu
12082012

2

Notes:	

Readiness Assessment

Rate on a scale of 5 (very willing) to 1 (not willing)

In order to improve your health, how willing are you to:

Significantly modify your diet	☐ 5 ☐ 4 ☐ 3 ☐ 2 ☐ 1
Take several nutritional supplements each day	☐ 5 ☐ 4 ☐ 3 ☐ 2 ☐ 1
Keep a record of everything you eat each day	☐ 5 ☐ 4 ☐ 3 ☐ 2 ☐ 1
Modify your lifestyle (e.g., work demands, sleep habits, exercise)	☐ 5 ☐ 4 ☐ 3 ☐ 2 ☐ 1
Practice a relaxation technique	☐ 5 ☐ 4 ☐ 3 ☐ 2 ☐ 1
Engage in regular exercise/physical activity	☐ 5 ☐ 4 ☐ 3 ☐ 2 ☐ 1
Have periodic lab tests to assess your progress	☐ 5 ☐ 4 ☐ 3 ☐ 2 ☐ 1

How much on-going support and contact (e.g., telephone, e-mail) from the nutritionist would be helpful to you as you implement your personal health program?

Allergy Information

Please list FOOD allergies	
Please list NON-FOOD allergies	
What type of allergic symptoms do you experience?	
Notes:	

The University of Kansas Medical Center | KU Integrative Nutrition | Leigh Wagner, MS, RD, LD | Integrative Nutritionist | http://integrativemed.kumc.edu
3901 Rainbow Blvd, MS 1017 | Kansas City, KS 66160 | (913) 588-6208 | Fax (913) 588-0012 | E-mail: integrativemedicine@kumc.edu
12082012

3

Medical History

	Height:	Weight:	Waist:

Please check those health conditions that your doctor has diagnosed (provide the date of onset)

GASTROINTESTINAL	INFLAMMATORY/AUTOIMMUNE
☐ Irritable Bowel Syndrome	☐ Chronic Fatigue Syndrome
☐ Inflammatory Bowel Disease	☐ Rheumatoid Arthritis
☐ Crohn's Disease	☐ Lupus SLE
☐ Ulcerative Colitis	☐ Poor Immune Function *(frequent infections)*
☐ Gastric or Peptic Ulcer Disease	☐ Severe Infectious Disease
☐ GERD (reflux/heartburn)	☐ Herpes-Genital
☐ Celiac Disease	☐ Multiple Chemical Sensitivities
☐ Hepatitis C or Liver Disease	☐ Gout
☐ Other Digestive:	☐ Other:
CARDIOVASCULAR	**METABOLIC/ENDOCRINE**
☐ Heart Disease (heart attack)	☐ Diabetes ☐ Type 1 or ☐ Type 2
☐ Stroke	☐ Metabolic Syndrome (insulin resistance)
☐ Elevated Cholesterol	☐ Hypoglycemia
☐ Irregular heart rate – Pacemaker	☐ Hypothyroidism (low thyroid)
☐ High Blood Pressure	☐ Hyperthyroidism (overactive thyroid)
☐ Mitral Valve Prolapse/heart murmur	☐ Polycystic Ovarian Syndrome (PCOS)
☐ Other Heart & Vascular:	☐ Genetic Disorder: ______________
	☐ Other:
RESPIRATORY	**MUSCULOSKELETAL/PAIN**
☐ Asthma ☐ Bronchitis	☐ Osteoarthritis ☐ Fibromyalgia
☐ Chronic Sinusitis ☐ Emphysema	☐ Chronic Pain ☐ Migraines
☐ Pneumonia ☐ Tuberculosis	☐ Other:
☐ Sleep Apnea ☐ Other:	

The University of Kansas Medical Center | KU Integrative Nutrition | Leigh Wagner, MS, RD, LD | Integrative Nutritionist | http://integrativemed.kumc.edu
3901 Rainbow Blvd, MS 1017 | Kansas City, KS 66160 | (913) 588-6208 | Fax (913) 588-0012 | E-mail: integrativemedicine@kumc.edu
12082012

4

Notes:

Medical History (continued)

Please note any past or current injuries:

NEUROLOGICAL/MOOD		CANCER
☐ Depression	☐ Bipolar Disorder	☐ Cancer *(please describe type and treatment)*
☐ Anxiety	☐ ADD/ADHD	
☐ Autism	☐ Multiple Sclerosis	
☐ Seizures	☐ Other:	

OTHER *(use separate sheet if necessary)*

☐ Kidney stones	☐ Anemia	Please any other diseases or health conditions
☐ Eczema	☐ Urinary (UTIs)	
☐ Psoriasis	☐ Frequent Yeast	Have you ever had genetic testing? ☐ Y ☐ N If yes, please note type and results.
☐ Acne	☐ OTHER:	

MEDICATIONS (Please list all prescribed medications you are taking and note reason.)

Name:	*Reason:*
Name:	*Reason:*
Name:	*Reason:*
Name:	*Reason:*
Name:	*Reason:*
Name:	*Reason:*
Name:	*Reason:*
Name:	*Reason:*

Have you had prolonged or regular use of Tylenol? ☐ Y ☐ N

Have you had prolonged or regular use of acid-blocking drugs (Tagamet, Zantac, etc.)? ☐ Y ☐ N

The University of Kansas Medical Center | KU Integrative Nutrition | Leigh Wagner, MS, RD, LD | Integrative Nutritionist | http://integrativemed.kumc.edu
3901 Rainbow Blvd, MS 1017 | Kansas City, KS 66160 | (913) 588-6208 | Fax (913) 588-0012 | E-mail: integrativemedicine@kumc.edu
12082012

5

Frequent antibiotics >3 times per year? ☐ Y ☐ N   Long term antibiotics? ☐ Y ☐ N

Environmental Information

Do you have known adverse food reactions or sensitivities? ☐ Y ☐ N	If yes, please describe symptoms.
Are you exposed regularly to any of the following? *(check all that apply)* ☐ Cigarette smoke ☐ Perfumes ☐ Auto exhaust/fumes ☐ Paint fumes ☐ Dry-cleaned clothes ☐ Mold ☐ Nail polish/hair dyes ☐ Pesticides ☐ Heavy metals ☐ Fertilizers ☐ Teflon Cookware ☐ Pet dander ☐ Aluminum Cookware ☐ Chemicals	What is your occupation? Please note any regular exposure to harmful chemical/substances. Please not any past exposure to harmful chemicals/substances.
Do you use any recreational drugs? If so, please note.	
Notes:	

Lifestyle Information

Do you engage in moderate cardiovascular physical activity at least 3 days a week, for a minimum of 20 minutes duration? (brisk walking, jogging, hiking, cardio exercise classes, cycling, stair-climbing, etc.)

☐ Y ☐ N

ACTIVITY	TYPE/INTENSITY *(low-moderate-high)*	# DAYS/WEEK	DURATION *(minutes)*
Stretching/Yoga			
Cardio/Aerobics			
Strength Training			
Sports or Leisure			

Rate your level of motivation for including exercise in your life? ☐ Low ☐ Med ☐ High

The University of Kansas Medical Center | KU Integrative Nutrition | Leigh Wagner, MS, RD, LD | Integrative Nutritionist | http://integrativemed.kumc.edu
3901 Rainbow Blvd, MS 1017 | Kansas City, KS 66160 | (913) 588-6208 | Fax (913) 588-0012 | E-mail: integrativemedicine@kumc.edu
12082012

6

Note any problems that limit your physical activity.

Lifestyle Information (continued)

Do you smoke? ☐ Y ☐ N	How many years?
Packs per day?	2nd hand smoke exposure? ☐ Y ☐ N
Excess stress in your life? ☐ Y ☐ N	Easily handle stress? ☐ Y ☐ N

Daily Stressors: *Rate on a scale of 1 (low) to 10 (high)*

☐ Work____ ☐ Family____ ☐ Social____ ☐ Finances____ ☐ Health____ ☐ Other:____

Do you feel your life has meaning and purpose? ☐ Y ☐ N ☐ unsure	Do you believe stress is presently reducing the quality of your life? ☐ Y ☐ N
Average number of hours you sleep per night **during the week**?	Average number of hours you sleep per night **on weekends**?
Trouble falling asleep? ☐ Y ☐ N	Rested upon waking? ☐ Y ☐ N

Do you wake up during the night? ☐ Y ☐ N If yes, how many times?

Note the approximate times you generally wake during the night.

How would you rate the overall quality of your sleep? *low quality* 1 2 3 4 5 *high quality*

Surgeries/Hospitalizations

Please list any surgeries or hospitalizations (include dates and your ages if known).

Family History

Please note any family history of the following diseases: *heart disease, cancer, stroke, high blood pressure, overweight, lung disease, kidney disease, diabetes, cancer, mental illness or addiction.*

Family Member:	*Health Condition:*
Family Member:	*Health Condition:*
Family Member:	*Health Condition:*
Family Member:	*Health Condition:*
Family Member:	*Health Condition:*

The University of Kansas Medical Center | KU Integrative Nutrition | Leigh Wagner, MS, RD, LD | Integrative Nutritionist | http://integrativemed.kumc.edu
3901 Rainbow Blvd, MS 1017 | Kansas City, KS 66160 | (913) 588-6208 | Fax (913) 588-0012 | E-mail: integrativemedicine@kumc.edu
12082012

7

Genetic Disorders Known:

Family History (continued)

Please complete the following information concerning your family's health history:

	If Living		If Deceased			If Living		If Deceased	
	Age	Health	Age at death	Cause		Age	Health	Age at death	Cause
Father					Spouse/Partner				
Mother					Children				
Siblings									

Notes:

Dental History

Do you have any silver/mercury amalgam fillings? ☐ Y ☐ N If **Y**, how many?

Do you have any ☐ Gold fillings ☐ Root canals ☐ Implants ☐ Bridges ☐ Crowns

Do you have any ☐ Tooth pain ☐ Bleeding gums ☐ Gingivitis ☐ Chewing problems

Do you visit a dentist regularly (twice per year)? ☐ Y ☐ N

Have you ever had an infection in your jawbone? ☐ Y ☐ N

TMJ: ☐ grinding teeth ☐ jaw clicking ☐ braces? If yes, what age ____ ☐ surgery ☐ jaw pain

Teeth: ☐ extraction? How many? _________ ☐ Which teeth are missing? (# or name)_ _________

The University of Kansas Medical Center | KU Integrative Nutrition | Leigh Wagner, MS, RD, LD | Integrative Nutritionist | http://integrativemed.kumc.edu
3901 Rainbow Blvd, MS 1017 | Kansas City, KS 66160 | (913) 588-6208 | Fax (913) 588-0012 | E-mail: integrativemedicine@kumc.edu
12082012

8

Medical Symptoms Questionnaire (MSQ)

Name: **Date:**

Rate each of the following symptoms based upon your typical health profile for:

☐ *Past 30 days* ☐ *Past 48 hours*

Point Scale

0 – *Never* or *almost never* have the symptom
1 – *Occasionally* have it, effect is *not severe*
2 – *Occasionally* have it, effect is *severe*
3 – *Frequently* have it, effect is *not severe*
4 – *Frequently* have it, effect is *severe*

HEAD

____ Headaches
____ Faintness
____ Dizziness
____ Insomnia

TOTAL ____

EYES

____ Watery or itchy eyes
____ Swollen, reddened/sticky eyelids
____ Bags, dark circles
____ Blurred or tunnel vision *(does not include near or far-sightedness)*

TOTAL ____

EARS

____ Itchy ears
____ Earaches, ear infections
____ Drainage from ear
____ Ringing /hearing loss

TOTAL ____

NOSE

____ Stuffy Nose
____ Sinus problems
____ Hay fever
____ Sneezing attacks
____ Excessive mucous

TOTAL ____

MOUTH/THROAT

____ Chronic coughing
____ Gagging/throat clearing
____ Sore throat, hoarseness
____ Swollen/discolored tongue, gums, lips
____ Canker sores

TOTAL ____

HEART

____ Irregular /skipped beats
____ Rapid/pounding beats
____ Chest pain

TOTAL ____

SKIN

____ Acne
____ Hives, rashes, dry skin
____ Hair loss
____ Flushing, hot flashes
____ Excessive sweating

TOTAL ____

LUNGS

____ Chest congestion
____ Asthma, bronchitis
____ Shortness of breath
____ Difficulty breathing

TOTAL ____

DIGESTIVE TRACT

____ Nausea, vomiting
____ Diarrhea
____ Constipation
____ Bloated feeling
____ Belching, passing gas
____ Heartburn
____ Intestinal/stomach pain

TOTAL ____

JOINTS/MUSCLE

____ Pain or aches in joints
____ Arthritis
____ Stiffness/limited movement
____ Pain or aches in muscles
____ Feeling of weakness or tiredness

TOTAL ____

MSQ TOTAL__________

WEIGHT

____ Binge eating/drinking
____ Craving certain foods
____ Excessive weight
____ Compulsive eating
____ Water retention
____ Underweight

TOTAL ____

ENERGY/ACTIVITY

____ Fatigue/sluggishness
____ Apathy, lethargy
____ Hyperactivity
____ Restless leg
____ Jetlag

TOTAL ____

MIND

____ Poor memory
____ Confusion, poor comprehension
____ Poor concentration
____ Poor physical coordination
____ Difficulty making decisions
____ Stuttering or stammering
____ Slurred speech
____ Learning disabilities

TOTAL ____

EMOTIONS

____ Mood swings
____ Anxiety, fear, nervousness
____ Anger, irritability, aggressiveness
____ Depression

TOTAL ____

OTHER

____ Frequent illness
____ Frequent or urgent urination
____ Genital itch or discharge
____ Bone pain

TOTAL ____

The University of Kansas Medical Center | KU Integrative Nutrition | Leigh Wagner, MS, RD, LD | Integrative Nutritionist | http://integrativemed.kumc.edu
3901 Rainbow Blvd, MS 1017 | Kansas City, KS 66160 | (913) 588-6208 | Fax (913) 588-0012 | E-mail: integrativemedicine@kumc.edu
12082012

10

INGESTION: Nutrition History

Have you ever had a nutrition consultation? ☐ Y ☐ N

Have you made any changes in your eating habits because of your health? ☐ Y ☐ N
Please describe.

Do you currently follow a special diet or nutritional program? ☐ Y ☐ N
Check all that apply.

☐ Low fat	☐ Low Carb	☐ High protein	☐ Low sodium
☐ No Gluten	☐ Vegetarian	☐ Vegan	☐ Diabetic
☐ No Dairy	☐ No Wheat	☐ Weight Loss	☐ Other ________

How often to you weigh yourself?

Have you had any recent history of weight loss or weight gain? If so, please describe.

How many meals per day do you eat? How many snacks?

Do you avoid any particular foods? *If yes, describe.*	
If you could only eat a few foods a week, what would they be?	
How many meals do you eat out per week?	☐ 0-1 ☐ 1-3 ☐ 3-5 ☐ more than 5 per week

Check all the factors that apply to your current lifestyle and eating habits:

☐ Fast eater	☐ Family member have different tastes
☐ Erratic eating patterns	☐ Love to Eat
☐ Eating too much	☐ Eat because I have to
☐ Late night eating	☐ Have a negative relationship to food
☐ Dislike healthy food	☐ Struggle with eating issues
☐ Time constraints	☐ Emotional eater (stress, bored, etc.)
☐ Travel frequently	☐ Confused about food/nutrition
☐ Do not plan meals or menus	☐ Frequently eat fast foods
☐ Rely on convenience items	☐ Poor snack choices

The University of Kansas Medical Center | KU Integrative Nutrition | Leigh Wagner, MS, RD, LD | Integrative Nutritionist | http://integrativemed.kumc.edu
3901 Rainbow Blvd, MS 1017 | Kansas City, KS 66160 | (913) 588-6208 | Fax (913) 588-0012 | E-mail: integrativemedicine@kumc.edu
12082012

Current Eating Habits

Mark the meals you eat regularly: ☐ Breakfast ☐ Lunch ☐ Dinner ☐ Snacks

Where do you obtain your food from: ☐ home prepared from whole foods ____% ☐ organic ___%

☐ home prepared convenience food ____% ☐ eat out ____%

Mark how many times you eat or drink the following items **PER WEEK**:

___ Soda (regular)
___ Soda (diet)
___ Alcohol
___ Hot tea
___ Cold tea
___ Coffee (regular)
___ Coffee (decaf.)
___ Sugar in coffee
___ Coffee drinks
___ Sweetened drinks
___ Sparkling water
___ Purified water
___ Tap water
___ Fruit juice
___ Lemonade
___ Milk (cow)
___ Milk (goat)
___ Soy Milk
___ Rice Milk
___ Nut Milk
___ Herbal teas

___ Fast food
___ Candy
___ Ice cream
___ Pudding
___ Refined sugars
___ Tuna fish
___ Swordfish
___ Sushi/sashimi
___ Salmon/other fish
___ Lunch meats
___ Bacon
___ Hot dogs
___ Whole eggs
___ Red meat
___ Poultry
___ Tofu
___ Tempeh/Miso

Sweeteners:

___ Equal/Nutrasweet (Aspartame)
___ Splenda (sucralose)
___ Saccharin
___ Stevia/Xylitol

___ Dried fruit
___ Canned fruit
___ Fresh Fruit
___ Jelly/jam
___ Sweets (cookies)
___ Green Salads
___ Raw veggies

What kind?

___ Cooked veggies

What kind?

___ Potatoes
___ Yams/Sweet Potatoes
___ Popcorn
___ Cereals
___ Oatmeal
___ Bagels/pretzels
___ White bread
___ Sprouted Br.
___ Wheat Bread

___ Crackers
___ Pasta
___ Brown rice
___ White rice
___ Corn tortillas
___ Flour tortillas
___ Potato Chips
___ Tortilla Chips
___ Pizza
___ Yogurt (plain)
___ Yogurt (sweet)
___ Prepared meals (Lean cuisine, etc.)
___ Microwave meals/soups
___ Restaurant meals (healthy)
___ Restaurant meals (unhealthy)
___ Airplane meals
___ Legumes (beans, lentils)

The University of Kansas Medical Center | KU Integrative Nutrition | Leigh Wagner, MS, RD, LD | Integrative Nutritionist | http://integrativemed.kumc.edu
3901 Rainbow Blvd, MS 1017 | Kansas City, KS 66160 | (913) 588-6208 | Fax (913) 588-0012 | E-mail: integrativemedicine@kumc.edu
12082012

12

Fats and Oils

Please indicate how many times PER WEEK you eat the following fats/oils.

OMEGA 9 *(stabilizer)*	___ Almond Oil	___ Olives
~50% of daily fat calories	___ Almonds/Cashews	___ Olive Oil
	___ Almond butter	___ Sesame Seeds/Tahini
Oleic Fatty Acid	___ Avocados	___ Hummus (tahini oil)
	___ Peanuts	___ Macadamia Nuts
	___ Peanut butter (natural/soft)	___ Pine Nuts
OMEGA 6 *(controllers)*	___ Eggs (whole), organic (AA)	___ Evening Primrose (GLA)
Essential Fatty Acid Family	___ Meats (commercial) (AA)	___ Black Currant Oil (GLA)
~30% of daily fat calories	___ Meats (grass-fed, org) (AA)	___ Borage Oil (GLA)
	___ Brazil nuts (raw)	___ Hemp Oil
LA → GLA → DGLA → AA	___ Pecan (raw)	___ Grapeseed Oil
	___ Hazelnuts/Filberts (raw)	___ Sunflower Seeds (raw)
	___ Hemp Seeds	___ Pumpkin seeds (raw)
OMEGA 3 *(fluidity/communicators)*	___ Fish Oil capsule: ↑DHA	___ Flax Oil
Essential Fatty Acid Family	___ Fish Oil capsule: ↑EPA	___ UDO's DHA Oil
~10% of daily fat calories	___ Fish (salmon/fin-fish)	___ Algae
	___ Fish (shellfish)	___ Greens Powder w/algae
ALA → EPA → DHA	___ Flax seeds/meal	___ Chia seeds
BENEFICIAL SATURATED *(structure)*	___ Coconut Oil	___ Meats, grass-fed
~10% of daily fat calories	___ Butter, organic	___ Wild game
	___ Ghee (clarified butter)	___ Poultry, organic
Short Chain/Medium-chain Triglycerides	___ Dairy, raw & organic	___ Eggs, whole organic
DAMAGED FATS/OILS (promoting stress to cells & tissues)	___ Margarine	___ Doughnuts (fried)
Should be <5% (try to avoid)	___ Reg. vegetable oils (corn, sunflower, canola)	___ Deep-fried foods
Trans Fats	___ Mayonnaise(Commercial)	___ Chips fried in oil
Acrylamides	___ Hydrogenated Oil (as an ingredient)	___ Reg. Salad dressing
Odd-Chain Fatty Acids	___ "Imitation" cheeses	___ Peanut Butter (JIF, etc)
VLCFA/damaged	___ Tempura	___ Roasted nuts/seeds
		___ Non-dairy products

The University of Kansas Medical Center | KU Integrative Nutrition | Leigh Wagner, MS, RD, LD | Integrative Nutritionist | http://integrativemed.kumc.edu
3901 Rainbow Blvd, MS 1017 | Kansas City, KS 66160 | (913) 588-6208 | Fax (913) 588-0012 | E-mail: integrativemedicine@kumc.edu
12082012

13

INGESTION: Nutrition History (continued)

What are the top three dietary changes do you think would make the most difference in your overall health?	**1.** **2.** **3.**
How committed are you to making dietary changes in order to improve your health?	*not committed* **1 2 3 4 5** *very committed*

Please list all **nutritional supplements** you currently take daily. Please include brand names and amounts as well as any herbs/botanical products.

Do you drink alcohol? ☐ Y ☐ N If yes, how many drinks per week?

Do you drink coffee or other caffeinated beverages? ☐ Y ☐ N If yes, # daily?

Do you use artificial sweeteners? ☐ Y ☐ N If yes, which ones?

DIGESTION

Do you feel like belching or are you bloated after eating? ☐ Y ☐ N

Do you have (or had) any eating disorders? ☐ Y ☐ N If yes, please describe.

Bowel Movements: How often? ___________ Color? ___________ Consistency? ___________

Your Birth: ☐ Natural/vaginal ☐ C-Section | Were you breastfed as an infant (if known)? ☐ Y ☐ N

Please note anything additional about your nutrition/eating habits.

The University of Kansas Medical Center | KU Integrative Nutrition | Leigh Wagner, MS, RD, LD | Integrative Nutritionist | http://integrativemed.kumc.edu
3901 Rainbow Blvd, MS 1017 | Kansas City, KS 66160 | (913) 588-6208 | Fax (913) 588-0012 | E-mail: integrativemedicine@kumc.edu
12082012

14

Authorization for the Release of Information

I, the patient, hereby authorize the use or disclosure of my health information from the listed Health practitioner as described below to the requesting practitioner.

Patient Information

Name ______________________________ Date of Birth ____________

Address ______________________________

City ____________________ State ____ Zip Code ____________

Phone ______________ Social Security Number ______________

Health Practitioner 1

Health Practitioner Name ______________________________

Address ______________________________

City ____________________ State ____ Zip Code ____________

Phone ______________ Fax Number ____________

I authorize for **[insert practitioner name here]** to release and/or disclose the medical information as indicated below to the health care provider, entity, or person I have indicated above.

DURATION: This authorization shall become effective immediately and shall remain in effect until ____________(date), or for one year from the date of signature if no date entered.

REVOCATION: This authorization may be revoked in writing by the undersigned at any time prior to the release of information from the disclosing party. Written revocation will not affect any action taken in reliance on this authorization before the written revocation was received.

INITIAL and check the box for which types of information are to be released and/or disclosed:

_____ General Medical Information from ____________ to ____________ (dates)

_____ Laboratory Tests (serum, urine) from ____________ to ____________ (dates)

_____ Information regarding specific diagnosis or treatment from ________ to ________.

_____Other ____ Nutrition and Dental ______________________

Requesting Practitioner Information

[insert practitioner name here]
[insert practitioner address, phone and fax here]

Patient Name (printed): ______________________

______________________________ Date: ______________

Signature of Patient

ALL PATIENT INFORMATION IS HANDLED UNDER THE HIPPA PRIVACY ACT
CONFIDENTIAL / HIPPA Approved Form

The University of Kansas Medical Center | KU Integrative Nutrition | Leigh Wagner, MS, RD, LD | Integrative Nutritionist | http://integrativemed.kumc.edu
3901 Rainbow Blvd, MS 1017 | Kansas City, KS 66160 | (913) 588-6208 | Fax (913) 588-0012 | E-mail: integrativemedicine@kumc.edu
12082012

15

Nutrition Intake Form – KU Integrative Medicine Referral

General Information	**Date:**		
Name			
Preferred Name			
Date of Birth	Age:	Gender: ☐ M ☐ F	Height __'__" Weight_____
Genetic Background	☐ African American ☐ Native American ☐ Mediterranean	☐ Hispanic ☐ Caucasian ☐ Northern European	☐ Asian ☐ Other *(please note)*
Family Status	Marital Status: M S	Do you have children: Y N	Children Ages:
ABO Blood Type	*(circle one)* **O A B AB**	Have you ever had a blood transfusion? **Y N**	
Address			
Home Phone			
Cell Phone			
Work Phone		Occupation:	
Fax			
Email			
Best Way to Reach?			
Primary Physician	*Name:*		
	City:	*Phone:*	
Secondary Physician	*Name:*		
	City:	*Phone:*	
Referred by			

The University of Kansas Medical Center | KU Integrative Nutrition | Leigh Wagner, MS, RD, LD | Integrative Nutritionist | http://integrativemed.kumc.edu
3901 Rainbow Blvd, MS 1017 | Kansas City, KS 66160 | (913) 588-6208 | Fax (913) 588-0012 | E-mail: integrativemedicine@kumc.edu
12082012

1

Complaints/Concerns

What do you hope to achieve in your visit?

If you had a magic wand and could erase three problems, what would they be?
(list you three main **health** concerns)

1	
2	
3	

If you had a magic wand and could erase three problems, what would they be?
(list you three main **nutrition** concerns)

1	
2	
3	

When was the last time you felt well?	

Did something trigger your change in health?

The biggest Challenge (s) to reaching my nutrition goals is/are?

In the past, I have tried the following techniques, diets, behaviors, etc. to reach my nutrition goals…

What makes you feel better?	
What makes you feel worse?	
What is the lowest body weight that you have been comfortably able to maintain for at least 2 years in your adult life, since around age 30?	

The University of Kansas Medical Center | KU Integrative Nutrition | Leigh Wagner, MS, RD, LD | Integrative Nutritionist | http://integrativemed.kumc.edu
3901 Rainbow Blvd, MS 1017 | Kansas City, KS 66160 | (913) 588-6208 | Fax (913) 588-0012 | E-mail: integrativemedicine@kumc.edu
12082012

2

Notes:	

Readiness Assessment

Rate on a scale of 5 (very willing) to 1 (not willing)

In order to improve your health, how willing are you to:

Significantly modify your diet	☐ 5 ☐ 4 ☐ 3 ☐ 2 ☐ 1
Take several nutritional supplements each day	☐ 5 ☐ 4 ☐ 3 ☐ 2 ☐ 1
Keep a record of everything you eat each day	☐ 5 ☐ 4 ☐ 3 ☐ 2 ☐ 1
Modify your lifestyle (e.g., work demands, sleep habits, exercise)	☐ 5 ☐ 4 ☐ 3 ☐ 2 ☐ 1
Practice a relaxation technique	☐ 5 ☐ 4 ☐ 3 ☐ 2 ☐ 1
Engage in regular exercise/physical activity	☐ 5 ☐ 4 ☐ 3 ☐ 2 ☐ 1
Have periodic lab tests to assess your progress	☐ 5 ☐ 4 ☐ 3 ☐ 2 ☐ 1

How much on-going support and contact (e.g., telephone, e-mail) from the nutritionist would be helpful to you as you implement your personal health program?

Allergy Information

Please list FOOD allergies	
Please list NON-FOOD allergies	
What type of allergic symptoms do you experience?	

Notes:	

The University of Kansas Medical Center | KU Integrative Nutrition | Leigh Wagner, MS, RD, LD | Integrative Nutritionist | http://integrativemed.kumc.edu
3901 Rainbow Blvd, MS 1017 | Kansas City, KS 66160 | (913) 588-6208 | Fax (913) 588-0012 | E-mail: integrativemedicine@kumc.edu
12082012

MEDICATIONS (Please list all prescribed medications you are taking and note reason.)	
Name:	*Reason:*
Name:	*Reason:*
Name:	*Reason:*
Name:	*Reason:*
Name:	*Reason:*
Name:	*Reason:*
Name:	*Reason:*
Name:	*Reason:*
Have you had prolonged or regular use of Tylenol? ☐ Y ☐ N	
Have you had prolonged or regular use of acid-blocking drugs (Tagamet, Zantac, etc.)? ☐ Y ☐ N	
Frequent antibiotics >3 times per year? ☐ Y ☐ N	Long term antibiotics? ☐ Y ☐ N

Environmental Information

Do you have known adverse food reactions or sensitivities? ☐ Y ☐ N		If yes, please describe symptoms.
Are you exposed regularly to any of the following? *(check all that apply)*		What is your occupation?
☐ Cigarette smoke ☐ Auto exhaust/fumes ☐ Dry-cleaned clothes ☐ Nail polish/hair dyes ☐ Heavy metals ☐ Teflon Cookware ☐ Aluminum Cookware	☐ Perfumes ☐ Paint fumes ☐ Mold ☐ Pesticides ☐ Fertilizers ☐ Pet dander ☐ Chemicals	Please note any regular exposure to harmful chemical/substances. Please not any past exposure to harmful chemicals/substances.
Do you use any recreational drugs? If so, please note.		

The University of Kansas Medical Center | KU Integrative Nutrition | Leigh Wagner, MS, RD, LD | Integrative Nutritionist | http://integrativemed.kumc.edu
3901 Rainbow Blvd, MS 1017 | Kansas City, KS 66160 | (913) 588-6208 | Fax (913) 588-0012 | E-mail: integrativemedicine@kumc.edu
12082012

4

Notes:

Lifestyle Information

Do you engage in moderate cardiovascular physical activity at least 3 days a week, for a minimum of 20 minutes duration? (brisk walking, jogging, hiking, cardio exercise classes, cycling, stair-climbing, etc.)

☐ Y ☐ N

ACTIVITY	TYPE/INTENSITY *(low-moderate-high)*	# DAYS/WEEK	DURATION *(minutes)*
Stretching/Yoga			
Cardio/Aerobics			
Strength Training			
Sports or Leisure			

Rate your level of motivation for including exercise in your life? ☐ Low ☐ Med ☐ High

Note any problems that limit your physical activity.

Do you smoke? ☐ Y ☐ N	How many years?
Packs per day?	2nd hand smoke exposure? ☐ Y ☐ N
Excess stress in your life? ☐ Y ☐ N	Easily handle stress? ☐ Y ☐ N

Daily Stressors: *Rate on a scale of 1 (low) to 10 (high)*

☐ Work____ ☐ Family____ ☐ Social____ ☐ Finances____ ☐ Health____ ☐ Other:____

Do you feel your life has meaning and purpose? ☐ Y ☐ N ☐ unsure	Do you believe stress is presently reducing the quality of your life? ☐ Y ☐ N
Average number of hours you sleep per night **during the week**?	Average number of hours you sleep per night **on weekends**?
Trouble falling asleep? ☐ Y ☐ N	Rested upon waking? ☐ Y ☐ N

Do you wake up during the night? ☐ Y ☐ N If yes, how many times?

Note the approximate times you generally wake during the night.

The University of Kansas Medical Center | KU Integrative Nutrition | Leigh Wagner, MS, RD, LD | Integrative Nutritionist | http://integrativemed.kumc.edu
3901 Rainbow Blvd, MS 1017 | Kansas City, KS 66160 | (913) 588-6208 | Fax (913) 588-0012 | E-mail: integrativemedicine@kumc.edu
12082012

5

How would you rate the overall quality of your sleep? *low quality* 1 2 3 4 5 *high quality*

Medical/Surgical Update

Please list any changes since your most recent Integrative Medicine appointment, including: changes in medications, symptoms, surgeries, and hospitalizations. (please include the date if known)

Dental History

Do you have any silver/mercury amalgam fillings? ☐ Y ☐ N If **Y**, how many?

Do you have any ☐ Gold fillings ☐ Root canals ☐ Implants ☐ Bridges ☐ Crowns

Do you have any ☐ Tooth pain ☐ Bleeding gums ☐ Gingivitis ☐ Chewing problems

Do you visit a dentist regularly (twice per year)? ☐ Y ☐ N

Have you ever had an infection in your jawbone? ☐ Y ☐ N

TMJ: ☐ grinding teeth ☐ jaw clicking ☐ braces? If yes, what age ____ ☐ surgery ☐ jaw pain

Teeth: ☐ extraction? How many? _________ ☐ Which teeth are missing? (# or name)_____________

The University of Kansas Medical Center | KU Integrative Nutrition | Leigh Wagner, MS, RD, LD | Integrative Nutritionist | http://integrativemed.kumc.edu
3901 Rainbow Blvd, MS 1017 | Kansas City, KS 66160 | (913) 588-6208 | Fax (913) 588-0012 | E-mail: integrativemedicine@kumc.edu
12082012

Medical Symptoms Questionnaire (MSQ)

Name: **Date:**

Rate each of the following symptoms based upon your typical health profile for:

☐ *Past 30 days* ☐ *Past 48 hours*

Point Scale

0 – *Never* or *almost never* have the symptom
1 – *Occasionally* have it, effect is *not severe*
2 – *Occasionally* have it, effect is *severe*
3 – *Frequently* have it, effect is *not severe*
4 – *Frequently* have it, effect is *severe*

HEAD

____ Headaches
____ Faintness
____ Dizziness
____ Insomnia

TOTAL ____

EYES

____ Watery or itchy eyes
____ Swollen, reddened/sticky eyelids
____ Bags, dark circles
____ Blurred or tunnel vision *(does not include near or far-sightedness)*

TOTAL ____

EARS

____ Itchy ears
____ Earaches, ear infections
____ Drainage from ear
____ Ringing /hearing loss

TOTAL ____

NOSE

____ Stuffy Nose
____ Sinus problems
____ Hay fever
____ Sneezing attacks
____ Excessive mucous

TOTAL ____

MOUTH/THROAT

____ Chronic coughing
____ Gagging/throat clearing
____ Sore throat, hoarseness
____ Swollen/discolored tongue, gums, lips
____ Canker sores

TOTAL ____

HEART

____ Irregular /skipped beats
____ Rapid/pounding beats
____ Chest pain

TOTAL ____

SKIN

____ Acne
____ Hives, rashes, dry skin
____ Hair loss
____ Flushing, hot flashes
____ Excessive sweating

TOTAL ____

LUNGS

____ Chest congestion
____ Asthma, bronchitis
____ Shortness of breath
____ Difficulty breathing

TOTAL ____

DIGESTIVE TRACT

____ Nausea, vomiting
____ Diarrhea
____ Constipation
____ Bloated feeling
____ Belching, passing gas
____ Heartburn
____ Intestinal/stomach pain

TOTAL ____

JOINTS/MUSCLE

____ Pain or aches in joints
____ Arthritis
____ Stiffness/limited movement
____ Pain or aches in muscles
____ Feeling of weakness or tiredness

TOTAL ____

MSQ TOTAL __________

WEIGHT

____ Binge eating/drinking
____ Craving certain foods
____ Excessive weight
____ Compulsive eating
____ Water retention
____ Underweight

TOTAL ____

ENERGY/ACTIVITY

____ Fatigue/sluggishness
____ Apathy, lethargy
____ Hyperactivity
____ Restless leg
____ Jetlag

TOTAL ____

MIND

____ Poor memory
____ Confusion, poor comprehension
____ Poor concentration
____ Poor physical coordination
____ Difficulty making decisions
____ Stuttering or stammering
____ Slurred speech
____ Learning disabilities

TOTAL ____

EMOTIONS

____ Mood swings
____ Anxiety, fear, nervousness
____ Anger, irritability, aggressiveness
____ Depression

TOTAL ____

OTHER

____ Frequent illness
____ Frequent or urgent urination
____ Genital itch or discharge
____ Bone pain

TOTAL ____

The University of Kansas Medical Center | KU Integrative Nutrition | Leigh Wagner, MS, RD, LD | Integrative Nutritionist | http://integrativemed.kumc.edu
3901 Rainbow Blvd, MS 1017 | Kansas City, KS 66160 | (913) 588-6208 | Fax (913) 588-0012 | E-mail: integrativemedicine@kumc.edu
12082012

7

INGESTION: Nutrition History

Have you ever had a nutrition consultation? ☐ Y ☐ N

Have you made any changes in your eating habits because of your health? ☐ Y ☐ N

Please describe.

Do you currently follow a special diet or nutritional program? ☐ Y ☐ N

Check all that apply.

☐ Low fat	☐ Low Carb	☐ High protein	☐ Low sodium
☐ No Gluten	☐ Vegetarian	☐ Vegan	☐ Diabetic
☐ No Dairy	☐ No Wheat	☐ Weight Loss	☐ Other ________

How often to you weigh yourself?

Have you had any recent history of weight loss or weight gain? If so, please describe.

How many meals per day do you eat? How many snacks?

Do you avoid any particular foods? *If yes, describe.*	
If you could only eat a few foods a week, what would they be?	
How many meals do you eat out per week?	☐ 0-1 ☐ 1-3 ☐ 3-5 ☐ more than 5 per week

Check all the factors that apply to your current lifestyle and eating habits:

- ☐ Fast eater
- ☐ Erratic eating patterns
- ☐ Eating too much
- ☐ Late night eating
- ☐ Dislike healthy food
- ☐ Time constraints
- ☐ Travel frequently
- ☐ Do not plan meals or menus
- ☐ Rely on convenience items
- ☐ Family member have different tastes
- ☐ Love to Eat
- ☐ Eat because I have to
- ☐ Have a negative relationship to food
- ☐ Struggle with eating issues
- ☐ Emotional eater (stress, bored, etc.)
- ☐ Confused about food/nutrition
- ☐ Frequently eat fast foods
- ☐ Poor snack choices

The University of Kansas Medical Center | KU Integrative Nutrition | Leigh Wagner, MS, RD, LD | Integrative Nutritionist | http://integrativemed.kumc.edu
3901 Rainbow Blvd, MS 1017 | Kansas City, KS 66160 | (913) 588-6208 | Fax (913) 588-0012 | E-mail: integrativemedicine@kumc.edu
12082012

9

Current Eating Habits

Mark the meals you eat regularly: ☐ Breakfast ☐ Lunch ☐ Dinner ☐ Snacks

Where do you obtain your food from: ☐ home prepared from whole foods ____% ☐ organic ___%
☐ home prepared convenience food ____% ☐ eat out ____%

Mark how many times you eat or drink the following items **PER WEEK**:

___ Soda (regular)
___ Soda (diet)
___ Alcohol
___ Hot tea
___ Cold tea
___ Coffee (regular)
___ Coffee (decaf.)
___ Sugar in coffee
___ Coffee drinks
___ Sweetened drinks
___ Sparkling water
___ Purified water
___ Tap water
___ Fruit juice
___ Lemonade
___ Milk (cow)
___ Milk (goat)
___ Soy Milk
___ Rice Milk
___ Nut Milk
___ Herbal teas

___ Fast food
___ Candy
___ Ice cream
___ Pudding
___ Refined sugars
___ Tuna fish
___ Swordfish
___ Sushi/sashimi
___ Salmon/other fish
___ Lunch meats
___ Bacon
___ Hot dogs
___ Whole eggs
___ Red meat
___ Poultry
___ Tofu
___ Tempeh/Miso

Sweeteners:

___ Equal/Nutrasweet (Aspartame)
___ Splenda (sucralose)
___ Saccharin
___ Stevia/Xylitol

___ Dried fruit
___ Canned fruit
___ Fresh Fruit
___ Jelly/jam
___ Sweets (cookies)
___ Green Salads
___ Raw veggies
What kind?

___ Cooked veggies
What kind?

___ Potatoes
___ Yams/Sweet Potatoes
___ Popcorn
___ Cereals
___ Oatmeal
___ Bagels/pretzels
___ White bread
___ Sprouted Br.
___ Wheat Bread

___ Crackers
___ Pasta
___ Brown rice
___ White rice
___ Corn tortillas
___ Flour tortillas
___ Potato Chips
___ Tortilla Chips
___ Pizza
___ Yogurt (plain)
___ Yogurt (sweet)
___ Prepared meals (Lean cuisine, etc.)
___ Microwave meals/soups
___ Restaurant meals (healthy)
___ Restaurant meals (unhealthy)
___ Airplane meals
___ Legumes (beans, lentils)

The University of Kansas Medical Center | KU Integrative Nutrition | Leigh Wagner, MS, RD, LD | Integrative Nutritionist | http://integrativemed.kumc.edu
3901 Rainbow Blvd, MS 1017 | Kansas City, KS 66160 | (913) 588-6208 | Fax (913) 588-0012 | E-mail: integrativemedicine@kumc.edu
12082012

10

Fats and Oils

Please indicate how many times PER WEEK you eat the following fats/oils.

OMEGA 9 *(stabilizer)* ~50% of daily fat calories Oleic Fatty Acid	___ Almond Oil ___ Almonds/Cashews ___ Almond butter ___ Avocados ___ Peanuts ___ Peanut butter (natural/soft)	___ Olives ___ Olive Oil ___ Sesame Seeds/Tahini ___ Hummus (tahini oil) ___ Macadamia Nuts ___ Pine Nuts
OMEGA 6 *(controllers)* *Essential Fatty Acid Family* *~30% of daily fat calories* **LA ➔** GLA **➔** DGLA **➔** AA	___ Eggs (whole), organic (AA) ___ Meats (commercial) (AA) ___ Meats (grass-fed, org) (AA) ___ Brazil nuts (raw) ___ Pecan (raw) ___ Hazelnuts/Filberts (raw) ___ Hemp Seeds	___ Evening Primrose (GLA) ___ Black Currant Oil (GLA) ___ Borage Oil (GLA) ___ Hemp Oil ___ Grapeseed Oil ___ Sunflower Seeds (raw) ___ Pumpkin seeds (raw)
OMEGA 3 *(fluidity/communicators)* *Essential Fatty Acid Family* *~10% of daily fat calories* ALA **➔** EPA **➔** DHA	___ Fish Oil capsule: ↑DHA ___ Fish Oil capsule: ↑EPA ___ Fish (salmon/fin-fish) ___ Fish (shellfish) ___ Flax seeds/meal	___ Flax Oil ___ UDO's DHA Oil ___ Algae ___ Greens Powder w/algae ___ Chia seeds
BENEFICIAL SATURATED *(structure)* *~10% of daily fat calories* Short Chain/Medium-chain Triglycerides	___ Coconut Oil ___ Butter, organic ___ Ghee (clarified butter) ___ Dairy, raw & organic	___ Meats, grass-fed ___ Wild game ___ Poultry, organic ___ Eggs, whole organic
DAMAGED FATS/OILS (promoting stress to cells & tissues) *Should be <5% (try to avoid)* Trans Fats Acrylamides Odd-Chain Fatty Acids VLCFA/damaged	___ Margarine ___ Reg. vegetable oils (corn, sunflower, canola) ___ Mayonnaise(Commercial) ___ Hydrogenated Oil (as an ingredient) ___ "Imitation" cheeses ___ Tempura	___ Doughnuts (fried) ___ Deep-fried foods ___ Chips fried in oil ___ Reg. Salad dressing ___ Peanut Butter (JIF, etc) ___ Roasted nuts/seeds ___ Non-dairy products

The University of Kansas Medical Center | KU Integrative Nutrition | Leigh Wagner, MS, RD, LD | Integrative Nutritionist | http://integrativemed.kumc.edu
3901 Rainbow Blvd, MS 1017 | Kansas City, KS 66160 | (913) 588-6208 | Fax (913) 588-0012 | E-mail: integrativemedicine@kumc.edu
12082012

INGESTION: Nutrition History (continued)

What are the top three dietary changes do you think would make the most difference in your overall health?	**1.** **2.** **3.**
How committed are you to making dietary changes in order to improve your health?	*not committed* **1 2 3 4 5** *very committed*

Please list all **nutritional supplements** you currently take daily. Please include brand names and amounts as well as any herbs/botanical products.

Do you drink alcohol? ☐ Y ☐ N If yes, how many drinks per week?

Do you drink coffee or other caffeinated beverages? ☐ Y ☐ N If yes, # daily?

Do you use artificial sweeteners? ☐ Y ☐ N If yes, which ones?

DIGESTION

Do you feel like belching or are you bloated after eating? ☐ Y ☐ N

Do you have (or had) any eating disorders? ☐ Y ☐ N If yes, please describe.

Bowel Movements: How often? ____________ Color? ____________ Consistency? ____________

Your Birth: ☐ Natural/vaginal ☐ C-Section	Were you breastfed as an infant (if known)? ☐ Y ☐ N

Please note anything additional about your nutrition/eating habits.

The University of Kansas Medical Center | KU Integrative Nutrition | Leigh Wagner, MS, RD, LD | Integrative Nutritionist | http://integrativemed.kumc.edu
3901 Rainbow Blvd, MS 1017 | Kansas City, KS 66160 | (913) 588-6208 | Fax (913) 588-0012 | E-mail: integrativemedicine@kumc.edu
12082012

12

Authorization for the Release of Information

I, the patient, hereby authorize the use or disclosure of my health information from the listed Health practitioner as described below to the requesting practitioner.

Patient Information

Name ______________________ Date of Birth ________

Address ______________________

City ______________ State ___ Zip Code ________

Phone __________ Social Security Number ______________

Health Practitioner 1

Health Practitioner Name ______________________

Address ______________________

City ______________ State ___ Zip Code ________

Phone __________ Fax Number __________

I authorize for **[insert practitioner name here]** to release and/or disclose the medical information as indicated below to the health care provider, entity, or person I have indicated above.

DURATION: This authorization shall become effective immediately and shall remain in effect until __________(date), or for one year from the date of signature if no date entered.

REVOCATION: This authorization may be revoked in writing by the undersigned at any time prior to the release of information from the disclosing party. Written revocation will not affect any action taken in reliance on this authorization before the written revocation was received.

INITIAL and check the box for which types of information are to be released and/or disclosed:

_____ General Medical Information from __________ to __________ (dates)

_____ Laboratory Tests (serum, urine) from __________ to __________ (dates)

_____ Information regarding specific diagnosis or treatment from _______ to _______.

_____Other ___ Nutrition and Dental ______________________

Requesting Practitioner Information

[insert practitioner name here]
[insert practitioner address, phone and fax here]

Patient Name (printed): ______________________

______________________ Date: ______________

Signature of Patient

ALL PATIENT INFORMATION IS HANDLED UNDER THE HIPPA PRIVACY ACT
CONFIDENTIAL / HIPPA Approved Form

The University of Kansas Medical Center | KU Integrative Nutrition | Leigh Wagner, MS, RD, LD | Integrative Nutritionist | http://integrativemed.kumc.edu
3901 Rainbow Blvd, MS 1017 | Kansas City, KS 66160 | (913) 588-6208 | Fax (913) 588-0012 | E-mail: integrativemedicine@kumc.edu
12082012

13

FUNCTIONAL MEDICINE MATRIX

Retelling the Patient's Story

Antecedents

Triggering Events

Mediators/Perpetuators

Physiology and Function: Organizing the Patient's Clinical Imbalances

Assimilation

Defense & Repair

Structural Integrity

Mental

Emotional

Spiritual

Energy

Communication

Biotransformation & Elimination

Transport

Modifiable Personal Lifestyle Factors

Sleep & Relaxation	Exercise & Movement	Nutrition	Stress	Relationships

Name:______________________ Date:__________ CC:__________

IFM®

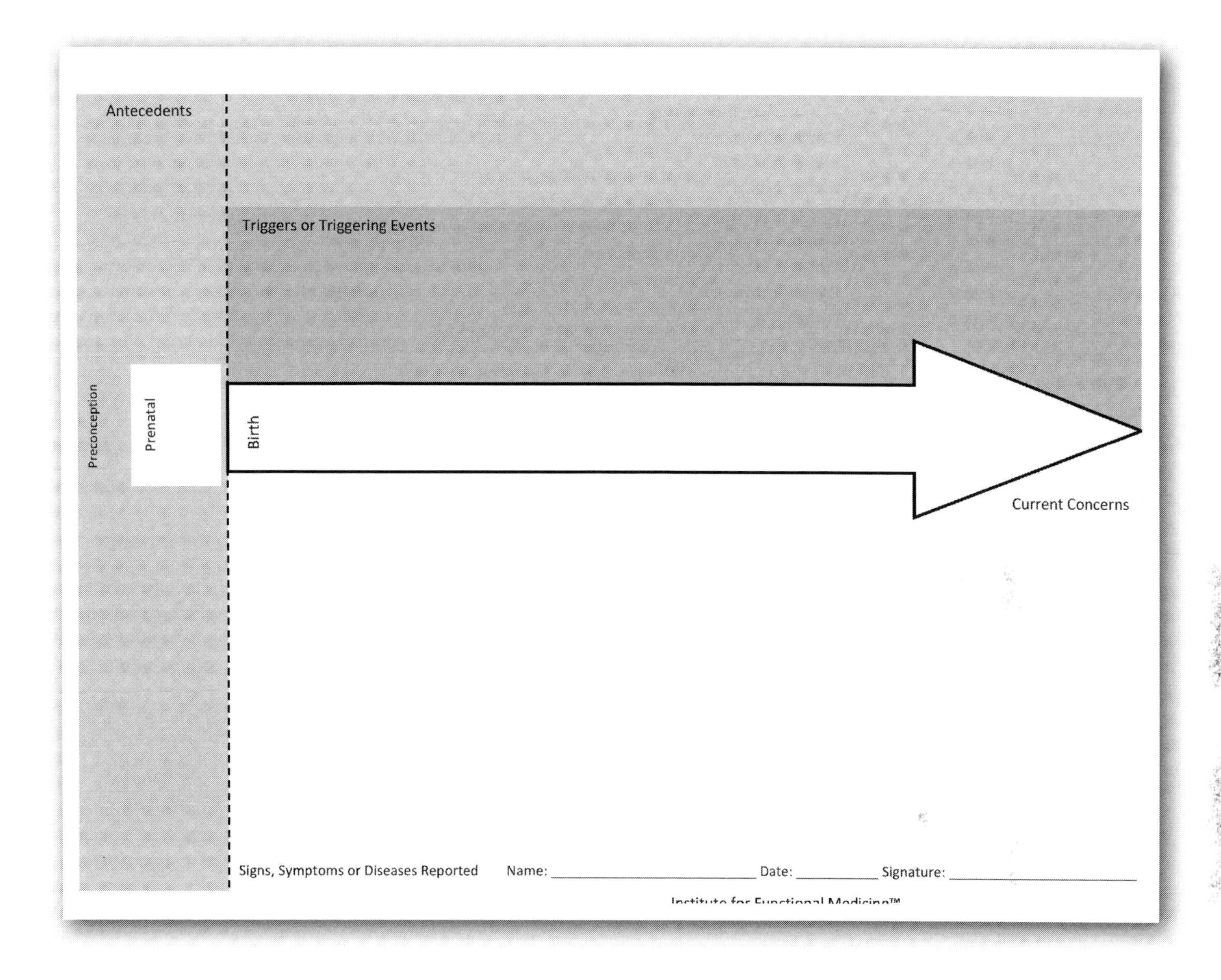
Antecedents
Triggers or Triggering Events
Preconception
Prenatal
Birth
Current Concerns
Signs, Symptoms or Diseases Reported
Name: ______________ Date: __________ Signature: ______________

GI TRACT SCREENING/ASSESSMENT

Subjective

- **Medical Symptoms Questionnaire**
  - GI symptoms: Constipation, diarrhea, stomach pain, etc.
  - Other themes in systems: headaches, sinuses/nasal, frequent illness, emotions...
- **Diet History**
  - Themes of diet (repetitive intake of foods + symptoms)
  - Foods → symptoms
  - Genomic risk
- **Patient report of food sensitivities**
- **Nutrition-focused physical**
  - Nails, hair, skin (rashes)
  - Abdominal exam: RUQ, LUQ, RLQ, LLQ
  - Oral cavity exam
- **Water balance (BIA, edema)**

Objective

- **Conventional labs**
  - Small bowel biopsy
  - IgE testing: Anaphylaxis
  - IgG: Primarily systemic symptoms
  - IgA: Primarily GI symptoms
  - Micronutrients: Suspected malabsorption, general screening (Fe, B12, Vit. D)
  - Hydrogen breath
  - Mannitol/lactulose
- **Genetic Testing**
- **Functional Labs**
  - CDSA
  - Neurotransmitters: Emotional indication, insomnia
  - Organic Acids
  - Stomach Acid Test

GI Tract

- **Mouth**
  - Saliva
  - Enzymes (amylase, lipase)
  - Mastication quality/time
  - Dental Health
- **Esophagus**
  - Eosinophilic esophagitis
  - Swallow difficulties
  - GERD or sensation of discomfort
- **Stomach**
  - pH (too high/low)
- **Biliary - Bile Acids**
- **Pancreas** - Elastase, amylase, etc.
- **Small Intestine**
  - Flora (Beneficial, imbalanced, dysbiotic)
  - Surgeries/disease (IBD/IBS)
- **Large Intestine**
  - Short chain fatty acids
  - Surgeries/disease (IBD/IBS)
  - β-glucaronidase
  - Inflammation (lactoferrin, calprotectin)

Leigh Wagner, KU Integrative Medicine – April, 2012

Dental Assessment

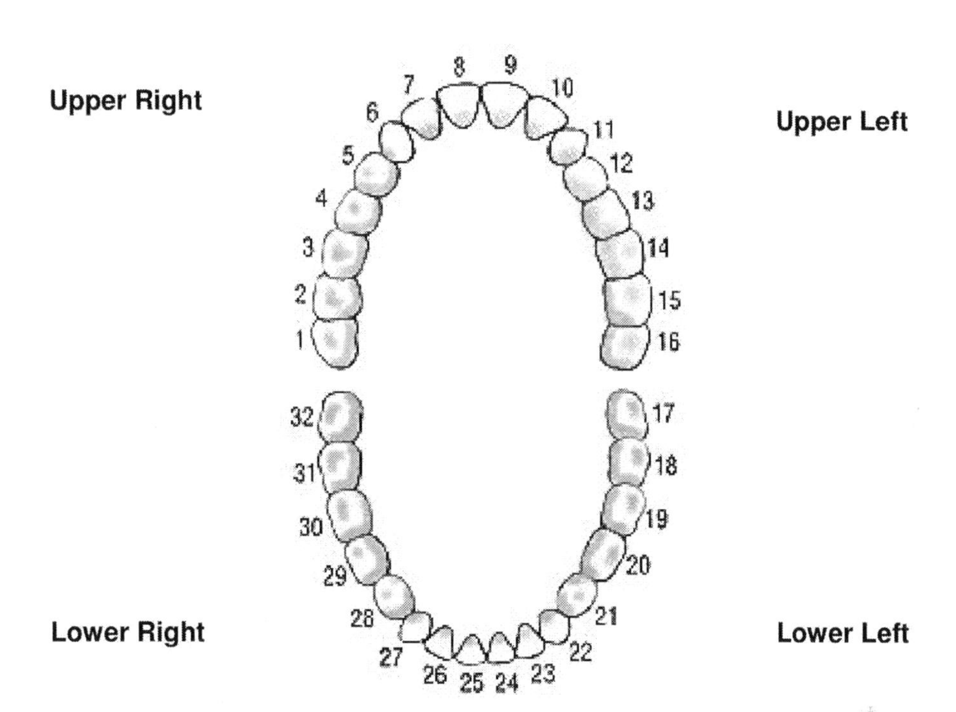

KEY:

Silver Amalgam Fillings - Yellow Highlight (Note S for small, M for medium and L for large sized fillings)
Root Canals – Circle in **RED** pen
Crowns – Make a **BLUE** square around the tooth
Bridges – Circle the affected teeth and connect with **GREEN** pen
Missing Teeth – Black out with a **BLACK** marker

Recommended Websites:

Tooth-Organ Relationships - http://www.secretofthieves.com/tooth-chart/tooth-meridian-14.cfm
Dams, Inc. - www.dams.cc
The International Academy of Oral Medicine and Toxicology - www.iaomt.org
Information on fluoride - www.fluoridealert.org
Information on mercury-free dentistry and fluoride - www.bioprobe.com

Medical Symptoms Questionnaire (MSQ)

Name: **Date:**

Rate each of the following symptoms based upon your typical health profile for:

☐ *Past 30 days* ☐ *Past 48 hours*

Point Scale

0 – *Never* or *almost never* have the symptom
1 – *Occasionally* have it, effect is *not severe*
2 – *Occasionally* have it, effect is *severe*
3 – *Frequently* have it, effect is *not severe*
4 – *Frequently* have it, effect is *severe*

HEAD

____ Headaches
____ Faintness
____ Dizziness
____ Insomnia TOTAL ____

EYES

____ Watery or itchy eyes
____ Swollen, reddened/sticky eyelids
____ Bags, dark circles
____ Blurred or tunnel vision *(does not include near or far-sightedness)*

TOTAL ____

EARS

____ Itchy ears
____ Earaches, ear infections
____ Drainage from ear
____ Ringing /hearing loss

TOTAL ____

NOSE

____ Stuffy Nose
____ Sinus problems
____ Hay fever
____ Sneezing attacks
____ Excessive mucous

TOTAL ____

MOUTH/THROAT

____ Chronic coughing
____ Gagging/throat clearing
____ Sore throat, hoarseness
____ Swollen/discolored tongue, gums, lips
____ Canker sores

TOTAL ____

HEART

____ Irregular /skipped beats
____ Rapid/pounding beats
____ Chest pain

TOTAL ____

SKIN

____ Acne
____ Hives, rashes, dry skin
____ Hair loss
____ Flushing, hot flashes
____ Excessive sweating

TOTAL ____

LUNGS

____ Chest congestion
____ Asthma, bronchitis
____ Shortness of breath
____ Difficulty breathing

TOTAL ____

DIGESTIVE TRACT

____ Nausea, vomiting
____ Diarrhea
____ Constipation
____ Bloated feeling
____ Belching, passing gas
____ Heartburn
____ Intestinal/stomach pain

TOTAL ____

JOINTS/MUSCLE

____ Pain or aches in joints
____ Arthritis
____ Stiffness/limited movement
____ Pain or aches in muscles
____ Feeling of weakness or tiredness

TOTAL ____

WEIGHT

____ Binge eating/drinking
____ Craving certain foods
____ Excessive weight
____ Compulsive eating
____ Water retention
____ Underweight

TOTAL ____

ENERGY/ACTIVITY

____ Fatigue/sluggishness
____ Apathy, lethargy
____ Hyperactivity
____ Restless leg
____ Jetlag

TOTAL ____

MIND

____ Poor memory
____ Confusion, poor comprehension
____ Poor concentration
____ Poor physical coordination
____ Difficulty making decisions
____ Stuttering or stammering
____ Slurred speech
____ Learning disabilities

TOTAL ____

`EMOTIONS

____ Mood swings
____ Anxiety, fear, nervousness
____ Anger, irritability, aggressiveness
____ Depression

TOTAL ____

OTHER

____ Frequent illness
____ Frequent or urgent urination
____ Genital itch or discharge
____ Bone pain

TOTAL ____

GRAND TOTAL___

Fats and Oils

Please indicate how many times PER WEEK you eat the following fats/oils.

OMEGA 9 *(stabilizer)* ~50% of daily fat calories Oleic Fatty Acid	___ Almond Oil ___ Almonds/Cashews ___ Almond butter ___ Avocados ___ Peanuts ___ Peanut butter (natural/soft)	___ Olives ___ Olive Oil ___ Sesame Seeds/Tahini ___ Hummus (tahini oil) ___ Macadamia Nuts ___ Pine Nuts
OMEGA 6 *(controllers)* *Essential Fatty Acid Family* *~30% of daily fat calories* LA → GLA → DGLA → AA	___ Eggs (whole), organic (AA) ___ Meats (commercial) (AA) ___ Meats (grass-fed, org) (AA) ___ Brazil nuts (raw) ___ Pecan (raw) ___ Hazelnuts/Filberts (raw) ___ Hemp Seeds	___ Evening Primrose (GLA) ___ Black Currant Oil (GLA) ___ Borage Oil (GLA) ___ Hemp Oil ___ Grapeseed Oil ___ Sunflower Seeds (raw) ___ Pumpkin seeds (raw)
OMEGA 3 *(fluidity/communicators)* *Essential Fatty Acid Family* *~10% of daily fat calories* ALA → EPA → DHA	___ Fish Oil capsule: ↑DHA ___ Fish Oil capsule: ↑EPA ___ Fish (salmon/fin-fish) ___ Fish (shellfish) ___ Flax seeds/meal	___ Flax Oil ___ UDO's DHA Oil ___ Algae ___ Greens Powder w/algae ___ Chia seeds
BENEFICIAL SATURATED *(structure)* *~10% of daily fat calories* Short Chain/Medium-chain Triglycerides	___ Coconut Oil ___ Butter, organic ___ Ghee (clarified butter) ___ Dairy, raw & organic	___ Meats, grass-fed ___ Wild game ___ Poultry, organic ___ Eggs, whole organic
DAMAGED FATS/OILS (promoting stress to cells & tissues) *Should be <5% (try to avoid)* Trans Fats Acrylamides Odd-Chain Fatty Acids VLCFA/damaged	___ Margarine ___ Reg. vegetable oils (corn, sunflower, canola) ___ Mayonnaise(Commercial) ___ Hydrogenated Oil (as an ingredient) ___ "Imitation" cheeses ___ Tempura	___ Doughnuts (fried) ___ Deep-fried foods ___ Chips fried in oil ___ Reg. Salad dressing ___ Peanut Butter (JIF, etc) ___ Roasted nuts/seeds ___ Non-dairy products

The University of Kansas Medical Center | KU Integrative Nutrition http://integrativemed.kumc.edu
3901 Rainbow Blvd, MS 1017 | Kansas City, KS 66160 | (913) 588-6208 | Fax (913) 588-0012 | E-mail: integrativemedicine@kumc.edu

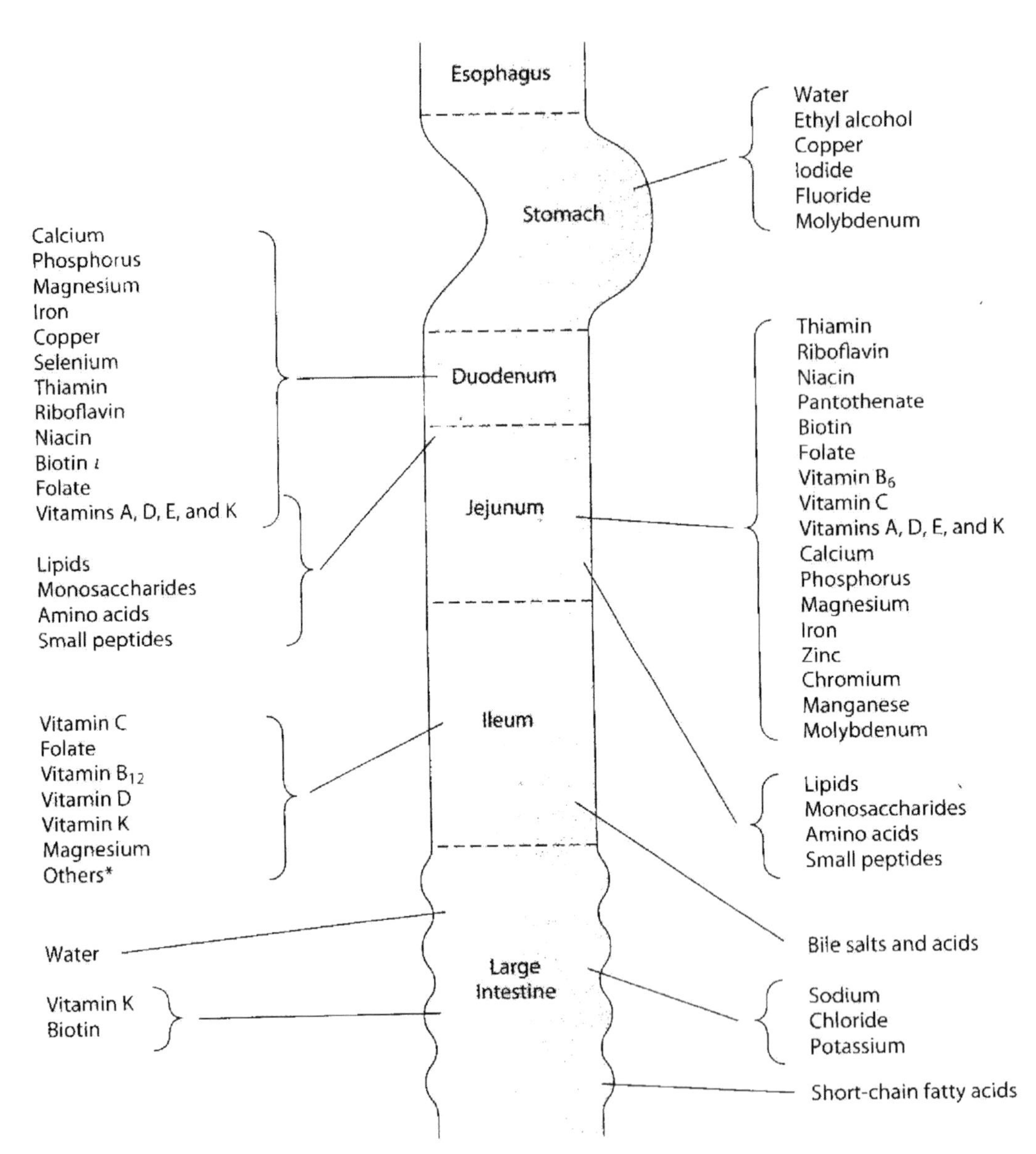

Figure 2.17 Sites of nutrient absorption in the gastrointestinal tract.

Anonymous source

Foods Withdrawn

Nutrition Assessment Summary Form

Reason for Nutrition Appointment or follow-up, "Chief Complaint" or relevant Medical Diagnoses

____

Age	Wt	Ht	Waist Circ:	Phase <	% IBW
Nutrition Physical Exam, Dental History (I, D, U)					

Subjective (Including Past Medical History (PMH) and History of Present Illness (HPI)):

Goal(s) of Appointment:

MSQ Summary (may use top ~3 categories)	Medications/Supplements
Digestion (BM frequency/form, symptoms) (D)	Labs: Abnormal or Meaningful "Normal" Values
Diet (I, D, U)	Lifestyle: Stress, Environmental Exposure, Physical Activity (I, D, U)
Assessment of Nutrition Status // Progress and Monitoring/Evaluation of previous plan	
Plan // Goals	

I: Ingestion D: Digestion U: Utilization

Patient Name ______________________ DOB___/___/____ DOS ___/___/___ Time ____:_____am/pm

End ____:_____am/pm

Dietetics and Integrative Medicine Nutrition Assessment Questionnaire

Intake - Dietary / Assess Toxin Load

Type of Cookware used □ Teflon □ Aluminum □ Glass / Ceramic □ Cast iron

Canned foods BPA lined? Y / N % canned ______ % fresh ______

Organic foods % organic ______ % not organic ______

Whole Foods / Processed – Packaged Food
% whole foods ________________
% processed foods ________________
Eating out / week ________________
Beverages □ water □ other ___________

Supplements
Y / N if yes, which ones?
______________________ ______________________
______________________ ______________________
______________________ ______________________

Medications (Rx and Over the counter)
______________________ ______________________

Digestion / Elimination

GI Health □ Indigestion □ GI Pain / cramping □ Bowel movements ____ / day

Do you use? □ Acid-reducers (e.g. Prilosec) □ Probiotics □ Cultured / fermented foods □ Other medications

Utilization of Nutrients

Symptoms □ Fatigue □ Pain □ Swelling

Nutrition Physical Exam

Hair

	Nutrient Influences
□ Skin – rash / eczema / redness	________________
□ Back of arms – dry / red bumps	________________
□ Mouth – pink / white / gums / cold sores	________________
□ Lips – dry / chapped / corner redness	________________
□ Hair – dry / breaks easy / lack-luster	________________
□ Eyes – poor vitality / crusty – mucus discharge	________________
□ Face – swelling / under eyes / cheeks	________________
□ Thighs & Buttocks – pimple like lesions	________________
□ Breast – sore & lumpy breast tissue	________________

Phenotype

Healthy Weight	*Overweight*	*Health risks*
□ Apple W/H < 0.7	□ Central Adiposity................... Hi waist circumference	overweight/visceral fat/MetSyn increased inflammation
□ Pear / spoon / bell W/H < 0.5	□ Hi hip/thigh circumference........ Smaller waist	risk hi estrogen
□ Banana	□ straight, rectangular, boxlike......	balance / Apple-Pear combo
□ Yam	□ large all over, strong................	excel at strong exercise, overweight

Waist Circumference ________in. [Reference - Adult: Male < 40 in. & Female < 38 in.]

Weight/Height ratio = weight ____ lbs ÷ height ____ in. = W/H ratio ____ [Reference - Adult: Male < 1.0 & Female < .8]

Lifestyle

Sleep
Average hours/night? _____
Wake feeling rested? Y / N
Wake feeling tired? Y / N

Activity Level
□ Sedentary
□ Mild physical activity
□ Moderate physical activity
□ Athletic

Emotional
Do you feel your life has purpose? Y / N
On a scale of 1 – 10 (1 being lowest 10 being highest)
-Happiness in your overall life? 1 2 3 4 5 6 7 8 9 10
-How happy are you currently? 1 2 3 4 5 6 7 8 9 10

KUMC DIM Dietetic Internship Workshop | Nutrition Assessment Questionnaire |

KUMC Clinical Nutrition Seminar

Integrative Approach to Nutrition-focused Physical Exam and Labs

"The art of the practice of medicine is to be learned only by experience, tis not an inheritance; it cannot be revealed. Learn to see, learn to hear, learn to feel, learn to smell and know that by practice alone can you become expert." William Osler, MD (1919)

NUTRITION-FOCUSED EXAM CHECKLIST/REFERENCE:

BODY AREA	LOCATION	MOST COMMON ABNORMAL EXAM FINDINGS	OTHER ABNORMAL FINDINGS	COMMON ABNOMAL LABS ASSOCIATED	OTHER ABNORMAL LABS TO CONSIDER
GENERAL	FACIAL EXPRESSION	↓ Affect	Depression	TSH T3-free TPO & TG Antibodies	
APPEARANCE	GAIT	Speed and Continuity	Stroke, Polio, Weakness, Arthritis	Mitochondrial functional test: Organic Acids RBC Fatty Acid Lipids	Toxicity testing
	CLOTHING	Unkempt; Unclean	Dementia, Poor living conditions	RBC Fatty Acids	
	STATURE	Dwarfism	Genetics	Genetic testing	
	POSTURE/MUSCLE TONE	Dowager's Hump	Bone status	DEXA Ca Metabolism: -Vit D25OH -Ca (serum & ionized), --RBC Mg -Osteocalcin -Vitamin A-retinol	Connective Tissue Testing
	ODOR/BREATH & BODY	Sweet/ketone/putrid	High blood sugar, GI tract overgrowth	Comprehensive Digestive Stool Analysis; FBS, Fasting Insulin ; HgbA1C	Nutritional testing, Intestinal Permeability Breath test
	BODY SHAPE/SIZE	Obese Emaciated ↑ Waist:Hip Ratio BMI	Intakes>Needs Needs>Intakes Overweight, Genetics Over/underweight	BIA: PA, Body Fat% Hydration; Lipids; Tot Protein/Alb/Glob; Vit D25OH	Toxicity (Dioxin, Heavy metals);
	CENTRAL ABDOMEN	↑ Waist:Hip Ratio Apple (Android)	Genetics/Obesity/ Overweight/Insulin resistance; ↑Inflammation	BIA: PA, Body Fat%, Hydration ; Lipids,; Tot Protein/Alb/Glob Vit D25OH; CRP-us	Liver enzymes

In Memoriam, Mary Ann Kight, PhD RD (1943-2011) Professor of Nutrition, University of Arizona, Pioneered the Nutrition Physical Examination and Diagnosis.

	LARGE HIPS/SMALL WAIST	Pear (Gynoid)	Genetics	Gonadal Hormone Panel	
HEAD	EYE	Corneal Arcus Xanthoma Inverted Lid Pallor Lid edema	Dyslipidema mid aged men Type IV LDL-C Hi Iron Deficiency Allergies	Lipids, RBC Fatty Acid ; Hgb/Hct/MCV/MCH ; Ferritin ; Sed Rate	RBC Fatty Acid; Carotenoid testing
	FACE/SKIN	↓Affect Acne/cysts Pallor Edematous Keratosis Moles Rash Rosacea Wrinkles	Depression ↓ Vitamin D Iron deficiency CHF ↓ Fatty Acid/ Vit A Cancer Allergies Inflammation Antioxidants	Zinc, serum; Alk Phos; Electrolytes; Vit D25OH; Ferritin; Allergy Test; Organic Acids; RBC Fatty Acids	Hormonal testing; Differential; Toxicity (dioxin);
	MOUTH/LIPS	Angular stomatitis Chelosis Undifferentiated mucocutaneous border (no lip prints) Pallor	B Vitamin defic B Vitamin defic B Vitamin defic Iron deficiency	CBC; Vit D25OH;F erritin; Lipids;	Nutritional testing: B2, MMA, FIGLU (urine)/Folate (serum);
	MOUTH/ORAL CAVITY/ TONGUE/TEETH	Inflammation Ulcerations Tora Abnormal tongue: Color Surface Papillae presence Odor Hygiene Poor teeth condition Hydration Ability to taste	Vitamin C and Antioxidants Genetics Iron, Folate, B12 Various nutrients Burns, taste, Hygiene, infection Habits Little dental care Poor fluid intake Zn nutriture	Organic Acids; Vit D25OH; Osteocalcin (K2) CoQ10 ; CBC; Zinc, serum; Alk Phos;	Nutritional testing: B2, MMA, FIGLU (urine)/Folate (serum); Biological Dentist Consult;
	HAIR/TOP OF /SCALP	Dry Dandruff Easily pluckable hair Sores Psoriasis	Omega 3:6 ratio, Vitamin A Protein, Perm Vitamin C, Zn, Cu Omega 3:6 ratio; Sulfur	Lipids; RBC fatty acids ; zinc, copper (serum); Vitamin A (retinol) Sed Rate; ANA Antibody Titer	RF Organic Acids;

The University of Kansas Medical Center Clinical Nutrition Seminar 2011, Department of Dietetics & Nutrition and Department of Integrative Medicine, Kansas City, KS. 2

	HEAD/FACE/NOSE	Hirsuitism/facial hair Beard Impaired smell	POCS, Hormones Allergies, sinus infection, cold, Zn	Gonadal hormone panel; TSH, T3-free, TPO & TG AB FBS, F-Insulin, HgbA1C; Zn	
	EARS	Rash Drainage Earlobe crease	Allergies Infection ↑ Cardiac risk	Sed Rate IgA; IgG & IgE Total Differential CRP-us Lipids	Toxicity testing; Cranial Sacral Exam; Biological Dental exam/TMJ;
NECK	THYROID	Enlarged/Goiter Nodules Palpated	Iodine or Endocrine system abnormalities	TSH, T3-free, TPO & TG AB Iodine Urine	Toxicity testing; Adrenal-HPA testing;
	GLANDS/NODES	Parotid Neck Nodes-bilateral	Inadequate intakes, inflammation	Biological Dental Exam; Zn CRP-us Sed Rate;	
	BACK	Dowager's Hump Loss of subcutaneous fat and/or muscle	Calcium, Vit D, Mg, Vit K2 Inadequate calorie &/or protein intake; inactivity; inflammation	BIA: Body Fat%, PA, Impedance, Hydration: Vit D25OH RBC Mg; Ca (serum & ionized) Osteocalcin (K2) Tot Prot/Alb/Glob Differential CRP-us Lipids	DEXA
SKIN	EXTREMITIES	Color Xanthoma Edema	Fe, B12, Folate, B6 Dyslipidemia, Cell membrane health, Omega 3, Extracellular Na++, Fluid overload	CBC;CMP; Lipids; BIA: Body Fat%, PA, Impedance, Hydration; RBC Fatty Acids;	Musculo-skeletal exam;
	HANDS/FEET	Open Areas/Pressure Sores	Inadequate calorie &/or protein, Hyperglycemia; Vit C, Zn insufficient	Tot Prot/Alb/Glob; Organic Acids (r/o Vit C def, etc); Zinc, serum; Differential;	Podiatry Consult; Toxicity; Candida Antibody; Diabetes Screening;
	HYDRATION	Edema Dehydration Oozing	Fluid or Na++, CHF Inadequate fluids/Na+2; Infection, Fluid overload	BIA: Body Fat%, PA, Impedance, Hydration; Electrolytes Urinalysis ; CBC	

The University of Kansas Medical Center Clinical Nutrition Seminar 2011, Department of Dietetics & Nutrition and Department of Integrative Medicine, Kansas City, KS. 3

	TRUNK	Moles Open Areas/Pressure Sores Rash	Cancer Inadequate Protein/Calorie intake Allergies, intolerances	Vit D25OH Tot Prot/Alb/Glob; Organic Acids (r/o Vit C def, etc); Zinc, serum; Differential; CRP-us; Sed Rate	
NAILS	NAILS/HANDS	Ridges/split nails White spots Loose cuticles Koilonychia Fungal growth	Accident, protein Zn defic, stressor Fe deficiency Microbial growth	Electrolytes; RBC Mg; Vit D25OH; Differential Ferritin; Zinc, serum; Tot Prot/Alb/Glob; Organic Acids (r/o Vit C def, etc); Zinc, serum; Differential;	Selenium, serum; Candida Antibody;
	NAILS/FEET	Fungal growth Ingrown nails Split nails/ridges	Microbial growth Poor pedicure Injuries, nutr. insult	Electrolytes; RBC Mg; Vit D25OH; Differential; Ferritin; Zinc, serum; Tot Prot/Alb/Glob; Organic Acids (r/o Vit C def, etc); Zinc, serum; Differential;	Selenium, RBC Candida Antibody TSH
BODY TEMP	HANDS/OVERALL BODY	Low body temps Fever	Hypothyroidism Infection, virus	TSH, T3-free, TPO & TG AB; Iodine Urine/blood	Nitric Oxide/ADMA (perfusion)

Lab recommendations are provided for today's preventive physician and integrative health professionals. They have been selected from those tests that have a high degree of sensitivity and relate to known mechanisms of chronic disease. The labs used by physicians for chronic disease care are from recommendations of respected resources and practice-based master integrative & functional medicine nutritionists, physicians, clinicians, microbiologists and physiologists. The use of this methodology is to better probe for the metabolic strengths and weaknesses of patients for prevention and total health, not the symptomatic treatment of disease.

Fischbach, Frances. *A Manual of Laboratory & Diagnostic Tests. Sixth Edition*. Lippincott 2000.
Lord RS, Bralley JA. *Laboratory Evaluations for Integrative and Functional Medicine, 2nd Edition*. 2008 Meta Metrix Institute
Libonati, CJ, *Recognizing Celiac Disease: Signs, Symptoms, Associated Disorders & Complications*. 2007. Gluten Free Works Publishing.
Queen S. *"The Basic 100" Third Review Edition* Institute for Health Realities 2001 www.healthrealities.org
Yanick P, Jaffe R. *Clinical Chemistry & Nutrition Guidebook: A Physician's Reference*, Volume One. 1988 T&H Publishing.
Gibson RS. *Principles of Nutritional Assessment, 2nd Edition*. 2005. Oxford University Press. pp. 375-376.
1 Floyd, R.A. Role of oxygen free radicals in carcinogenesis and brain ischemia. FASEB J 4 2587-2597 (1990).
2 Beckman, K.B., Ames, B.N. Oxidative decay of DNA. J Biol Chem 272 19633-19636 (1997).
3 Spencer, J.P.E., Jenner, A., Chimel, K., et al. DNA strand breakage and base modification induced by hydrogen peroxide treatment of human respiratory tract epithelial cells. FEBS Lett 374 233-236 (1995).
4 Epe, B., Ballmaier, D., Roussyn, I., et al. DNA damage by peroxynitrite characterized with DNA repair enzymes. Nucleic Acids Res 24 4105-4110 (1996).

Specialized Diets for GI Healing: Allowed Foods & Forbidden Foods *(italics = none)*							
	Comprehensive Elimination Diet	**Gluten Free/ Casein Free**	**Specific Carbohydrate Diet**	**Gut & Psychology Syndrome Diet**	**Anti-Fungal Diet**	**FODMAP Diet**	**Restoration Diet**
Protein	ALL unprocessed meats: chicken, turkey, duck, goose, quail, ostrich, fish, shellfish, lamb, venison, rabbit, eggs. Wild game.	ALL unprocessed meats	ALL unprocessed meats: beef, pork, chicken, turkey, duck, goose, quail, ostrich, fish, shellfish, lamb, venison, rabbit, eggs. Processed meats that do not have any SCD forbidden ingredients	Eggs, fresh (if tolerated) Fresh meats (not preserved), fish, shellfish Broths with every meal. Canned fish in oil or water only	ALL unprocessed meats: beef, pork, chicken, turkey, duck, goose, quail, ostrich, fish, shellfish, lamb, venison, rabbit, eggs. Tofu, tempeh, Texturized vegetable protein	All unprocessed meats Eggs	All unprocessed meats in small amounts: Pureed, well-cooked, stews, soups.
Dairy Products & Dairy Alternatives	NONE Dairy alternatives are allowed: coconut, hemp, rice	NONE Dairy alternatives are allowed: nut, coconut, hemp, rice, soy.	All natural cheeses ***except for: ricotta, mozzarella, cottage cheese, cream cheese, feta, processed cheeses and spreads.*** Homemade yogurt cultured 24 hours.	All natural cheeses Yogurt-homemade	Eggs, plain yogurt (cow, sheep, goat) with live cultures, organic soy milk, soy cheese, coconut milk, unaged goat cheese	Lactose-free dairy products: milk, cottage cheese Rice milk, almond milk, hemp milk	Goat milk or sheep milk kefir. Dairy alternatives as coconut kefir
Fats & Oils	Sunflower, olive, flax, ghee, coconut, avocado, nut oils.	ALL	Avocados, olive oil, coconut oil, corn oil, avocado oil, etc.	Butter, ghee, coconut, avocado oil, olive	ALL	ALL	Ghee, coconut, olive, Sam Queen's restorative ghee
Nuts & Seeds	Coconut, pine nuts, chia seeds, flaxseeds, almonds, Brazil nuts, walnuts, chestnuts, filberts, pecans, nut flours, and meals	ALL that are non-processed with dairy or gluten.	Almonds, Brazil nuts, walnuts, chestnuts, filberts, pecans, nut flours and meals	Almonds, avocado, Brazil nuts, coconut, filberts, walnuts, chestnuts, pecans, nut flours and meals, peanuts, nut butters	ALL raw. Can roast at home or cook them.	***Nuts & Seeds in moderation*** ***Nut butters in moderation,*** Psyllium	***Nut butters in tiny amounts***

The University of Kansas Medical Center | KU Integrative Nutrition | Leigh Wagner, MS, RD, LD | Integrative Nutritionist | http://integrativemed.kumc.edu
3901 Rainbow Blvd, MS 1017 | Kansas City, KS 66160 | (913) 588-6208 | Fax (913) 588-0012 | E-mail: integrativemedicine@kumc.edu 1

	Comprehensive Elimination Diet	Gluten Free/ Casein Free	Specific Carbohydrate Diet	Gut & Psychology Syndrome Diet	Anti-Fungal Diet	FODMAP Diet	Restoration Diet
Non-Starchy Vegetables	ALL	ALL	Most: Fresh, frozen, raw or cooked. Asparagus, broccoli, cauliflower, artichokes, beets, Brussels sprouts, cabbage carrots, celery, cucumbers, eggplant, zucchini, summer squash, rhubarb, peppers, garlic, lettuce, spinach, mushrooms(unless Candidiasis), onions, turnips, watercress. NO canned vegetables.	Most: Fresh, mostly cooked, some raw	ALL	Alfalfa, avocado, bamboo shoots, bean shoot, beets, bok choy, broccoli, chili peppers, carrots, celery, chive, corn, cucumber, eggplant, fennel, kohlrabi, lettuce, olive, parsnip, mushroom, snow peas, spinach, squash, water chestnut, watercress	Well-cooked
Starchy Vegetables	ALL except corn	ALL	***NONE: potatoes, yams***	Beets, winter squash ***NONE: potatoes, yams***	***NONE: Exclude corn, yams, potatoes***	peas, potato, sweet potato, taro, turnip, pumpkin,	Well-cooked
Legumes	ALL	ALL	Dried navy beans, lentils, peas, split peas, unroasted cashews, peanuts in shell, natural peanut butter, lima beans, string beans	***Lima beans, peas (dried split, fresh green) These are consumed in later stages of the diet only, best sprouted***	Small amounts, not more than 1 cup cooked per day	Sweet peas, peanuts, peanut butter	Dahl
Fruits	ALL	ALL	ALL.	ALL, fresh and	***Restricted: Only***	RESTRICTED	Cooked,

The University of Kansas Medical Center | KU Integrative Nutrition | Leigh Wagner, MS, RD, LD | Integrative Nutritionist | http://integrativemed.kumc.edu 2
3901 Rainbow Blvd, MS 1017 | Kansas City, KS 66160 | (913) 588-6208 | Fax (913) 588-0012 | E-mail: integrativemedicine@kumc.edu

			Juices with no additives.	dried	***whole/fresh or frozen in protein smoothie***	QUANTITY: ½ cup serving/ no more often than every 2 hours Berries, citrus fruits, Cantaloupe, Banana, jackfruit, kiwi, grapes, passionfruit, pineapple, rhubarb, guava, pawpaw, lychee,	smoothies
	Comprehensive Elimination Diet	**Gluten Free/ Casein Free**	**Specific Carbohydrate Diet**	**Gut & Psychology Syndrome Diet**	**Anti-Fungal Diet**	**FODMAP Diet**	**Restoration Diet**
Grains	Quinoa, millet, amaranth, teff*, oat*, tapioca, rice, sorghum	Quinoa, millet, amaranth, teff*, oat*, tapioca, rice, sorghum	***NONE***	***NONE***	***NONE***	Barley, oats, quinoa millet, teff*, oat*, tapioca, rice, sorghum, seitan, amaranth, buckwheat, arrowroot, sago, oat bran, barley bran NO: WHEAT/RYE	Rice Congee
Herbs & Spices	All pure spices, fresh or dried	All pure spices, fresh or dried	All pure spices, fresh or dried	All pure spices, fresh or dried	Fresh only.	All pure spices, fresh or dried. ***No onion, Minor amts of garlic tolerated***	Not at first, then add: turmeric, ginger, cumin, coriander, and other spices
Beverages	Water, broths. un-caffeinated herbal teas, seltzer, mineral	ALL without dairy or gluten	Water, Tea, weak, freshly made Water Broths	Water, Tea, weak, freshly made Water Broths	Water, herbal tea	Tea, herbal teas, herbal infusions, hot water, coconut water	Broths Water Herbal teas Seltzer, mineral

	Comprehensive Elimination Diet	Gluten Free/ Casein Free	Specific Carbohydrate Diet	Gut & Psychology Syndrome Diet	Anti-Fungal Diet	FODMAP Diet	Restoration Diet
	water Diluted juices, vegetable juices					Coffee: < 2 cups daily Chicory/roasted	water, diluted juices, diluted vegetable juices
Sweeteners	Use Sparingly: Brown rice syrup, agave nectar, honey, stevia, fruit sweetener, blackstrap molasses	ALL	Honey if tolerated Saccharine	Honey	Stevia	Maple syrup, Rice syrup, Treacle, Golden syrup, glucose syrup, nutrasweet, sucralose, aspartame, stevia, saccharine	Use sparingly
	Comprehensive Elimination Diet	**Gluten Free/ Casein Free**	**Specific Carbohydrate Diet**	**Gut & Psychology Syndrome Diet**	**Anti-Fungal Diet**	**FODMAP Diet**	**Restoration Diet**
Miscellaneous	Broths Medical foods (non dairy, soy, or gluten-containing) Fermented and cultured foods Vinegar (not white vinegar)	Broths Medical foods (non dairy, soy, or gluten-containing) Fermented and cultured foods Vinegar	Broths Gelatin Pickles (without additives)	Soups Stews Cellulose in supplements Gin, Scotch occasionally Pickles (without additives) Tea, weak, freshly made Vinegar Wine (dry)	Lemon and lime and vitamin C crystals as replacements for vinegar. Herbal tea ***Tequila & Mead in small amounts***	Jam, marmalade, vegemite, marmite Alcohol: clear refined spirits such as gin and vodka in moderation	Medical Foods Broths Herbal Infusions Coconut kefir Coconut water

- ***Certified Gluten Free**
- **Comprehensive Elimination Diet: IFM Tool Kit**
- **Specific Carbohydrate Diet: http://www.breakingtheviciouscycle.info/**
- **Gut and Psychology Syndrome Diet: http://gapsdiet.com/The_Diet.html**
- **Restoration Diet: *Digestive Wellness,* 4th ed.**
- **Anti-Fungal Diet: IFM Tool Kit**
- **Yeast Questionnaire: http://cassia.org/candida.htm**
- **Fodmaps Diet: http://www.fodmapsdiet.com**

The University of Kansas Medical Center | KU Integrative Nutrition | Leigh Wagner, MS, RD, LD | Integrative Nutritionist | http://integrativemed.kumc.edu
3901 Rainbow Blvd, MS 1017 | Kansas City, KS 66160 | (913) 588-6208 | Fax (913) 588-0012 | E-mail: integrativemedicine@kumc.edu

KU Integrative Medicine

KU Integrative Nutrition

Healthy Proteins with Estimated Serving Sizes

Why are Proteins Important?

- Proteins make up healthy cell membranes
- Proteins provide energy
- Proteins support immune defense
- Bile Salts contain proteins needed for nutrient absorption & detoxification
- Proteins are a major part of muscle tissue
- Proteins supply essential amino acids our body cannot make
- Some hormones/chemical messengers are proteins
- Enzymes are proteins required proper metabolism

** Include protein with every meal and start your meals with 2 bites of protein**		
Plant-Based Protein	**Example**	**#Servings**
Grains & Beans Canned, Dry, Frozen Organic when possible Look for BPA-free cans	GF Grains: Quinoa, Rice, Amaranth, Teff, Rice, Buckwehat, Millet Legumes/Beans: Kidney, Black, Lima, Navy, Pinto, White, etc., Lentils, Green Peas, Black Eyed Peas, Split Peas Soy Beans & Soy Products: Soy Beans, Tofu, Tempeh, Soy Milk Vegetable Protein Powders	
Seeds & Seed Butters Raw, Unsalted, preferable Sealed & Refrigerated	Seeds: Pumpkin Seeds, Sesame Seeds, Sunflower Seeds, Chia Seeds, Flax Seeds Seed Butters: Sesame Tahini	
Nuts & Nut Butters Raw, Unsalted, preferable Sealed & Refrigerated	Nuts: Almonds, Cashews, Hazelnuts, Peanuts, Pecans, Pistachios, Walnuts, Macadamia Nuts Nut Butters: Peanut, Almond, and Cashew Butters *Excluding peanut butter, nuts are not a primary protein source	
Clean Animal Protein	**Example**	**#Servings**
Lean Red Meat Organic, Free Range/Grass Fed	Beef: Medallions, Filet Mignon, Steaks – Flank, Skirt, Top Round Pork: Tenderloin Lamb & Game Meats: Lamb Shoulder & Shoulder Steak, Bison	
Poultry Lean, Organic, Free Range	Lean Cuts include the Breast and Dark Meat Chicken, Duck, Goose, Turkey	
Fish/Seafood Fresh, Cold Water	Wild-caught, Northern Pacific Fish and Seafood Sardines and Anchovies Scallops, Mussels, Oysters	
Egg White Organic, free range Omega 3-Rich Eggs	Purchase locally if possible: Campo Lindo Farms, Good Natured Family Farms Chicken Eggs, Duck Eggs	
Organic Dairy Grass fed, GMO-, Pesticide-, Hormone- & antibiotic-free	Purchase locally if possible: Good Natured Family Farms, Shatto Dairy Milk, Cheese, Yogurt, Cream, Butter, Cottage Cheese, Cream Cheese, Sour Cream, Ice Cream	

Type of Protein	Serving Size Estimate	Protein Grams
Grains	½ cup	6 grams
Beans & Lentils	¾ - 1 cup	7 grams
Whole Egg/Egg White	2 each	12 grams/8 grams
Meat, Poultry, Seafood	3-6 ounces	7 grams/ounce
Seeds/Peanut butter	¼ cup/2 Tbsp	8 grams
Protein Powders	Variable	10-15 grams per ~2 tablespoons

The University of Kansas Medical Center | KU Integrative Nutrition | Leigh Wagner, MS, RD, LD | Integrative Nutritionist | http://integrativemed.kumc.edu
3901 Rainbow Blvd, MS 1017 | Kansas City, KS 66160 | (913) 588-6208 | Fax (913) 588-0012 | E-mail: integrativemedicine@kumc.edu
06282012

KU Integrative Medicine

KU Integrative Nutrition

Healthy Carbohydrates with Estimated Serving Sizes

Why Are Carbohydrates Important?

- Complex carbohydrates (carbs) are the body's primary energy source and preferred source for the brain and nervous system.
- Complex carbs provide essential vitamins and minerals needed for good health
- Complex carbs contain many phytonutrients ("phyto" = plant, nutrients) known to help our bodies remove toxins, fight infection and prevent disease
- Complex carbs provide fiber and bulk to our diet, promoting satiety and healthy digestion.
- Complex carbs help remove toxins, slow absorption and promote colon health
- **Choose mostly complex carbs: Low-starchy vegetables (Raw, Fermented, Steamed, Sautéed, Boiled, Pureed)**

Carbohydrate Category	Example	#Servings
Low-Starchy Vegetables Organic, Fresh, Local - When Possible Fresh, Raw, Cooked, Frozen (when cooking add oil/fats just before serving)	Artichoke, Asparagus, Baby Corn, Bamboo Shoots, Bean Sprouts, Beets, Broccoli, Brussels sprouts, Cabbage, Carrot, Cauliflower, Celery*, Cucumber, Greens* - Collard, Kale, Mustard, Turnip, Kohlrabi, Lettuce*, Leeks, Mushrooms, Okra, Onions, Pea Pods, Rhubarb, Radish, Rutabaga, Sauerkraut, Spinach*, Summer & Spaghetti Squash, Sugar Snap Peas, Swiss Chard, Turnips, Water chestnuts Nightshades: Tomatoes, Sweet & Hot Peppers*, Eggplant, Tomatillos, Pepinos, Pimentos, Paprika, Cayenne Peppers	
Starchy Vegetables Organic, Fresh, Local –When Possible Fresh, Raw, Cooked, Frozen These can fill ¼ of your plate	Beans/Lentils: Garbanzo Beans, Kidney Beans, Black Beans, Lentils, Lima Beans, Navy Beans, Pinto Beans, White Beans Peas: Black Eyed Peas, Green Peas, Split Peas, Chick Peas Corn, Parsnips, Plantains, Sweet potatoes, Taro, Yams, Pumpkin, Squash Nightshades: Potatoes*	
Starchy Grains Organic, Non GMO These can fill ¼ of your plate	Rice: Wild, Brown, Long Grain, Basmati, Abborio Quinoa, Amaranth, Teff, Buckwheat, Millet, Corn, Oats Wheat, Barley, Rye, Spelt (avoid if gluten free)	
Fruit Organic, Fresh Local Eat with Meals Fresh, Dried, Frozen	Grapefruit, Apples*, Apricots, Blueberries*, Pears, Plums, Strawberries*, Oranges, Nectarines*, Peaches*, Pineapple, Grapes*, Bananas, Kiwi, Papaya, Figs, Raisins, Cantaloupe, Watermelon	
Carbs & Sweeteners to Avoid	High-Fructose Corn Syrup Artificial Sweeteners: Splenda, Equal, Sweet 'N Low (Sucralose, Aspartame, Saccharin, Acesulfame, etc.) Avoid Processed, Packaged Carbohydrates Limit 100% Fruit Juices to 3-4 Ounces and Only with Meals Avoid Sugar-Sweetened Drinks	

Type of Carbohydrate	Serving Size Estimate
Low-Starchy Vegetables, Spaghetti Squash	1 cup or 2 cups lettuces
Starchy Vegetables & Grains	½ cup or 1 small potato
Fruit (Apple, Orange, Melon, Berries)	1 small or ½ cup

*Organic When Possible

The University of Kansas Medical Center | KU Integrative Nutrition | Leigh Wagner, MS, RD, LD | Integrative Nutritionist | http://integrativemed.kumc.edu
3901 Rainbow Blvd, MS 1017 | Kansas City, KS 66160 | (913) 588-6208 | Fax (913) 588-0012 | E-mail: integrativemedicine@kumc.edu

06282012

KU Integrative Medicine

KU Integrative Nutrition

Fats and Oils Servings

Why are Fats & Oils Important?

- Fats provide energy
- Fats build healthy cell membranes
- Fats make hormones
- Fats help absorb fat soluble vitamins
- Fats make up a large portion of our brain and nervous system
- Dietary fats supply essential fatty acids our body cannot make
- Fats make bile salts for nutrient absorption & detoxification
- Fats insulate, protect and cushion our organs

Fat or Oil Category	Example	#Servings
Omega 9s Oleic Fatty Acids *Stabilizers* ~50% daily fat calories	Raw Nuts & Seeds: Almonds, Cashews, Peanuts, Sesame Seeds, Walnuts, Macadamia Nuts, Pine Nuts Peanut Butter(natural, oil on top), Almond Butter, Tahini (sesame seed butter), Olives Almond Oil, Olive Oil, Avocado, Hummus	
Omega 6s Linoleic Acid *Controllers* ~30% daily fat calories	Eggs (whole, organic) Meats (commercial, grass-fed) Raw Nuts & Seeds: Brazil nuts, Pecans, Hazelnuts, Filberts, Walnuts, Hemp Seeds, Sunflower Seeds, Pumpkin Seeds Oils: Evening Primrose, Black Currant, Borage, Hemp, Grapeseed	
Omega 3s Alpha-Linolenic Acid *Fluidity/communicators* ~10% daily fat calories	Fish Oil (High DHA or EPA), 3-6-9 Balanced or DHA oils Fish (salmon/fin-fish), Fish (shellfish) Flax Seeds (ground/meal), Chia Seeds Flax Oil Algae	
Beneficial Saturated Fats SCT & MCT *Structure* ~10% daily fat calories	Butter (organic, pasture), Ghee (clarified butter–Indian cuisine) Dairy (preferably organic, raw) Meats (preferably grass-fed) Wild Game, Poultry (preferably organic) Coconut Oil & Butter, MCT Oil (Medium Chain Triglyceride) Eggs (whole, organic)	
Fats to Avoid Trans fats & Damaged LCFA *Stressors* <5% daily fat calories	Most packaged foods and fast foods Margarine, Vegetable Oils (corn, sunflower, canola), Mayonnaise (commercial), Hydrogenated Oil (as an ingredient), "imitation" cheeses, Tempura, Doughnuts (fried), Deep-Fried Foods, Chips, Regular Salad Dressing, Peanut Butter (Jif, Skippy, etc.), Roasted Nuts/Seeds, Dairy Substitutes (not including almond, coconut milk, etc.) Avoid acrylamides formed with high temperature cooking - browning during grilling, baking, frying or deep-frying will produce acrylamide	**Zero** (Less than 5%)

Type of Fat or Oil	Serving Size Estimate
Hummus	⅓ cup
Nuts, Seeds, Ground Flaxseeds, Olives	¼ cup
Nut butters (peanut butter, almond butter, cashew, coconut butter, etc.)	2 tablespoons
Oils (olive oil, almond oil, avocado oil, etc.)	1 tablespoon
Butter or Ghee (clarified butter – Indian cuisine)	1 teaspoon
Eggs	2 each
Fatty Ocean Fish, Meat, Poultry	3-4 ounces
Avocado	½ avocado

Adapted from Fats & Oils Survey, Diana Noland, MPH RD CCN. The University of Kansas Medical Center | KU Integrative Nutrition | Leigh Wagner, MS, RD, LD | Integrative Nutritionist | http://integrativemed.kumc.edu 3901 Rainbow Blvd, MS 1017 | Kansas City, KS 66160 | (913) 588-6208 | Fax (913) 588-0012 | E-mail: integrativemedicine@kumc.edu 06282012

Keeping a Food Diary

Instructions

The information you record in your food diary will help you and your doctor or dietitian identify patterns in your diet that may correlate to your health condition. This information can help them to design an eating program to meet your special needs.

These instructions will help you get the most out of your food diary. Generally, food diaries are meant to be used for a whole week, but studies have shown that keeping track of what you eat for even 1 day can help you make changes in your diet.

Date and Time:
Write the date and time of day you ate the food.

Food or Beverage Consumed:
In this column, write down the type of food you ate or drank. Be as specific as you can. Don't forget to write down "extras," such as butter, oils, salad dressing, mayonnaise, sour cream, sugar and ketchup. Please include brand names when possible, or indicate if an item was homemade.

How much:
In this space indicate the amount of the particular food item you ate. Give your best estimate of the size (2" x 1" x 1"), the volume (1/2 cup), the weight (2 ounces) and/or the number of items (12) of that type of food.

Where:
Write what room or part of the house you were in when you ate. If you ate in a restaurant, fast-food chain, your desk, or your car, write that location down.

Activity while eating:
In this column, list any activities you were doing while you were eating (for example, working on the computer, driving, watching TV, sitting at the dinner table).

Mood:
How were you feeling while you were eating (for example, sad, happy, rushed, stressed, bored)?

Symptoms:
In this column, make a note of any symptoms (good or bad) you experience throughout the day to help tune into how certain foods make you feel. Include: bowel/urine habits such as formed stool, loose stool, hard stool, scant urination, or frequent urination; feelings of discomfort such as gas, bloating, heartburn, headaches, brain fog, low energy, or sinus congestion; feelings of wellness such as increased energy, mental clarity, and/or relief of previous symptoms. Try to correlate the entries as closely as possible with the times listed to the left on the diet diary form.

Helpful Hints:

- Do not change your eating habits while you are keeping your food diary, unless your doctor or dietitian has given you specific instructions to do so.
- Tell the truth. Your doctor or dietitian can help only if you record what you really eat.
- Record what you eat on all days your doctor or dietitian recommends.
- Be sure to bring the completed forms back with you to your next appointment.

The University of Kansas Medical Center | KU Integrative Nutrition http://integrativemed.kumc.edu
3901 Rainbow Blvd, MS 1017 | Kansas City, KS 66160 | (913) 588-6208 | Fax (913) 588-0012 | E-mail: integrativemedicine@kumc.edu

Some basic rules to remember:

Write everything down:
Keep your form with you all day, and do your best to write down everything you eat or drink. A piece of candy, a handful of pretzels, a can of soda pop or a small donut may not seem like much at the time, but over a week these foods may add up!

Do it now:
Don't depend on your memory at the end of the day. Record your eating as you go.

Be specific:
Make sure you include "extras," such as gravy on your meat or cheese on your vegetables. Do not generalize. For example, record French fries as French fries, not as potatoes.

Estimate amounts:
If you had a piece of cake, estimate the size (2" x 1" x 2") or the weight (3 ounces). If you had a vegetable, record how much you ate (1/4 cup). When eating meat, remember that a 3-ounce cooked portion is about the size of a deck of cards.

If you have any questions, contact your doctor or dietitian.

Sample Food Diary Entry

Date	Time	Food or Drink: What kind	How much	Where	Activity	Mood	Symptoms
1/3/08	8am	Quaker instant oatmeal made with water	1 cup	car	Driving to work	Rushed/anxious	Loose bowel at 7am
		Wyman's frozen blueberries	½ cup				
		Starbucks Coffee with half and half	20 oz 2 tbsp				

The University of Kansas Medical Center | KU Integrative Nutrition http://integrativemed.kumc.edu
3901 Rainbow Blvd, MS 1017 | Kansas City, KS 66160 | (913) 588-6208 | Fax (913) 588-0012 |
E-mail: integrativemedicine@kumc.edu

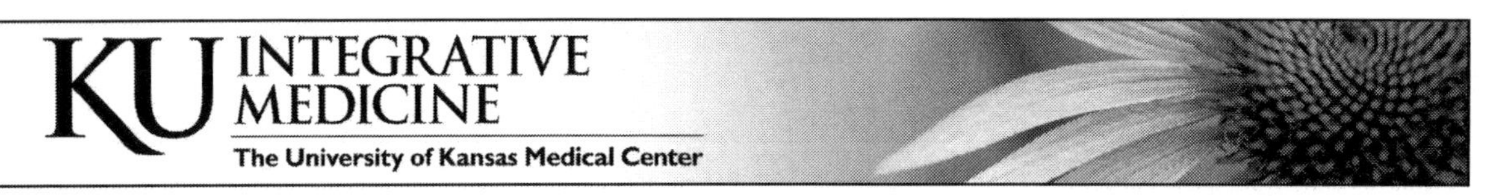

Diet Diary

Name:					
Date/Time	**Location/ Activity**	**Food or Beverage Consumed**	**Amount (cup, etc)**	**Mood**	**Symptoms**

Was this a typical day for you? Yes_ No If no, why not:

Reviewed by____________________________________ **Date/Time**______________

KU Integrative Nutrition | 3901 Rainbow Blvd, MS 1017 | Kansas City, KS 66160 | (913) 588-6208 | Fax (913) 588-0012
Leigh Wagner, MS, RD, LD | Integrative Nutritionist | http://integrativemed.kumc.edu | E-mail: integrativemedicine@kumc.edu
12312012

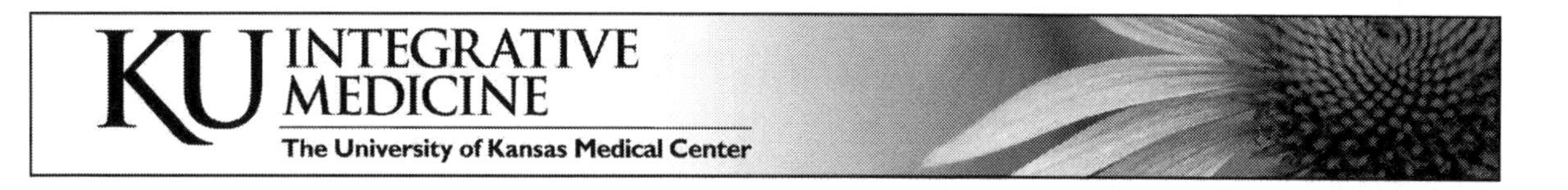

Dietary Withdrawal and Challenge Guidelines

The doctor or nutritionist has recommended you complete a food withdrawal trial to determine whether or not certain foods may be affecting your health. A Food Withdrawal trial (or "Elimination Diet") is prescribed to:

1) alleviate any potential stress or inflammation in your body or
2) determine which foods/food groups may be affecting your health.

By withdrawing these foods you may alleviate stress on your whole body and immune system. This dietary plan will help minimize symptoms, promote vitamin and mineral absorption, and generally calm down your immune system and overall decrease inflammation.

Did you know that an estimated 60-70% of your immune system is associated with your digestive tract? When we consistently consume foods that we are unable digest and absorb, then our immune system is constantly on high-alert. This stress makes our body vulnerable to other illness or disease: depression, anxiety, diabetes, cancer, cardiovascular disease, and others.

With that said, it is very important to remain 100% committed to this plan. Keep in mind that you have been eating these foods for 10, 20, 30 and more years. It takes a lot of time (months and ***years***) for your body to recover from these offending foods. Since it takes time, patience and commitment, we suggest you set aside a 5-6 week period that gives you freedom to prepare or plan meals and/or menus. Depending on the time you have available and your comfort in the kitchen, you may want to prepare meals each night of the week or cook large batches on weekends to eat throughout the week.

Common foods that all people are asked to eliminate during the trial are caffeine (for certain individuals, 2 cups green tea or organic coffee daily may be beneficial), alcohol, and added sugars. Plus, the two proteins that are difficult for many bodies to process are gluten and casein. Gluten is a protein formed when water mixes with certain grains (wheat, rye, barley, etc.) and their flours. Casein is a major protein in dairy foods.

For the next ______ days/weeks/months/lifelong, you will remove gluten and casein as well as ________ ______________________ from your diet. Consuming these "offending foods" can be associated with symptoms including:

- Joint/muscle pain, aches or twitching
- Fatigue/low energy
- Digestive upset: Bloating, gas, diarrhea, constipation, reflux, abdominal pain, etc.
- Headaches/migraines (may be brief or prolonged)
- Sore throat, stuffy nose, runny nose, itchy nose or eyes
- Skin rash or redness
- Lower back pain
- Anemia or low iron levels
- Vitamin/Mineral imbalances
- Brain "fog", lack of focus and/or concentration
- Sleepiness, insomnia, fatigue, apathy
- Mood disturbances: irritability, depression, anxiety
- Excitability (feeling hyper or "buzzed")
- Inflammation of any kind

✱ **Symptoms** associated with the food "reintroduction" or "challenge" period may not be the same symptoms experienced before the food withdrawal trial. For example, before the diet, a person's symptom may be chronic sinus pain. Once the food is reintroduced / challenged, their main symptom may be abdominal pain or diarrhea. This does not mean that the food group being challenged was not causing the sinus pain. It means the body and immune system react differently when the offending agent is removed and then reintroduced.

KU Integrative Medicine | 3901 Rainbow Blvd, MS 1017 | Kansas City, KS 66160 | (913) 588-6208 | Fax (913) 588-0012
http://integrativemed.kumc.edu | E-mail: integrativemedicine@kumc.edu
03252013

General Guidelines: What can I Eat and Drink?

Food withdrawal recommendations are based on an individual assessment which evaluates specific symptoms, lab values and medical recommendations. Food withdrawal and specific nutrition recommendations are necessary to allow the GI tract to heal while providing optimal levels of nutrients to support metabolism, reduce inflammation and promote healing. The types and amounts of carbohydrates, protein and fats recommended for each individual will vary based on the individual's GI tract ability to digest and absorb nutrients. For impaired GI tracts elemental forms of food may be used (simple sugars, amino acids, oils) while a more functional GI tract will allow consumption of whole foods (fruits, vegetables, meats). Instead of focusing on those foods you *can't* eat, we will focus on those you *can enjoy!* The following is a summary of whole, pure foods, supplemental support and beverages that you will enjoy during you trial:

Cleansing Beverages

Water, Mineral Water, Green & Herbal Tea: Keep a *glass* or *stainless steel* water bottle or other container to keep you supplied with water and clean liquids throughout the day. Water helps deliver nutrients to your cells, and subsequently water helps remove waste and toxins from the body. In other words, drinking water and green or herbal teas helps you take out the body's trash!
Organic Coffee: If you tolerate coffee and caffeine, 1-2 cups daily (8 ounces).

Healthy Carbohydrates

Guidelines: Organic, when possible (Dirty Dozen/Clean 15), Varied colors and types
Avoid/Minimize: High fructose corn syrup, processed/packaged foods, simple sugars and drinks

Low-starch Vegetables: Should make up 50% of your plate at each meal
Starchy Vegetables and Fruits: Sweet potatoes, potatoes, corn, fresh or frozen (not canned) fruit
Beans/legumes: All dried beans/green/waxed beans.
Soy may or may not be recommended or tolerated by all people. Thus, ask your dietitian or physician whether or not soy should be consumed
Peanuts should be organic
Whole Grains: Quinoa, rice, amaranth, millet, teff, buckwheat, and others.
Nut, Seed Milks: Almond, Hazelnut, Coconut, Soy (if tolerated), Oat (if tolerated), Rice or other non-dairy milks.
Supplemental carbohydrates/fiber: Ground flaxseed, psyllium, modified citrus pectin, oat bran

Clean Protein

Guidelines: Organic meats, BPA free canned beans, Raw nuts and seeds
Avoid: High temperature cooking or grilling, charred meats, improperly stored meats, processed meats, roasted nuts, processed nut butters

Poultry, Meat, Seafood: Free-range/organic (if possible) poultry, wild game (bison/buffalo, deer/venison, lamb, etc.), wild Alaskan salmon, protein powders.
Eggs: Pasture raised, omega-3, organic are preferable choices.
Beans/legumes, lentils: Plant-based protein
Nuts and seeds: Plant-based protein
Supplemental Protein: Whey protein powder, Amino Acid Complex, other protein powders

Balanced Fats and Oils

Guidelines: Organic meats, Cold pressed oils, Temperature resistant cooking oils, Organic butters
Avoid: Damaged fats and oils (see handout), trans fats (packaged foods), processed butters, fast food

Nuts and Seeds: All, peanuts should be organic. Pistachios may or may not be recommended.
Fats & Oils: Olive oil, avocado, organic pasture butter, coconut oil. See Fats & Oils Handout, which lists options: Healthy *Omega 9, 6, 3, and beneficial saturated fats*
Supplemental Fats & Oils: On an individual basis: MCT oil, Fish oil, Evening primrose, Borage oil, Black currant oil

KU Integrative Medicine | 3901 Rainbow Blvd, MS 1017 | Kansas City, KS 66160 | (913) 588-6208 | Fax (913) 588-0012
http://integrativemed.kumc.edu | E-mail: integrativemedicine@kumc.edu
03252013
2

Preparation

Week 1:

1. Clean the Cupboards: When possible, clear your cupboards and refrigerator of foods that are not "approved" on your particular withdrawal trial. Read labels, looking for added sugars, high-fructose corn syrup, and any of the "red flag" words we discussed.

2. Shop for foods and stock your pantry: Make sure that your refrigerator and cupboards are prepared with "approved" items so that you're always able to make a safe choice.

3. Supplements: Order any supplements or protein powders recommended by your doctor or dietitian.

4. Caffeine and Your Genes: Individuals with SNP's CYP1A1, CYP1A2 and CYP1B1 should avoid caffeine or consume no caffeine after noon.

5. Wean off caffeine, if necessary:
   - Begin on a weekend so you're able to take naps, as needed
   - For the first 3 days, cut down to ½ normal amount of coffee, soda, black tea, or other caffeinated beverages
   - For the next 4 days, drink 1 cup caffeinated green tea steeped in boiling water for 5 minutes
   - You may consider taking 1000 to 2000 mg buffered vitamin C powder (Emergen-C is one brand that would be ok, even though it has added sugar, it would still help you adjust to decreased caffeine intake).
   - Drink a minimum of 6-8 glasses filtered water daily

6. Diet Diary: You will need to keep a diet diary for the 3 days prior to reintroduction or "challenge" period, and throughout the reintroduction process. This is time consuming, but it is very important. You want to make your efforts worth it by noting any symptom changes. This helps determine next steps for continued healing.

KU Integrative Medicine | 3901 Rainbow Blvd, MS 1017 | Kansas City, KS 66160 | (913) 588-6208 | Fax (913) 588-0012
http://integrativemed.kumc.edu | E-mail: integrativemedicine@kumc.edu

Diet Snapshot

Yes: These items are gluten/dairy-free

Naturally Gluten and Dairy-Free Foods

Vegetables and Fruits
Beans (lentils, navy, kidney, black beans, garbanzo beans/chickpeas, etc.)
Nuts/Seeds (almonds, walnuts, pecans, cashews, sunflower seeds, etc.)
Meat, Poultry, Seafood

Gluten-Free grains and gluten alternatives (not recommended if grain-free)

Amaranth	GF Oats (generally, not recommended for celiac disease)	Rice (brown, wild, white)	Tapioca
Arrowroot	Millet	Rice bran	Teff
Buckwheat	Organic, Non-GMO Corn	Sago	
Flax	Quinoa	Sorghum	
Flours made from nuts, beans & seeds		Soy	

Dairy-Free Alternatives

Almond milk*	Coconut milk yogurt	Hazelnut milk*	Rice milk
Cocoa butter	Daiya (tapioca-based cheese shreds)	Hempseed milk*	*So Delicious* brand yogurts, desserts, milks
Coconut butter and oil	Ghee (if guaranteed casein-free)	100% Fruit Sorbet	
Coconut milk*		Imagine brand soups	
Coconut milk creamer		Oat milk*	

For those who avoid dairy, kosher "pareve" products are considered milk-free under kosher dietary law; however, they may contain a very small amount of milk protein. Individuals who have a dairy allergy will want to look closer at the ingredients list for confirmation of safety before consuming the product.

Make sure to read labels. If there is insufficient information on the label to make an informed decision, avoid the food. You can also call food companies to gather manufacturing information.

*Preferably unsweetened version

KU Integrative Medicine | 3901 Rainbow Blvd, MS 1017 | Kansas City, KS 66160 | (913) 588-6208 | Fax (913) 588-0012
http://integrativemed.kumc.edu | E-mail: integrativemedicine@kumc.edu
03252013

4

No: These items contain gluten or dairy and must be avoided			
Gluten-Containing Food Items		**Dairy or Casein-Containing Food Items**	
Barley	Matzo flour/meal	Butter	Recaldent®
Barley malt/extract	Pastas (wheat-based)	Cheeses (most, except some soy brands)	Rennet casein
Bran	Panko	Cream	Sherbet
Bread crumbs	Rye	Creamed soups and vegetables	Soup bases
Bulgur	Seitan	Curds	Sour cream
Cereal extract	Semolina	Custards	Tagatose
Club wheat	Spelt	Diacetyl	Whey
Couscous	Sprouted wheat	Ghee	White or milk chocolate
Durum	Triticale	Half & half	Yogurt
Einkorn	Vital wheat gluten	Ice cream	
Emmer	Udon	Ice milk	
Farina	Wheat	Lactose, lactulose, lactoferrin, lactalblumin	
Faro	Wheat bran	Milk	
Graham flour	Wheat germ/germ oil	Puddings	
Hydrolyzed wheat protein	Wheat grass		
Kamut	Wheat protein isolate		
Malt vinegar/flavoring	Wheat starch		
	Whole wheat berries		
Maybe: These food items require further inspection. They may or may not contain gluten or dairy			
Items that May Contain Gluten		**Foods that May Contain Casein**	
Ales, beers, lagers	Marinades/thickeners	Artificial flavorings	Tuna fish
Breading mixes	Pasta	Bacterial cultures	*Many non-dairy foods contain casein proteins. Avoid foods that contain any ingredient with casein or caseinate.
Brown rice syrup	Roux	Caramel candies	
Brown sugar	Sauces	Cosmetics, medicines	
Caramel coloring	Soup Bases & broths	Dairy-free cheese (most brands)	
Coating mixes	Stuffing	Dairy-free may contain casein*	
Communion wafers	Self-basting poultry	Ghee	
Condiments (mustard, ketchup, BBQ sauce, etc.)	Soy sauce (wheat-free Tamari is gluten-free)	Hot dogs	
Croutons	Medications	Lactic acid	
Candy	Modified food/veg. starch	Lunch meats	
Deli/luncheon meats	Over the counter meds	Margarine	
Herbal supplements	Prescription meds	Nisin	
Imitation bacon/seafood	Surim	Nougat	
Lotions, body care	Vitamin & mineral supplements	Sausage	
		Semi-sweet chocolate	

<u>Condiments:</u> Any condiments made from apple cider vinegar are safe; Heinz and Organicville brands are gluten-free.
<u>Deli Meats:</u> Applegate Farms, Boar's Head, Hormel Naturals are gluten-free.
<u>Cosmetics:</u> Shampoos and others: Dessert Essence and Burt's Bees are gluten-free
<u>Medications:</u> Celiac Central website: celiaccentral.org/resources

- http://www.glutenfreedrugs.com/
- Ingredients in medications that may indicate gluten: Wheat, Modified starch (source not specified), Pregelatinized starch (source not specified), Pregelatinized modified starch (source not specified), Dextrates (source not specified), Dextrimaltose (when barley malt is used), Caramel coloring (when barley malt is used), Dextrin (source not specified, but usually by corn or potato)

KU Integrative Medicine | 3901 Rainbow Blvd, MS 1017 | Kansas City, KS 66160 | (913) 588-6208 | Fax (913) 588-0012
http://integrativemed.kumc.edu | E-mail: integrativemedicine@kumc.edu
03252013

5

Breakfast Ideas

- Eggs and Greens: Two Omega 3 or organic eggs with 2 cups sautéed greens with onions in vegetable or chicken broth. Drizzle with olive oil after sautéed. Add poached or sliced hard-boiled egg over the greens and season with sea salt, pepper or other spices as desired.
- Warm Apple Cinnamon Quinoa: ½ cup cooked Quinoa with diced apples, ½ teaspoon cinnamon, and ¼ cup almonds/walnuts or drizzle of natural peanut butter or almond butter
- Nutty Cereal: 1 ½ cups Gluten-free cereal with 1 cup unsweetened soy milk or other unsweetened milk alternative, ¼ cup nuts or 2 tablespoons nut butter (peanut, almond, etc.), 1 tablespoon ground flaxseed.
- Protein Smoothie: 1 cup unsweetened milk alternative with 1 serving hempseed protein, RAW Protein, or egg protein powder (Jay Robb brand is a staple at Whole Foods), 1 cup frozen or fresh berries, 1 cup fresh spinach or other green or 2-3 stems from leafy greens, 1 tablespoon olive oil or Balance 3-6-9 oil or flaxseed oil (depending on those recommended by your healthcare practitioner), however, you can always default to olive oil, ¼ avocado or 1 tablespoon ground flax or flaxseed oil.
- Breakfast Roll-Up: 3.5 ounces Leftover fish or chicken wrapped in a gluten-free rice or teff tortilla filled with 2 tablespoons guacamole, 3 tablespoons salsa. Enjoy with 1 cup fresh fruit such as cubed cantaloupe.
- Rice Cakes or Crackers with Hummus & a side of Chicken Sausage or Nut Butter: Two rice cakes topped with hummus and 3 ounces leftover meat or gluten-free turkey or chicken sausage (1 link Applegate Farms Chicken Sausage) or spread with 2 tablespoons almond or organic peanut butter. Serve with a whole grapefruit or 1 cup fresh berries or mixed fruit.

Lunch/Dinner Ideas

- Hummus and Veggies with Gluten-Free Crackers: ¼ cup hummus (chick peas/garbanzo bean garlic dip) or baba ghanouj (same as hummus only with eggplant instead of chick peas). Dip the fresh vegetables and/or gluten-free crackers. Choose a variety of brightly colored and flavored vegetables: Bell peppers, carrots, celery, snap peas, mini-sweet peppers, cucumber, broccoli, cauliflower, zucchini, etc.
- Lentil Tacos with Mixed Greens: Sauté onions and garlic and add cooked lentils. Season with Mexican seasoning, lime juice and a pinch of salt, and serve with a brown rice tortilla or corn tortilla (make sure the corn tortilla is 100% gluten-free – no added wheat).
- Gluten-Free Pasta with Veggie-Boosted Sauce and Side Salad: Sauté ½ to one whole onion (chopped), ¼ cup zucchini, 2 cloves garlic with 1-2 tablespoons olive oil, pinch of salt and Italian seasoning with 3 ounces of chicken. Add ½ cup Classico brand (or other brand with no sugar added) marinara sauce and ¼ cup white, black or garbanzo beans. Serve over ¾ cup brown rice, gluten-free pasta. Serve with a side salad.
- Salmon Salad 4-Ways: Mix canned wild Alaska salmon (Bear & Wolf or Kirkland brands from Costco, for example) or chunk light tuna in water mixed with 1-2 tablespoons light mayonnaise or vegannaise, 2 teaspoons lemon or lime juice, ¼ cup diced grapes or apples and 1 tablespoon walnuts; season with pepper to taste.
    - Make as a sandwich with GF bread
    - Serve over a bed of greens and mixed vegetables
    - Dip or top gluten-free crackers
    - Dip with vegetables: carrots, broccoli, cucumber, etc.
- Salad with Herbs: 2 cups mixed salad greens: Romaine, leaf lettuce, spinach, cabbage; herbs: basil, cilantro, parsley, mint; top with your favorite chopped vegetables: tomatoes, onions, bell peppers, asparagus, shredded beets, sprouts, broccoli, cauliflower. Add ¼ cup quinoa or brown rice and ½ beans and sprinkle with raw nuts and 1 tablespoon dried fruit (raisins, cranberries, diced figs, etc.). Dress with a citrus or balsamic vinaigrette or vinegar and extra virgin olive oil. Optional: Top with 2-3 ounces leftover chicken, canned or fresh cooked salmon or canned chunk-light tuna in water.

KU Integrative Medicine | 3901 Rainbow Blvd, MS 1017 | Kansas City, KS 66160 | (913) 588-6208 | Fax (913) 588-0012
http://integrativemed.kumc.edu | E-mail: integrativemedicine@kumc.edu
03252013

Lunch/Dinner Ideas with Recipes: See Recipe Packet

- Turkey Spinach Meatloaf with Mashed Cauliflower
- Gluten & Dairy-Free Fajita/Burrito Bowls
- Asian Chicken Salad
- Italian Tuscan Vegetable Soup
- Grilled Citrus Trout Crunchy Mediterranean Slaw
- Whole Roast Chicken with Sweet Apple Walnut Kale
- Black Bean Cakes with Mango Salsa
- Quinoa Cabbage Soup
- Curry Chicken Breast with Tomato and Coconut Milk served over brown rice or quinoa
- Chicken Salad Wraps/Roll-Ups
- Quick Lemon and Garlic Quinoa Salad and Spiced Collard Greens
- Spaghetti Squash
- Quick Sautéed Chicken with Sautéed Vegetables with Cashews
- Ginger Peanut or Almond Chicken with Sweet Potatoes & Snap Peas
- Fish Tacos with Citrus Slaw
- Salmon Salad
- Quick Turkey Pasta Sauce
- Cumin Crusted Salmon and Cauliflower Rice

Snacks

- Hummus & Veggies or Gluten Free Crackers/Chips (Beanitos - Bean chips)
- Trail Mix
- Hard Boiled Eggs
- Apple or Pear with Almonds/Nut Butter
- Cinnamon Mixed Nuts
- Roasted Chickpeas
- Quick Easy Kale Chips
- Chocolate Avocado Pudding
- Whipped Sweet Potatoes

KU Integrative Medicine | 3901 Rainbow Blvd, MS 1017 | Kansas City, KS 66160 | (913) 588-6208 | Fax (913) 588-0012
http://integrativemed.kumc.edu | E-mail: integrativemedicine@kumc.edu

Gluten and Dairy-Free Shopping List

Vegetables				
Artichoke	Cabbage	Kale	Potatoes	Sweet Potatoes
Asparagus	Carrots	Kohlrabi	Pumpkin	Swiss Chard
Avocado	Cauliflower	Leeks	Radishes	Tomatoes
Beets & Beet greens	Celery	Mushrooms	Romaine Lettuce	Turnips
	Collard Greens	Mustard Greens	Rutabaga	Winter Squash
Bell Peppers	Cucumber	Okra	Salad Greens	Yams
Bok Choy	Eggplant	Olives	Snap Peas	Yellow Squash
Broccoli	Fennel	Onions	Snow Peas	Zucchini
Brussels Sprouts	Green Beans	Parsnips	Spinach	

Herbs & spices

Fresh or dried herbs and spices

Italian (blends of basil, oregano, marjoram, parsley, thyme, sage, and rosemary)

Fruits				
Apples	Currants	Lemons	Peaches	Raspberries
Apricots	Dates	Limes	Pears	Strawberries
Bananas	Dried fruits	Mango	Pineapple	Tangerines
Blackberries	Figs	Melons	Plums	Watermelon
Blueberries	Grapes	Nectarines	Pluots	
Cherries	Grapefruit	Oranges	Pomegranate	
Cranberries	Kiwi	Papaya	Prunes	

Dairy Alternatives

Unsweetened almond milk, coconut milk, hempseed milk, hazelnut milk, etc.

Daiya tapioca-based cheese shreds

Meat, Fish, Poultry, Protein

Fresh or frozen Poultry (turkey, chicken, etc.)

Wild Game (deer (venison), elk, duck, buffalo, etc.)

Grass-fed beef

Wild Alaskan Salmon or other wild Pacific seafood

Eggs (preferably pasture raised, organic)

Clean Deli Meats:

Boar's Head (found at Hen House)

Applegate Farms Deli Meats (Hy-Vee, Whole Foods)

Beverages

Water

Green, white, and herbal teas (chamomile, peppermint, ginger, tulsi)

Coconut water

Vegetable juice, up to 8-16 oz. daily

Mineral water (still or sparkling)

Organic Coffee 1-2 cups daily (8 oz. cups)

Fats and Oils

Nuts, nut butters and nut flours (e.g. almond butter, cashew butter, pumpkin butter)

Organic Peanuts and Peanut butters

Extra Virgin Olive Oil

Unrefined Coconut Oil

Organic, pasture butter

Grapeseed oil, flaxseed oil, etc.

Frozen Foods

Variety of frozen vegetables, fruits (preferably organic)

KU Integrative Medicine | 3901 Rainbow Blvd, MS 1017 | Kansas City, KS 66160 | (913) 588-6208 | Fax (913) 588-0012
http://integrativemed.kumc.edu | E-mail: integrativemedicine@kumc.edu
03252013

8

Snacks	
Terra Brand Vegetable Chips (Sweet potato, taro, yuca, batata, parsnip, and ruby taro)	
Baby carrots, celery sticks or other veggies	
Hummus made with Olive Oil	
Rice crackers	
Mary's Gone Crackers Brand Gluten-Free Crackers	
Fresh Fruit	
Nuts and trail mixes (without yogurt/chocolate-covered pieces)	
Cereals, Grains and Beans/Legumes	
Amaranth	Brown or White Rice
Beans/Legumes: Lentils, peanuts, soybeans, black, navy, garbanzo (aka chickpeas), black-eyed peas, great northern, kidney, etc.	Cream of Rice Brown Rice Tortillas Rice Crackers
Buckwheat	Rice Cakes
Quinoa	La Tortilla Brand Teff Tortillas
Quinoa Flakes	Corn
100% Buckwheat Soba Noodles	Corn Tortillas
Buckwheat Kasha	Polenta
Cream of Buckwheat	Millet
Wild Rice (not the same as rice)	Tapioca
Enjoy Life Brand Cereals (Nutty Flax and Rice Cereals, GF Granolas)	Sorghum Flax seed
Condiments	
Condiments made with apple cider vinegar	
Vinegars, oils	

Food Reintroduction or "Challenge" Guidelines

The length of the withdrawal/elimination period will vary based on your individual needs and the amount of digestive healing that needs to occur.

After the trial period, you will begin to reintroduce each food/food group in a systematic manner with the following guidelines:

1) Choose **one** food group (e.g. gluten, dairy, corn, egg...). Eat a minimum of 2-3 servings of that food daily for 3 days, *as long as you do not experience any symptom changes.* If you experience symptoms, proceed to step 2 below. If you experience no symptoms, proceed to step 3 below.

2) **If you experience symptom changes at any time during the 3 days**:
   a. Immediately remove the food group and wait until symptoms subside/disappear (you may notice symptoms as soon as 3 hours after eating a serving or 2 of the food, or it may take a full 3 days to experience symptoms). It is best to remove the food for another 2-3 months, then challenge it again.
   b. After removing the food, wait until you're symptom-free to move to the next food group. When you are symptom-free, choose the next food group and complete the 3-day challenge (Step 1) above: eat minimum of 2-3 servings of the food per day for 3 days as long as you do not experience any symptoms.

3) **If you do not experience symptoms for 3 days of the reintroduction/challenge:**
   a. Leave the food group in your diet, and move on to the next food group.
   b. Continue through each food and food group until you've reintroduced each one to determine your tolerance.
   c. I would advise starting with either gluten or dairy.

KU Integrative Medicine | 3901 Rainbow Blvd, MS 1017 | Kansas City, KS 66160 | (913) 588-6208 | Fax (913) 588-0012
http://integrativemed.kumc.edu | E-mail: integrativemedicine@kumc.edu

Gluten-Free Resources

ORGANIZATIONS	
• Celiac Sprue Association	www.csaceliacs.org
WEB RESOURCES	
• Celiac Sprue Association	www.csaceliacs.org
• Celiac Sprue Association of Greater Kansas City	www.csakansascity.org/
• Elana's Pantry: Gluten free recipes	www.elanaspantry.com
• Gluten Intolerance Group of North America	www.gluten.net
• *The Gluten Connection* by Shari Lieberman	www.glutenconnection.com
• Celiac Disease and Gluten-Free Diet Information	www.celiac.com
• *The Whole Life Nutrition Cookbook and Blog* by Alissa Segersten & Tom Malterre	www.nourishingmeals.com
• A Gluten-Free Day	http://glutenfreeday.com/
• Grocery: Whole Foods Market: download list of gluten-free products:	http://www.wholefoodsmarket.com/service/gluten-free-products-list
• Grocery: Whole Foods Market: download list of gluten-free and casein-free products:	http://www.wholefoodsmarket.com/service/gluten-casein-free-products-list
• Grocery: HyVee: download of gluten-free product listing:	http://www.hy-vee.com/webres/File/Gluten-Free-Listing0211.pdf
• The Whole Life Nutrition Kitchen	www.nourishingmeals.com
• Restaurants: Urban Spoon website: Link to Gluten-Friendly Restaurants	www.urbanspoon.com/t/34/1/Kansas-City/Gluten-free-friendly-restaurants

BOOK & MAGAZINE RESOURCES

- *The Ultimate Food Allergy Cookbook and Survival Guide* by Nicolette Dumke
- *The Gluten-Free Gourmet Cooks Fast and Healthy* by Betty Hagman
- *The Gluten-Free Gourmet, Living Well without Wheat* by Betty Hagman
- *Gluten-Free Diet: A Comprehensive Resource Guide* by Shelley Case
- *The Gluten Connection* by Shari Lieberman
- *Gluten-Free Quick & Easy* by Carol Fenster, PhD (Avery, 2007)
- *The Allergy Self-Help Cookbook* by Majorie Hurt Jones
- *The Wheat-Free Cook* by Jacqueline Mallorca (William Morrow, 2007)
- *The Whole Life Nutrition Cookbook and Blog* by Alissa Segersten & Tom Malterre
- *Nourishing Meals cookbook by Alissa Segersten & Tom Malterre*
- *Complete Gluten-Free Cookbook* by Donna Washburn and Heather Butt (Robert Rose, 2007)
- *Gluten-Free Diet* by Shelley Case, RD (Case Nutrition Consulting Inc., Expanded Edition, 2006)
- *Gluten-Free 101* by Carol Fenster, PhD (Savory Palate, 2006)
- *Cooking Free* by Carol Fenster, PhD (Avery, Penguin Group, 2005)
- *Best Gluten-Free Family Cookbook* by Donna Washburn and Heather Butt (Robert Rose, 2005)
- *Wheat-Free Recipes & Menus* by Carol Fenster, PhD (Avery, Penguin Group, 2004)
- *Food Allergy Survival Guide* by Vesanto Melina, MS, RD, Jo Stepaniak, MSEd, Dina Aronson, MS, RD (Healthy Living Publications, 2004)
- *Gluten-Free Friends* by Nancy Patin Falini, RD (Savory Palate, 2003) - for kids
- *Living Without Gluten-Free & Dairy-Free magazine,* Living Without®, Inc.

The University of Kansas Medical Center | KU Integrative Nutrition | Leigh Wagner, MS, RD, LD | Integrative Nutritionist | http://integrativemed.kumc.edu
3901 Rainbow Blvd, MS 1017 | Kansas City, KS 66160 | (913) 588-6208 | Fax (913) 588-0012 | E-mail: integrativemedicine@kumc.edu

KU Integrative Medicine

KU Integrative Nutrition

Meal Guide

This meal guide will help you choose servings per meal. The ultimate goal is for you to meet your nutritional and health needs with real, *whole* foods. If your body is accustomed to eating more convenience, processed or packaged foods, with time, your body will begin to crave these whole foods your body *needs to live*. Eventually, you will be able to listen to your body's cravings and signals of hunger or fullness decide when and how much to eat.

Please refer to the tan handouts for [A] Protein, [B] Carbohydrate, and [C] Fats & Oils. If you need to avoid dairy foods (casein), please eat two servings daily of the calcium-rich dairy-free foods (see handout).

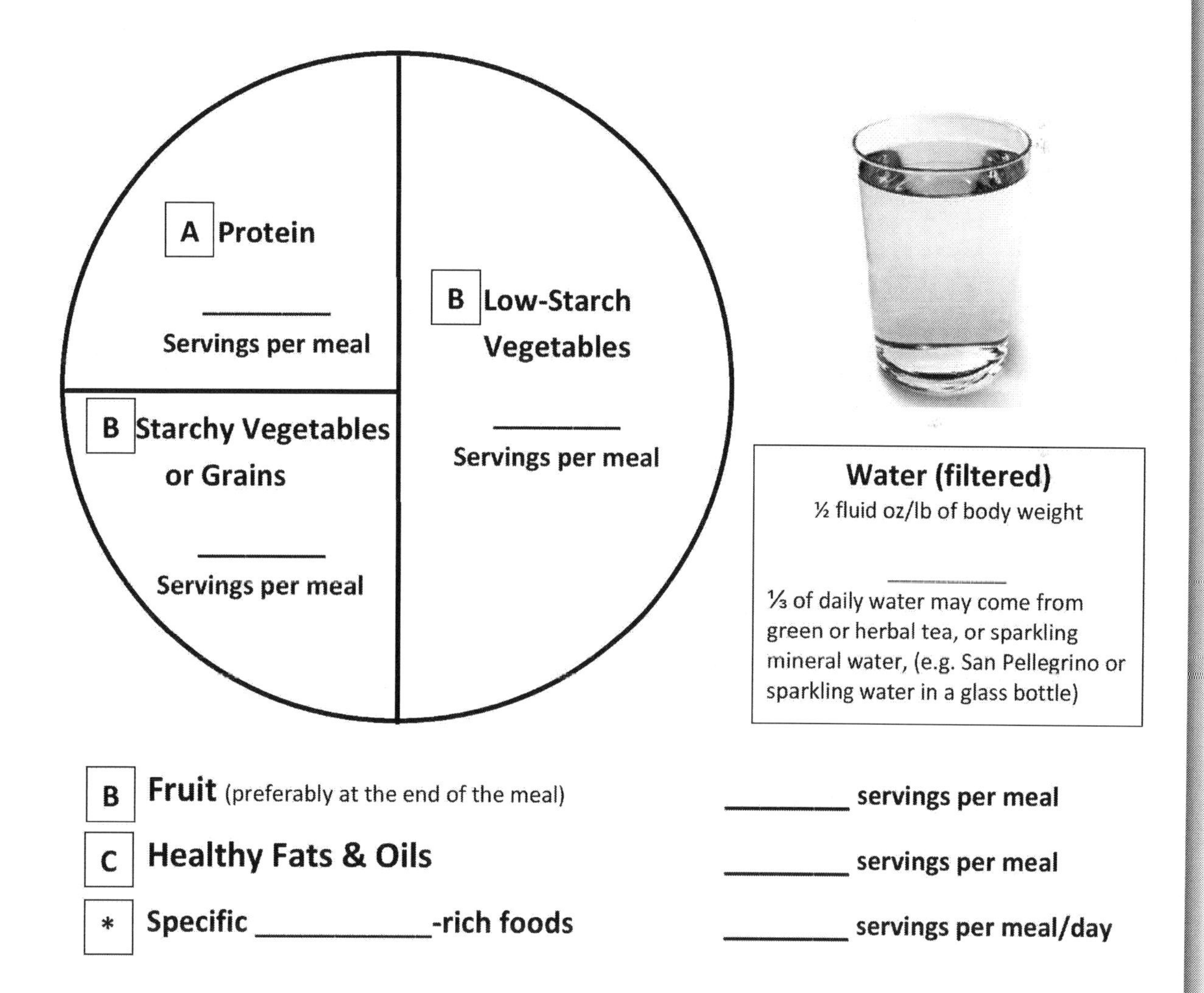

The University of Kansas Medical Center | KU Integrative Nutrition | Leigh Wagner, MS, RD, LD | Integrative Nutritionist | http://integrativemed.kumc.edu
3901 Rainbow Blvd, MS 1017 | Kansas City, KS 66160 | (913) 588-6208 | Fax (913) 588-0012 | E-mail: integrativemedicine@kumc.edu

12102012

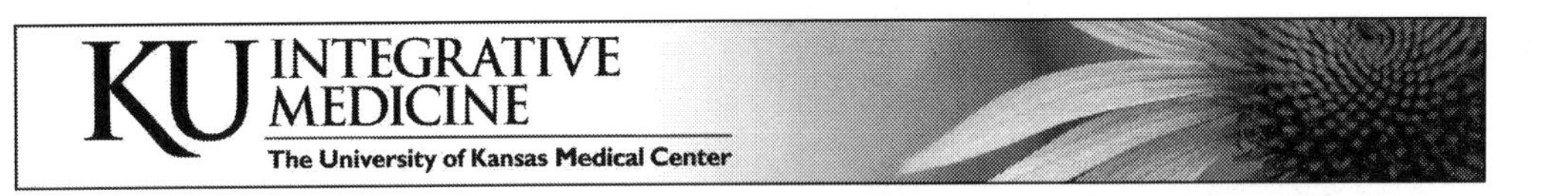

Criteria for students/interns of Dietetics and Integrative Medicine research project

Students in the Dietetics and Integrative Medicine program at KU Medical Center must ask a research question or questions that investigates, in depth, one of the 7 principles of nutrition and dietetics from an integrative medicine perspective. An easy way to ensure your topic is Integrative is ensuring you include one of the 7 principles of Dietetics and Integrative Medicine:

1. Biochemical Individuality

Chornic Disease Pathophysiology

2. Nutritional influence on Inflammation
3. Nutritional influence on Immune Regulation
4. Long Latency Nutrient Insufficiencies
5. Nutritional Toxicology and Epigenetics
6. Energy Metabolism: Cell to Body Composition
7. Lifestyle: Diet, Physical Activity/Exercise, Sleep, Beliefs, Community/Relationships, Environment

Each of the above can be expanded upon and outlined/supported with the following articles/publications.

- Ford, D., Raj, S., Batheja, R. K., Debusk, R., Grotto, D., Noland, D., Redmond, E., et al. (2011). American Dietetic Association: standards of practice and standards of professional performance for registered dietitians (competent, proficient, and expert) in integrative and functional medicine. *Journal of the American Dietetic Association*, *111*(6), 902–913.e1–23. doi:10.1016/j.jada.2011.04.017
- Jones DS, Hofmann L, Quinn S. 21st century medicine: A new model for medical education and practice. Gig Harbor, WA:The Institute for Functional Medicine, 2009;p1-35. (Consortium of Academic Health Centers for Integrative Medicine definition of Integrative Medicine), http://www.imconsortium.org
- Sears, B., & Ricordi, C. (2011). Anti-inflammatory nutrition as a pharmacological approach to treat obesity. *J Obes, 2011*. doi:10.1155/2011/431985
- McCann, J. C., & Ames, B. N. (2009). Vitamin K, an example of triage theory: is micronutrient inadequacy linked to diseases of aging? *Am J Clin Nutr*, *90*(4), 889–907. doi:10.3945/ajcn.2009.27930
- Heaney, R. P. (2012). The nutrient problem. *Nutr Rev*, *70*(3), 165–169. doi:10.1111/j.1753-4887.2011.00469.x
- Diamanti-Kandarakis, E., Bourguignon, J.-P., Giudice, L. C., Hauser, R., Prins, G. S., Zoeller, R. T., & Gore, A. C. (2009). Endocrine disrupting chemicals. *Endocirine reviews*.
- Lacey, K., & Pritchett, E. (2003). Nutrition Care Process and Model: ADA adopts road map to quality care and outcomes management. *Journal of the American Dietetic Association*, *103*(8), 1061–72. doi:10.1053/jada.2003.50564
- Heaney, R. P. (2003). Long-latency deficiency disease: insights from calcium and vitamin D. *The American journal of clinical nutrition*, *78*(5), 912–9. Retrieved from http://www.ncbi.nlm.nih.gov/pubmed/14594776

KU Integrative Medicine | 3901 Rainbow Blvd, MS 1017 | Kansas City, KS 66160 | (913) 588-6208 | Fax (913) 588-0012
http://integrativemed.kumc.edu | E-mail: integrativemedicine@kumc.edu
05032013

Research Projects for Interns

1. Review charts, compile and organize data related to food sensitivities
    a. Relate to diabetes or pre-diabetes: Gluten sensitivity/Celiac Disease related to diabetes.
    b. Relate to Medical Symptoms Questionnaire
    c. Relate food sensitivities and gluten/dairy sensitivities
    d. Other ideas related to food sensitivities
2. BIA phase angle related to
    a. Neurofeedback data
    b. RBC fatty acids
    c. Minerals/electrolyte levels
    d. Cancer survivorship
3. Work with on of the KU IM doctors and/or fellows on research projects
4. DN department projects/activities
5. Review literature using the Nutrition EBL on Mendeley

The University of Kansas Medical Center | KU Integrative Nutrition | Leigh Wagner, MS, RD, LD | Integrative Nutritionist | http://integrativemed.kumc.edu
3901 Rainbow Blvd, MS 1017 | Kansas City, KS 66160 | (913) 588-6208 | Fax (913) 588-0012 | E-mail: integrativemedicine@kumc.edu 06282012

Community Nutrition Resources, Keywords and Websites

National Organizations and Resources

Organization	Website
Local Harvest	www.localharvest.org
Sustainable Table	www.sustainabletable.org
Community Supported Agriculture	http://www.localharvest.org/csa/ http://www.nal.usda.gov/afsic/pubs/csa/csa.shtml
The Real Food Challenge	http://www.realfoodchallenge.org
Cook for your Life	http://www.cookforyourlife.org
Price-Pottenger Nutrition Foundation	http://ppnf.org
Academy Dietetic Practice Groups (DPGs)	
Dietetics and Integrative Medicine (DIFM) DPG	www.integrativerd.org
Food and Culinary Professionals DPG	http://www.foodculinaryprofs.org
Hunger and Environmental Nutrition	http://www.hendpg.com
Nutrition Entrepreneurs	http://www.nedpg.org

Kansas City Organizations and Resources

Organization	Website
Greater Kansas City Food Policy Coalition	http://www.kcfoodpolicy.org
Kansas City Food Circle	www.kcfoodcircle.org
Cultivate KC	www.cultivatekc.org
Kansas City Community Gardens	http://www.kccg.org

The University of Kansas Medical Center | KU Integrative Nutrition | Leigh Wagner, MS, RD, LD | Integrative Nutritionist | http://integrativemed.kumc.edu
3901 Rainbow Blvd. MS 1017 | Kansas City, KS 66160 | (913) 588-6208 | Fax (913) 588-0012 | E-mail: integrativemedicine@kumc.edu 06282012

Bibliography

Evidenced Based

Practice Based

Science Based

BIBLIOGRAPHY | REFERENCES CITED

1. Adams K, Kohlmeier M, Powell M, Zeisel S. Nutrition in medicine: nutrition education for medical students and residents. Nutrition In Clinical Practice 2010;25.

2. Adams K, Kohlmeier M, Zeisel S. Nutrition education in U.S. medical schools: latest update of a national survey. . Acad Med 2010;85:1537–42.

3. Frantz DJ, Munroe C, McClave SA, Martindale R. Current perception of nutrition education in U.S. medical schools. Current Gastroenterology Reports 2011;13:376-9.

4. Definition of Integrative Medicine. 2013. (Accessed 7-20-2013, 2013, at http://www.imconsortium.org/about/.)

5. Integrative Medicine: Improving Health Care for Patients and Health Care Delivery for Providers and Payors. The Bravewell Collaborative, 2010. (Accessed March, 2014, at http://www.bravewell.org/content/pdf/IntegrativeMedicine2.pdf.)

6. Brown AC, Valiere A. Probiotics and medical nutrition therapy. Nutrition in Clinical Care 2004;7:56-68.

7. Brown AC, Medical Nutrition Therapy as a Potential Complementary Treatment for Psoriasis - Five Case Reports. Alternative Medicine Review 2004;9:297-307.

8. Pietzak M. Celiac disease, wheat allergy, and gluten sensitivity: when gluten free is not a fad. JPEN Journal of Parenteral & Enteral Nutrition 2012;36:68S-75s.

9. Staudacher HM, Whelan K, Irving PM, Lomer MCE. Comparison of symptom response following advice for a diet low in fermentable carbohydrates (FODMAPs) versus standard dietary advice in patients with irritable bowel syndrome. Journal of Human Nutrition & Dietetics 2011;24:487-95.

10. Hao L, Kim JJH. Immigration and the American Obesity Epidemic. International Migration Review 2009;43:237-62.

11. Murray S. Doubling the burden: chronic disease. CMAJ: Canadian Medical Association Journal 2006;174:771-.

12. Popkin BM, Adair LS, Ng S. Global nutrition transition and the pandemic of obesity in developing countries. Nutrition Reviews 2012;70:3-21.

13. Satia JA. Dietary acculturation and the nutrition transition: an overview. Applied Physiology, Nutrition & Metabolism 2010;35:219-23.

14. Sharma S, Gittelsohn J, Rosol R, Beck L. Addressing the public health burden caused by the nutrition transition through the Healthy Foods North nutrition and lifestyle intervention programme. Journal of Human Nutrition & Dietetics 2010;23:120-7.

15. Boeing H, Bechthold A, Bub A, Ellinger S, Haller D. Critical review: vegetables and fruit in the prevention of chronic diseases. European Journal of Nutrition 2012;51:637-63.

16. Fitzgerald N, Morgan KT, Slawson DL. Practice paper of the Academy of Nutrition and Dietetics abstract: the role of nutrition in health promotion and chronic disease prevention. Journal of the Academy of Nutrition and Dietetics 2013;113:983-.

17. Slawson D, Fitzgerald N, Morgan K. Position of the academy of nutrition and dietetics: the role of nutrition in health promotion and chronic disease prevention. Journal of the Academy of Nutrition and Dietetics 2013;113:972-9.

18. Chiurchiù V, M. M. Chronic inflammatory disorders and their redox control: From molecular mechanisms to therapeutic opportunities. . Antioxid Redox Signal 2011;15:2605–41.

19. Glantz S, Gonzalez M. Effective tobacco control is key to rapid progress in reduction of non-communicable diseases. Lancet 2012;379:1269-71.

20. Hudson NL, Mannino DM. Tobacco Use: A Chronic Illness? Journal of Community Health 2010;35:549-53.

21. Reuter S, Gupta S, Chaturvedi M, Aggarwal B. Oxidative stress, inflammation, and cancer: How are they linked? Free Radical Biology & Medicine 2010;49:1603–16.

22. Midlife exercise: the gift (to yourself) that keeps on giving. University of California at Berkeley Wellness Letter 2013;29:6-.

23. Danese A, McEwen B. Adverse childhood experiences, allostasis, allostatic load, and age-related disease. Physiology & Behavior 2012;106:29–39.

24. McEwen B. Stress, Adaptation, and Disease: Allostasis and Allostatic Load. . Annals of the New York Academy of Sciences 1998;840:33–44.

25. McEwen B. Protective and Damaging Effects of the Mediators of Stress and Adaptation: Allostasis and Allostatic Load. In: Schulkin J, ed. Allostasis, homeostasis, and the costs of physiological adaptation. New York, NY US: Cambridge University Press; 2004:65-98.

26. McEwen B, Wingfield J. What is in a name? Integrating homeostasis, allostasis and stress. Hormones And Behavior 2010;57:105-11.

27. Romero LM, Dickens M, Cyr N. The Reactive Scope Model - a new model integrating homeostasis, allostasis, and stress. Hormones And Behavior 2009;55:375-89.

28. Hayes DP. Nutritional hormesis. European Journal of Clinical Nutrition 2007;61:147-59.

29. Hayes DP. Adverse effects of nutritional inadequacy and excess: a hormetic model. The American Journal Of Clinical Nutrition 2008;88:578S-81S.

30. Lindsay DG. Nutrition, hormetic stress and health. Nutrition Research Reviews 2005;18:249-58.

31. Clifton PM. Dietary fatty acids and inflammation. Nutrition & Dietetics 2009;66:7-11.

32. Ji Y, Sakata Y, Tso P. Nutrient-induced inflammation in the intestine. Current Opinion in Clinical Nutrition & Metabolic Care 2011;14:315-21.

33. Sears B, Ricordi C. Anti-inflammatory nutrition as a pharmacological approach to treat obesity. Journal Of Obesity 2011;2011.

34. Sears B, Ricordi C. Role of fatty acids and polyphenols in inflammatory gene transcription and their impact on obesity, metabolic syndrome and diabetes. European Review For Medical And Pharmacological Sciences 2012;16:1137-54.

35. Vasquez A. Reducing pain and inflammation naturally part I: new insights into fatty acid biochemistry and the influence of diet. Nutritional Perspectives: Journal of the Council on Nutrition 2004;27:5-, 7-10, 2 passim.

36. Vasquez A. Reducing pain and inflammation naturally. Part II: new insights into fatty acid supplementation and its effect on eicosanoid production and genetic expression. Nutritional Perspectives: Journal of the Council on Nutrition 2005;28:5.

37. Wall R, Ross RP, Fitzgerald GF, Stanton C. Fatty acids from fish: the anti-inflammatory potential of long-chain omega-3 fatty acids. Nutrition Reviews 2010;68:280-9.

38. Palmer S. Foods that Fuel the Immune System. Environmental Nutrition 2010;33:1-4.

39. Public policy statements. Position of dietitians of Canada and the American Dietetic Association: nutrition intervention in the care of persons with human immunodeficiency virus infection. Canadian Journal of Dietetic Practice & Research 2000;61:77-87.

40. Young JS. HIV and medical nutrition therapy. Journal of the AMERICAN DIETETIC ASSOCIATION 1997;97:S161-S6.

41. Rad A, Torab R, Ghalibaf M, Norouzi S, Mehrabany E. Might patients with immune-related diseases benefit from probiotics? Nutrition 2013;29:583-6.

42. Fau A, Ahern P, Griffin N, Goodman A, Gordon J. Human nutrition, the gut microbiome and the immune system. Nature 2011;474:327-35.

43. Indrio F, Neu J. The intestinal microbiome of infants and the use of probiotics. Current Opinion in Pediatrics 2011;23:145-50.

44. Kau A, Ahern P, Griffin N, Goodman A, Gordon J. Human nutrition, the gut microbiome and the immune system. Nature 2011;474:327-36.

45. Kelly D, Mulder I. Microbiome and immunological interactions. Nutrition Reviews 2012;70:S18-S30.

46. Lomax AR, Calder PC. Probiotics, immune function, infection and inflammation: a review of the evidence from studies conducted in humans. Current Pharmaceutical Design 2009;15:1428-518.

47. Ahmadieh H, A. A. Vitamins and bone health: beyond calcium and vitamin D. Nutrition Reviews 2011;69:584-98.

48. Baker H. Nutrition in the elderly. Nutritional aspects of chronic diseases. Geriatrics 2007;62:21.

49. Heaney RP. Long-latency deficiency disease: insights from calcium and vitamin D. American Journal of Clinical Nutrition 2003;78:912-9.

50. Georgieff MK. Long-term brain and behavioral consequences of early iron deficiency. Nutrition Reviews 2011;69:S43-S8.

51. Lucock M. Folic Acid: Beyond Metabolism. Journal of Evidence-Based Complementary & Alternative Medicine 2011;16:102-13.

52. Bondi C, Taha A, Tock J, et al. Adolescent behavior and dopamine availability are uniquely sensitive to dietary omega-3 fatty acid deficiency. Biological Psychiatry 2013.

53. Gordon E, Bond J, Gordon R, Denny M. Zinc deficiency and behavior: A developmental perspective. Physiology & Behavior 1982;28:893-7.

54. Hegarty BDPGB. Marine omega-3 fatty acids and mood disorders - linking the sea and the soul. Acta Psychiatrica Scandinavica 2011;124:42-51.

55. Innis SM, Novak EM, Keller BO. Long chain omega-3 fatty acids: micronutrients in disguise. Prostaglandins, Leukotrienes, And Essential Fatty Acids 2013;88:91-5.

56. Lafourcade M, al e. Nutritional omega-3 deficiency abolishes endocannabinoid-mediated neuronal functions. Nature Neuroscience 2011;14:345-50.

57. McNamara R, Carlson S. Role of omega-3 fatty acids in brain development and function: potential implications for the pathogenesis and prevention of psychopathology. Prostaglandins, Leukotrienes, And Essential Fatty Acids 2006;75:329-49.

58. Ames BN. Low micronutrient intake may accelerate the degenerative diseases of aging through allocation of scarce micronutrients by triage. Proceedings Of The National Academy Of Sciences Of The United States Of America 2006;103:17589-94.

59. Ames BN. Prevention of mutation, cancer, and other age-associated diseases by optimizing micronutrient intake. Journal Of Nucleic Acids 2010;2010.

60. Ames BN. Optimal micronutrients delay mitochondrial decay and age-associated diseases. Mechanisms Of Ageing And Development 2010;131:473-9.

61. McCann JC, Ames BN. Vitamin K, an example of triage theory: is micronutrient inadequacy linked to diseases of aging? American Journal of Clinical Nutrition 2009;90:889-907.

62. McCann JC, Ames BN. Adaptive dysfunction of selenoproteins from the perspective of the triage theory: why modest selenium deficiency may increase risk of diseases of aging. FASEB Journal: Official Publication Of The Federation Of American Societies For Experimental Biology 2011;25:1793-814.

63. McKay JAMJC. Diet induced epigenetic changes and their implications for health. Acta Physiologica 2011;202:103-18.

64. Hanley B, Djiane J, Fewtrell M, Grynberg A, Hummel S. Metabolic imprinting, programming and epigenetics -- a review of present priorities and future opportunities. British Journal of Nutrition 2010;104:S1-25.

65. Neustadt J, Pieczenik S. Biochemical individuality. Integrative Medicine: A Clinician's Journal 2007;6:30-2.

66. Neustadt J, Pieczenik S. The important role of biochemical individuality. Integrative Medicine: A Clinician's Journal 2007;6:34-5.

67. Simmons R. Epigenetics and maternal nutrition: nature v. nurture. Proceedings of the Nutrition Society 2011;70:73-81.

68. Simmons RA. Developmental origins of diabetes: the role of epigenetic mechanisms. Current Opinion In Endocrinology, Diabetes, And Obesity 2007;14:13-6.

69. Verma M. Cancer control and prevention: nutrition and epigenetics. Current Opinion in Clinical Nutrition & Metabolic Care 2013;16:376-84.

70. Vucetic Z, Carlin J, Totoki K, Reyes T. Epigenetic dysregulation of the dopamine system in diet-induced obesity. Journal of Neurochemistry 2012;120:891-8.

71. Wang J, Wu Z, Li D, et al. Nutrition, epigenetics, and metabolic syndrome. Antioxidants & Redox Signaling 2012;17:282-301.

72. Xu X-f, Du L-z. Epigenetics in neonatal diseases. Chinese Medical Journal 2010;123:2948-54.

73. Curtis L, Patel K. Nutritional and Environmental Approaches to Preventing and Treating Autism and Attention Deficit Hyperactivity Disorder (ADHD): A Review. Journal of Alternative & Complementary Medicine 2008;14:79-85.

74. TRANSCRIPT. The Secret Life of Fat, with Michele La Merrill. Environmental Health Perspectives 2013;121:1-4.

75. Allen J, Montalto M, Lovejoy J, . WW. Detoxification in naturopathic medicine: a survey. . The Journal of Alternative and Complementary Medicine 2011;17:1175-80.

76. Axtell S, Birr A, Halvorson C, et al. Detoxification diets: Three pilot studies. Townsend Letter 2013:97.

77. Crinnion WJ. The CDC Fourth National Report of Human Exposure to Environmental Chemicals: what it tells us about our toxic burden and how it assists environmental medicine physicians. Alternative Medicine Review 2010;15:101-8.

78. Morrison JA, lannucci AL. Symptom Relief and Weight Loss From Adherence to a Meal Replacement-enhanced, Low-calorie Detoxification Diet. Integrative Medicine: A Clinician's Journal 2012;11:42-7.

79. Richardson J. Toxins and immunity in chronic fatigue syndrome. JOURNAL OF CHRONIC FATIGUE SYNDROME 2002;10:43-50.

80. Rountree R. Roundoc Rx: a functional approach to environmental toxins. Alternative & Complementary Therapies 2009;15:216-20.

81. Soderland P, Lovekar S, Weiner DE, Brooks DR, Kaufman JS. Chronic kidney disease associated with environmental toxins and exposures. Advances in Chronic Kidney Disease 2010;17:254-64.

82. Outline for a National Action Plan for the prevention, detection and management of infertility. 2010. (Accessed 9/10, 2013, at http://www.cdc.gov/art/PDF/NationalActionPlan.pdf)

83. Hughes K. Advanced Metabolic Detoxification Strategies. Townsend Letter 2013:45-52.

84. Anderson OS, Sant KE, Dolinoy DC. Nutrition and epigenetics: an interplay of dietary methyl donors, one-carbon metabolism and DNA methylation. Journal of Nutritional Biochemistry 2012;23:853-9.

85. Burdge G, Lillycrop K. Bridging the gap between epigenetics research and nutritional public health interventions. Genome Med 2010;2:80.

86. Burdge GC, Hoile SP, Lillycrop KA. Epigenetics: are there implications for personalised nutrition? Current Opinion in Clinical Nutrition & Metabolic Care 2012;15:442-7.

87. Burdge GC, Lillycrop KA. Nutrition, Epigenetics, and Developmental Plasticity: Implications for Understanding Human Disease. Annual Review of Nutrition 2010;30:315-39.

88. Supic G, Jagodic M, Magic Z. Epigenetics: a new link between nutrition and cancer. Nutrition And Cancer 2013;65:781-92.

89. Ball L, Johnson C, Desbrow B, Leveritt M. General practitioners can offer effective nutrition care to patients with lifestyle-related chronic disease. Journal of Primary Health Care 2013;5:59-69.

90. Butcher L. The root of disease. Lifestyle interventions take aim at chronic ailments. Modern Healthcare 2012;42:30-2.

91. Centre for R, Dissemination. Nurse delivered lifestyle interventions in primary health care to treat chronic disease risk factors associated with obesity: a systematic review (Provisional abstract). In: Sargent GM, Forrest LE, Parker RM, eds.; 2012:1148-71.

92. Kushner RF, Sorensen KW. Lifestyle medicine: the future of chronic disease management. Current Opinion In Endocrinology, Diabetes, And Obesity 2013;20:389-95.

93. Lind L, Elmståhl S, Bergman E, Englund M, Lindberg E. EpiHealth: a large population-based cohort study for investigation of gene-lifestyle interactions in the pathogenesis of common diseases. European Journal Of Epidemiology 2013;28:189-97.

94. Sassone-Corsi P. When Metabolism and Epigenetics Converge. Science 2013;339:148-50.

95. Rowen L, Milner JA, Ross S. Obesity, cancer and epigenetics. Bariatric Nursing & Surgical Patient Care 2010;5:275-83.

96. Academy of Nutrition and Dietetics. Position and practice paper update for 2014. Journal of the Academy of Nutrition and Dietetics 2014;114:297-8.

97. Badawi A, El-Sohemy A. Nutrigenetics and Modulation of Oxidative Stress. Annals Of Nutrition & Metabolism 2012;60:27-36.

98. Gruber L, Lichti P, Rath E, Haller D. Nutrigenomics and nutrigenetics in inflammatory bowel diseases. Journal of Clinical Gastroenterology 2012;46:735-47.

99. Liu B, Qian S-B. Translational regulation in nutrigenomics. Advances In Nutrition (Bethesda, Md) 2011;2:511-9.

100. Lovegrove JA, Gitau R. Personalized nutrition for the prevention of cardiovascular disease: a future perspective. Journal Of Human Nutrition And Dietetics: The Official Journal Of The British Dietetic Association 2008;21:306-16.

101. Minihane AM. Nutrient gene interactions in lipid metabolism. Current Opinion in Clinical Nutrition & Metabolic Care 2009;12:357-63.

102. Phillips CM. Nutrigenetics and metabolic disease: current status and implications for personalised nutrition. Nutrients 2013;5:32-57.

103. Pizzorno L. Nutrigenomics: the potential to optimize chronic disease with SNP-based dietary recommendations. Integrative Medicine: A Clinician's Journal 2009;8:44-9.

104. Raqib R, Cravioto A. Nutrition, immunology, and genetics: future perspectives. Nutrition Reviews 2009;67:S227-36.

105. Riso P, Klimis-Zacas D, Bo C, et al. Effect of a wild blueberry (Vaccinium angustifolium) drink intervention on markers of oxidative stress, inflammation and endothelial function in humans with cardiovascular risk factors. European Journal of Nutrition 2013;52:949-61.

106. PLoS Medicine Series on Big Food: The Food Industry is Ripe for Scrutiny. 2012. (Accessed at https://www.plos.org/media/press/2012/plme-09-06-editorial.pdf)

107. Frantz D, Munroe C, McClave S, Martindale R. Current perception of nutrition education in U.S. medical schools. Current Gastroenterology Reports 2011;13:376-9.

108. Maeshiro R, Johnson I, Koo D, Parboosingh J, Carney J. Medical education for a healthier population: Reflections on the Flexner report from a public health perspective. Academic Medicine 2010;85:211-9.

109. Daghigh F, Vettori DJ, Harris J. Nutrition in medical education: history, current status, and resources. Topics in Clinical Nutrition 2011;26:147-57.

110. Stambolliu E, Bogataj J, Monteiro Grillo I, Camilo M, Ravasco P. International research program between medical schools: The relevance of clinical research training in nutrition. Nutritional Therapy & Metabolism 2012;30:129-36.

111. Orimo H, Ueno T, Yoshida H, Sone H, Tanaka A, Itakura H. Nutrition education in Japanese medical schools: a follow-up survey. Asia Pacific Journal of Clinical Nutrition 2013;22:144-9.

112. Ray S, Udumyan R, Rajput-Ray M, Thompson B, Lodge K-M. Evaluation of a novel nutrition education intervention for medical students from across England. BMJ Open 2012;2:e000417-e.

113. Chronic Diseases and Health Promotion. 2012. (Accessed 7/29, 2013, at http://www.cdc.gov/chronicdisease/overview/index.htm.)

114. Cody M, Tuma P. The Academy of Nutrition and Dietetics' Public Policy Priorities Overview. Journal of the Academy of Nutrition & Dietetics 2013;113:392-5.

115. Di Noia J, Furst G, Park K, Byrd-Bredbenner C. Designing culturally sensitive dietary interventions for African Americans: review and recommendations. Nutrition Reviews 2013;71:224-38.

116. Grantham C, Whitelaw S, Coulton T, Walker G. An enhanced dietetic service to care homes can improve appropriate prescribing of oral nutritional supplements. Journal of Human Nutrition & Dietetics 2011;24:388-9.

117. Neelemaat F. Short-Term Oral Nutritional Intervention with Protein and Vitamin D Decreases Falls in Malnourished Older Adults. Journal of the American Geriatrics Society 2012;60:691-9.

118. Oostdam N. Interventions for Preventing Gestational Diabetes Mellitus: A Systematic Review and Meta-Analysis. Journal of Women's Health (15409996) 2011;20:1551-63.

119. Perry KJ, Hickson M, Thomas J. Factors enabling success in weight management programmes: systematic review and phenomenological approach. Journal of Human Nutrition & Dietetics 2011;24:301-2.

120. Wong SY, Lau EM, Lau WW, Lynn HS. Is dietary counselling effective in increasing dietary calcium, protein and energy intake in patients with osteoporotic fractures? A randomized controlled clinical trial. Journal of Human Nutrition & Dietetics 2004;17:359-64.

121. Burke JD. Bridging the Sustainability Gap: Food Systems and the Nutrition Professional. Nutrition Today 2012;47:155-60.

122. Yeatman H. Window of opportunity – positioning food and nutrition policy within a sustainability agenda. Australian & New Zealand Journal of Public Health 2008;32:107-9.

123. Bertmann F, Ohri-Vachaspati P, Buman M, Wharton C. Implementation of Wireless Terminals at Farmers' Markets: Impact on SNAP Redemption and Overall Sales. American Journal of Public Health 2012;102:e53-e5.

124. Cortes F, Steeples M, Stone M. Promoting Healthy Eating: Contra Costa County's Food Policy. American Journal of Public Health 1995;85:1449-50.

125. Dannefer R, Williams D, Baronberg S, Silver L. Healthy Bodegas: Increasing and Promoting Healthy Foods at Corner Stores in New York City. American Journal of Public Health 2012;102:e27-e31.

126. Nutrition and You: Trends 2011 Webinar. 2013. (Accessed 7/29, 2013, at http://www.eatright.org/nutrition-trends/#.UfmZ_e_n9Ms)

127. Jacobs Jr DR, Tapsell LC. Food, Not Nutrients, Is the Fundamental Unit in Nutrition. Nutrition Reviews 2007;65:439-50.

128. Resolution adopted by the General Assembly:Political Declaration of the High-level Meeting of the General Assembly on the Prevention and Control of Non-communicable Diseases. WHO, 2012. (Accessed 9/6, 2013, at http://www.who.int/nmh/events/un_ncd_summit2011/political_declaration_en.pdf

129. Jones D, Bland JS, Quinn S. What is Functional Medicine. In: Jones DS, Quinn S, eds. Textbook of Functional Medicine. Gig Harbor, WA, USA: Institute of Functional Medicine; 2010:5.

130. Jones DS, Bland JS. History of Functional Medicine. In: Jones DS, ed. Textbook of Functional Medicine. Gig Harbor, WA, USA: Institute for Functional Medicine; 2010.

131. Jones DS, Hofmann L, Quinn S. 21st Century Medicine: A New Model for Medical Education and Practice. Gig Harbor: Institute for Functional Medicine; 2009.

132. Banz MF, Most PV, Banz WJ. A Workshop Designed to Educate Dietetics Professionals about the Cardiovascular Benefits of Soyfoods. Journal of Nutrition Education & Behavior 2004;36:103-4.

133. Centre for R, Dissemination. Cost-effectiveness of medical nutrition therapy and therapeutically designed meals for older adults with cardiovascular disease (Provisional abstract). Journal of the AMERICAN DIETETIC ASSOCIATION 2010;110:1840-51.

134. Galasso P, Amend A, Melkus GD, Nelson GT. Barriers to medical nutrition therapy in black women with type 2 diabetes mellitus. Diabetes Educator 2005;31:719-25.

135. Mead A, Atkinson G, Albin D, et al. Dietetic guidelines on food and nutrition in the secondary prevention of cardiovascular disease – evidence from systematic reviews of randomized controlled trials (second update, January 2006). Journal of Human Nutrition & Dietetics 2006;19:401-19.

136. Psota TL, Lohse B, West SG. Associations between eating competence and cardiovascular disease biomarkers. Journal of Nutrition Education and Behavior 2007;39:S171-S8.

137. Troyer JL, McAuley WJ, McCutcheon ME. Cost-effectiveness of medical nutrition therapy and therapeutically designed meals for older adults with cardiovascular disease. Journal of the AMERICAN DIETETIC ASSOCIATION 2010;110:1840-51.

138. White S, Bissell P, Anderson C. A qualitative study of cardiac rehabilitation patients' perspectives on making dietary changes. Journal of Human Nutrition & Dietetics 2011;24:122-7.

139. Racine E, Troyer J, Warren-Findlow J, McAuley W. The effect of medical nutrition therapy on changes in dietary knowledge and DASH diet adherence in older adults with cardiovascular disease. Journal of Nutrition, Health & Aging 2011;15:868-76.

140. Craven K, Messenger J, Kolasa KM. What dietitians need to know about medical nutrition therapy and pharmacotherapy for type 2 diabetes. Nutrition Today 2010;45:240-9.

141. Daly A, Michael P, Johnson EQ, Harrington CC, Patrick S, Bender T. Diabetes white paper: Defining the delivery of nutrition services in Medicare medical nutrition therapy vs Medicare diabetes self-management training programs. Journal of the AMERICAN DIETETIC ASSOCIATION 2009;109:528-39.

142. Daly A, Warshaw H, Pastors JG, Franz MJ, Arnold M. Diabetes medical nutrition therapy: practical tips to improve outcomes. Journal of the American Academy of Nurse Practitioners 2003;15:206-11.

143. Franz MJ, Powers MA, Leontos C, et al. The evidence for medical nutrition therapy for type 1 and type 2 diabetes in adults. Journal of the AMERICAN DIETETIC ASSOCIATION 2010;110:1852-89.

144. McCabe-Sellers BJ, Skipper A. Position of the American Dietetic Association: integration of medical nutrition therapy and pharmacotherapy [corrected] [published erratum appears in J AM DIET ASSOC 2010 Nov;110(11):1761]. Journal of the AMERICAN DIETETIC ASSOCIATION 2010;110:950-6.

145. Morris SF, Wylie-Rosett J. Medical nutrition therapy: a key to diabetes management and prevention. Clinical Diabetes 2010;28:12-8.

146. Perichart-Perera O, Balas-Nakash M, Parra-Covarrubias A, et al. A medical nutrition therapy program improves perinatal outcomes in Mexican pregnant women with gestational diabetes and type 2 diabetes mellitus. Diabetes Educator 2009;35:1004-13.

147. Vetter M, Volger S. Medical nutrition therapy for the management of diabetes. Journal of Clinical Outcomes Management 2010;17:175-91.

148. Oncology Nutrition DPG member spotlight. Oncology Nutrition Connection 2009;17:15-6.

149. Cranganu A, Camporeale J. Nutrition aspects of lung cancer. Nutrition in Clinical Practice 2009;24:688-700.

150. Hejl A, Furze AD. Transforming care for head and neck cancer patients: a multidisciplinary approach. Support Line 2010;32:3-9.

151. Isenring E, Capra S, Bauer J. Nutrition support, quality of life and clinical outcomes. Journal of Human Nutrition and Dietetics 2012;25:505-6.

152. Isenring EA, Bauer JD, Capra S. Nutrition support using the American Dietetic Association medical nutrition therapy protocol for radiation oncology patients improves dietary intake compared with standard practice. Journal of the AMERICAN DIETETIC ASSOCIATION 2007;107:404-12.

153. Nguyen A, Nadler E. Head and neck cancer: defining effective medical nutrition therapy for nutritional phases observed during chemoradiation. Oncology Nutrition Connection 2012;20:3-16.

154. Petzel M, Meddles J. Medical nutrition therapy for patients with pancreatic cancer. Oncology Nutrition Connection 2005;13:15.

155. Potter JD. Vegetables, fruit, and cancer. Lancet 2005;366:527-30.

156. Rose DJ, DeMeo MT, Keshavarzian A, Hamaker BR. Influence of Dietary Fiber on Inflammatory Bowel Disease and Colon Cancer: Importance of Fermentation Pattern. Nutrition Reviews 2007;65:51-62.

157. Vainio H, Weiderpass E. Fruit and Vegetables in Cancer Prevention. Nutrition & Cancer 2006;54:111-42.

158. Burden S. Dietary treatment of irritable bowel syndrome: current evidence and guidelines for future practice. Journal of Human Nutrition & Dietetics 2001;14:231-41.

159. Hess JR, Greenberg NA. The role of nucleotides in the immune and gastrointestinal systems: potential clinical applications. Nutrition In Clinical Practice: Official Publication Of The American Society For Parenteral And Enteral Nutrition 2012;27:281-94.

160. McKenzie YA, Alder A, Anderson W, et al. British Dietetic Association evidence-based guidelines for the dietary management of irritable bowel syndrome in adults. Journal of Human Nutrition & Dietetics 2012;25:260-74.

161. Siener R, Alteheld B, Terjung B, et al. Change in the fatty acid pattern of erythrocyte membrane phospholipids after oral supplementation of specific fatty acids in patients with gastrointestinal diseases. European Journal of Clinical Nutrition 2010;64:410-8.

162. Suneson JE. Irritable bowel syndrome: a practical approach to medical nutrition therapy. Support Line 1999;21:11.

163. Werbach MR. A Nutritional Approach to Treating Irritable Bowel Syndrome. Townsend Letter for Doctors & Patients 2004:160-59.

164. Williams L, Slavin JL. Dietary fiber and other alternative therapies and irritable bowel syndrome. Topics in Clinical Nutrition 2009;24:262-71.

165. Wolf BW, Wheeler KB, Ataya DG, Garleb KA. Safety and tolerance of Lactobacillus reuteri supplementation to a population infected with the human immunodeficiency virus. Food and chemical toxicology : an international journal published for the British Industrial Biological Research Association 1998;36:1085-94.

166. Position of the American Dietetic Association and the Canadian Dietetic Association: nutrition intervention in the care of persons with human immunodeficiency virus infection. Journal of the AMERICAN DIETETIC ASSOCIATION 1994;94:1042-5.

167. Shoaf LR, Mitchell MC. Nutrition for the older adult. Topics in Clinical Nutrition 1996;11:70-6.

168. Beto JA, Bansal VK. Medical nutrition therapy in chronic kidney failure: integrating clinical practice guidelines. Journal of the AMERICAN DIETETIC ASSOCIATION 2004;104:404-9.

169. Cotton AB. Issues in renal nutrition: focus on nutritional care for nephrology patients. Medical nutrition therapy when kidney disease meets liver failure. Nephrology Nursing Journal 2007;34:661-2.

170. Kalista-Richards M. Invited Review: The Kidney: Medical Nutrition Therapy—Yesterday and Today. Nutrition in Clinical Practice 2011;26:143-50.

171. Munson L. Strategies for setting medical nutrition therapy priorities for patients with stage 3 and 4 chronic kidney disease. Journal Of Renal Nutrition: The Official Journal Of The Council On Renal Nutrition Of The National Kidney Foundation 2013;23:e43-e6.

172. Sheean P, Peterson S, Zhao W, Gurka D, Braunschweig C. Intensive Medical Nutrition Therapy: Methods to Improve Nutrition Provision in the Critical Care Setting. Journal of the Academy of Nutrition & Dietetics 2012;112:1073-9.

173. McCloud E, Papoutsakis C. A medical nutrition therapy primer for childhood asthma: current and emerging perspectives. Journal of the AMERICAN DIETETIC ASSOCIATION 2011;111:1052-64.

174. Sachdev HPS, Kapil U, Vir S. Consensus Statement National Consensus Workshop on Management of SAM Children through Medical Nutrition Therapy. Indian Pediatrics 2010;47:661-5.

175. Carey S, Ling H, Ferrie S. Nutritional management of patients undergoing major upper gastrointestinal surgery: A survey of current practice in Australia. Nutrition & Dietetics 2010;67:219-23.

176. Kulick D, Hark L, Deen D. The bariatric surgery patient: a growing role for registered dietitians. Journal of the AMERICAN DIETETIC ASSOCIATION 2010;110:593-9.

177. Rinaldi Schinkel E, Pettine S, Adams E, Harris M. Impact of varying levels of protein intake on protein status indicators after gastric bypass in patients with multiple complications requiring nutritional support. Obesity Surgery 2006;16:24-30.

178. Scutt S, Hellman Z. A review into the use of 'light diets' for patients on surgical wards. Journal of Human Nutrition & Dietetics 2008;21:401-2.

179. Shapiro J. Surgical management of oropharyngeal dysphagia... proceedings of the fourth annual Ross Medical Nutrition and Device Roundtable, Charleston, SC, April 26-28, 1999. Nutrition in Clinical Practice 1999;14:S37-40.

180. Allmer C, Ventegodt S, Kandel I, Merrick J. Positive effects, side effects, and adverse events of clinical holistic medicine. A review of Gerda Boyesen's nonpharmaceutical mind-body medicine (biodynamic body-psychotherapy) at two centers in the United Kingdom and Germany. International Journal of Adolescent Medicine & Health 2009;21:281-97.

181. Jonas WB, Crawford CC. The healing presence: can it be reliably measured? Journal of Alternative & Complementary Medicine 2004;10:751-6.

182. Perez JC. Healing presence. Care Management Journals 2004;5:41-6.

183. Reynolds A. Patient-centered care. Radiologic Technology 2009;81:133-47.

184. Ripinsky-Naxon M. The nature of shamanism: Substance and function of a religious metaphor. . Albany, NY.: State University of New York Press; 1993.

185. Snyderman R, Williams R. Prospective medicine: The next health care transformation. . Acad Med 2003;78:1079-84.

186. Snyderman R, Yoediono Z. Prospective health care and the role of academic medicine: lead, follow, or get out of the way. . Acad Med 2008;83:707-14.

187. Ferguson LR. Nutrigenomics approaches to functional foods. Journal of the AMERICAN DIETETIC ASSOCIATION 2009;109:452-8.

188. Grayson M. Nutrigenomics. Nature 2010;468:S1-S.

189. Smith CE, Ordovás JM. Fatty acid interactions with genetic polymorphisms for cardiovascular disease. Current Opinion in Clinical Nutrition & Metabolic Care 2010;13:139-44.

190. Williams SF. Nutrigenomics: a new approach to personalized nutrition. Nutritional Perspectives: Journal of the Council on Nutrition 2008;31:9.

191. Lavebratt C, Almgren M, Ekström TJ. Epigenetic regulation in obesity. International Journal of Obesity 2012;36:757-65.

192. Link A, Balaguer F, Goel A. Cancer chemoprevention by dietary polyphenols: promising role for epigenetics. Biochem Pharmacol 2010;80:1771–92.

193. Miller W, Rollnick S. Ten things that motivational interviewing is not. Behav Cogn Psychother 2009;37:129-40.

194. Godfrey K, Sheppard A, Gluckman P. Epigenetic gene promoter methylation at birth is associated with child's later adiposity. . Diabetes 2011; 60:1528–34.

195. Roseboom T, Van Der Meulen J, Ravelli A. Effects of prenatal exposure to the Dutch famine on adult disease in later life: an overview. . Mol Cell Endocrinol 2001;185:93-8.

196. Kussmann M, Krause L, Siffert W. Nutrigenomics: where are we with genetic and epigenetic markers for disposition and susceptibility? Nutrition Reviews 2010;68:S38-47.

197. Ryan-Harshman M, Vogel E, Jones-Taggart H, et al. Nutritional genomics and dietetic professional practice. Canadian Journal of Dietetic Practice & Research 2008;69:177-82.

198. Stryjecki C, Mutch DM. Fatty acid-gene interactions, adipokines and obesity. European Journal of Clinical Nutrition 2011;65:285-97.

199. Goldner WS, Sandler DP, Yu F, Hoppin JA, Kamel F, LeVan TD. Pesticide use and thyroid disease among women in the Agricultural Health Study. American Journal of Epidemiology 2010;171:455-64.

200. van Bemmel DM, Visvanathan K, Freeman LEB, Coble J, Hoppin JA, Alavanja MCR. S-Ethyl-N, N-dipropylthiocarbamate exposure and cancer incidence among male pesticide applicators in the Agricultural Health Study: a prospective cohort. Environmental Health Perspectives 2008;116:1541-6.

201. Singh M, Bhardwaj N, Kaur A, Singh K. Biochemical, DNA and Electron Microscopic Changes in Carbamate Exposed Workers. Journal of Human Ecology 2009;28:161-6.

202. Cha ES, Lee YK, Moon EK, et al. Paraquat application and respiratory health effects among South Korean farmers. Occupational & Environmental Medicine 2012;69:398-403.

203. Crinnion WJ. Do Environmental Toxicants Contribute to Allergy and Asthma? Alternative Medicine Review 2012;17:6-18.

204. Hoppin JA, Umbach DM, London SJ, Lynch CF, Alavanja MCR, Sandler DP. Pesticides associated with wheeze among commercial pesticide applicators in the Agricultural Health Study. American Journal of Epidemiology 2006;163:1129-37.

205. Brouwer M, Kromhout H, Nijssen P, Huss A, Vermeulen R. Is Pesticide Use Related to Parkinson Disease? Some Clues to Heterogeneity in Study Results. Environmental Health Perspectives 2012;120:340-7.

206. Schultz C, Richard F. The impact of chronic pesticide exposure on neuropsychological functioning. Psychological Record 2013;63:175-84.

207. Starks S, Hoppin J, Kamel F, et al. Peripheral Nervous System Function and Organophosphate Pesticide Use among Licensed Pesticide Applicators in the Agricultural Health Study. Environmental Health Perspectives 2012;120:515-20.

208. Lifang H, Andreotti G, Baccarelli A, et al. Lifetime Pesticide Use and Telomere Shortening among Male Pesticide Applicators in the Agricultural Health Study. Environmental Health Perspectives 2013;121:1-24.

209. Ross MK, Bonner MR. Increased cancer burden among pesticide applicators and others due to pesticide exposure. CA: A Cancer Journal for Clinicians 2013;63:120-42.

210. Corsini E, Liesivuori J, Vergieva T, Van Loveren H, Colosio C. Effects of pesticide exposure on the human immune system. Human & Experimental Toxicology 2008;27:671-80.

211. Corsini E, Sokooti M, Galli CL, Moretto A, Colosio C. Pesticide induced immunotoxicity in humans: a comprehensive review of the existing evidence. Toxicology 2013;307:123-35.

212. Marchese M. Autoimmune Disease and the Environment. Townsend Letter 2011:95-6.

213. Parks C, Walitt B, Pettinger M, Chen J-C, de Roos A. Insecticide use and risk of rheumatoid arthritis and systemic lupus erythematosus in the Women's Health Initiative Observational Study. Arthritis Care & Research 2011;63:184-94.

214. Campbell AW. Pesticides: Our Children in Jeopardy. Alternative Therapies in Health & Medicine 2013;Sect. 8-10.

215. Crowe KM, Francis C. Position of the Academy of Nutrition and Dietetics: Functional Foods. Journal of the Academy of Nutrition & Dietetics 2013;113:1096-103.

216. Cani PD, Neyrinck AM, Fava F, et al. Selective increases of bifidobacteria in gut microflora improve high-fat-diet-induced diabetes in mice through a mechanism associated with endotoxaemia. Diabetologia 2007;50:2374-83.

217. Guarner F. Inulin and oligofructose: impact on intestinal diseases and disorders. The British Journal Of Nutrition 2005;93 Suppl 1:S61-S5.

218. Guarner F. Studies with inulin-type fructans on intestinal infections, permeability, and inflammation. The Journal of nutrition 2007;137:2568S-71S.

219. O'Keefe S, Ou J, Delany J, et al. Effect of fiber supplementation on the microbiota in critically ill patients. World Journal Of Gastrointestinal Pathophysiology 2011;2:138-45.

220. Pimentel G, Micheletti T, Pace F, Rosa J, Santos R, Lira F. Gut-central nervous system axis is a target for nutritional therapies. Nutrition Journal 2012;11:22-.

221. Scholz-Ahrens KE, Schrezenmeir J. Inulin and oligofructose and mineral metabolism: the evidence from animal trials. The Journal of nutrition 2007;137:2513S-23S.

222. Bastarache JA, Ware LB, Girard TD, Wheeler AP, Rice TW. Markers of inflammation and coagulation may be modulated by enteral feeding strategy. JPEN Journal of Parenteral & Enteral Nutrition 2012;36:732-40.

223. Franz MJ. Diabetes mellitus nutrition therapy: beyond the glycemic index. Archives Of Internal Medicine 2012;172:1660-1.

224. Hubbard RE, O'Mahony MS, Calver BL, Woodhouse KW. Nutrition, inflammation, and leptin levels in aging and frailty. Journal of the American Geriatrics Society 2008;56:279-84.

225. Jarvandi S, Davidson NO, Jeffe DB, Schootman M. Influence of lifestyle factors on inflammation in men and women with type 2 diabetes: results from the national health and nutrition examination survey, 1999-2004. Annals of Behavioral Medicine 2012;44:399-407.

226. Long H, Yang H, Lin Y, Situ D, Liu W. Fish Oil-Supplemented Parenteral Nutrition in Patients Following Esophageal Cancer Surgery: Effect on Inflammation and Immune Function. Nutrition & Cancer 2013;65:71-5.

227. Lubbers T, Kox M, de Haan J-J, et al. Continuous administration of enteral lipid- and protein-rich nutrition limits inflammation in a human endotoxemia model. Critical Care Medicine 2013;41:1258-65.

228. Pereira RF, Franz MJ. From research to practice. Prevention and treatment of cardiovascular disease in people with diabetes through lifestyle modification: current evidence-based recommendations. Diabetes Spectrum 2008;21:189-93.

229. Trapp C, Levin S. Nutrition FYI. Preparing to Prescribe Plant-Based Diets for Diabetes Prevention and Treatment. Diabetes Spectrum 2012;25:38-44.

230. Weichselbaum E, Coe S, Buttriss J, Stanner S. Fish in the diet: A review. Nutrition Bulletin 2013;38:128-77.

231. Larsen L, Ritz C, Hellgren L, Michaelsen K, Vogel U, Lauritzen L. FADS genotype and diet are important determinants of DHA status: a cross-sectional study in Danish infants. American Journal of Clinical Nutrition 2013;97:1403-10.

232. Koletzko B, Lattka E, Zeilinger S, Illig T, Steer C. Genetic variants of the fatty acid desaturase gene cluster predict amounts of red blood cell docosahexaenoic and other polyunsaturated fatty acids in pregnant women: findings from the Avon Longitudinal Study of Parents and Children. American Journal of Clinical Nutrition 2011;93:211-9.

233. Lattka E, Illig T, Heinrich J, Koletzko B. Do FADS genotypes enhance our knowledge about fatty acid related phenotypes? Clinical Nutrition 2010;29:277-87.

234. Martinelli N, Girelli D, Malerba G, et al. FADS genotypes and desaturase activity estimated by the ratio of arachidonic acid to linoleic acid are associated with inflammation and coronary artery disease. American Journal of Clinical Nutrition 2008;88:941-9.

235. Standl M, Sausenthaler S, Lattka E, et al. FADS gene cluster modulates the effect of breastfeeding on asthma. Results from the GINIplus and LISAplus studies. Allergy 2012;67:83-90.

236. Baïlara KM, Henry C, Lestage J, et al. Decreased brain tryptophan availability as a partial determinant of postpartum blues. Psychoneuroendocrinology 2006;31:407-13.

237. Binder EB, Jeffrey Newport D, Zach EB, et al. A serotonin transporter gene polymorphism predicts peripartum depressive symptoms in an at-risk psychiatric cohort. Journal Of Psychiatric Research 2010;44:640-6.

238. Sanjuan J, Martin-Santos R, Garcia-Esteve L, et al. Mood changes after delivery: Role of the serotonin transporter gene. The British Journal of Psychiatry 2008;193:383-8.

239. Shapiro GDFWDSJR. Emerging Risk Factors for Postpartum Depression: Serotonin Transporter Genotype and Omega-3 Fatty Acid Status. Canadian Journal of Psychiatry 2012;57:704-12.

240. Brenseke B, Prater MR, Bahamonde J, Gutierrez JC. Current thoughts on maternal nutrition and fetal programming of the metabolic syndrome. Journal Of Pregnancy 2013;2013:368461-.

241. Chmurzynska A. Fetal programming: link between early nutrition, DNA methylation, and complex diseases. Nutrition Reviews 2010;68:87-98.

242. Remacle C, Bieswal F, Bol V, Reusens B. Developmental programming of adult obesity and cardiovascular disease in rodents by maternal nutrition imbalance. The American Journal Of Clinical Nutrition 2011;94:1846S-52S.

243. Yajnik C. Obesity epidemic in India: intrauterine origins? . Proc Nutr Soc 2004;63:387-96.

244. Yajnik C, Deshmukh U. Fetal programming: maternal nutrition and role of one-carbon metabolism. Reviews In Endocrine & Metabolic Disorders 2012;13:121-7.

245. Bowron A, Scott J, Stansbie D. The influence of genetic and environmental factors on plasma homocysteine concentrations in a population at high risk for coronary artery disease. Annals Of Clinical Biochemistry 2005;42:459-62.

246. del Río Garcia C, Torres-Sánchez L, Chen J, et al. Maternal MTHFR 677C>T genotype and dietary intake of folate and vitamin B12: their impact on child neurodevelopment. Nutritional Neuroscience 2009;12:13-20.

247. Gilbody S, Lewis S, Lightfoot T. Methylenetetrahydrofolate reductase (MTHFR) genetic polymorphisms and psychiatric disorders: a HuGE review. American Journal of Epidemiology 2007;165:1-13.

248. Lewis SJ, Ebrahim S, Davey Smith G. Meta-analysis of MTHFR 677C--->T polymorphism and coronary heart disease: does totality of evidence support causal role for homocysteine and preventive potential of folate? BMJ: British Medical Journal (International Edition) 2005;331:1053-6.

249. Lewis SJLDADSGARTNDINMS. The thermolabile variant of MTHFR is associated with depression in the British Women's Heart and Health Study and a meta-analysis. Molecular Psychiatry 2006;11:352-60.

250. Oterino A. The Relationship Between Homocysteine and Genes of Folate-Related Enzymes in Migraine Patients. Headache: The Journal of Head & Face Pain 2010;50:99-168.

251. Ramsay S. Folate's role further revealed at the population and molecular levels. Lancet 1999;353:1247.

252. Rossi GP, Maiolino G, Seccia TM, et al. Hyperhomocysteinemia predicts total and cardiovascular mortality in high-risk women. Journal of Hypertension 2006;24:851-9.

253. Wilcken DEL. MTHFR 677C...T mutation, folate intake, neural-tube defect, and risk of cardiovascular disease. Lancet 1997;350:603.

254. Young-In K. 5,10-Methylenetetrahydrofolate Reductase Polymorphisms and Pharmacogenetics: A New Role of Single Nucleotide Polymorphisms in the Folate Metabolic Pathway in Human Health and Disease. Nutrition Reviews 2005;63:398-407.

255. Agodi A, Barchitta M, Valenti G, Marzagalli R, Frontini V, Marchese AE. Increase in the prevalence of the MTHFR 677 TT polymorphism in women born since 1959: potential implications for folate requirements. European Journal of Clinical Nutrition 2011;65:1302-8.

256. Bogolub C. Elevated homocysteine? Consider testing for folate metabolism gene variants. Minnesota Medicine 2012;95:39-42.

257. Boyles AL, Billups AV, Deak KL, et al. Neural tube defects and folate pathway genes: family-based association tests of gene-gene and gene-environment interactions. Environmental Health Perspectives 2006;114:1547-52.

258. Crider KS, Zhu J-H, Hao L, et al. MTHFR 677C->T genotype is associated with folate and homocysteine concentrations in a large, population-based, double-blind trial of folic acid supplementation. American Journal of Clinical Nutrition 2011;93:1365-72.

259. Deb R, Arora J, Meitei SY, et al. Folate supplementation, MTHFR gene polymorphism and neural tube defects: A community based case control study in North India. Metabolic Brain Disease 2011;26:241-6.

260. Ericson UC, Ivarsson MIL, Sonestedt E, et al. Increased breast cancer risk at high plasma folate concentrations among women with the MTHFR 677T allele. American Journal of Clinical Nutrition 2009;90:1380-9.

261. Frankenburg FR. The Role of One-Carbon Metabolism in Schizophrenia and Depression. Harvard Review of Psychiatry 2007;15:146-60.

262. Galván-Portillo MV, Cantoral A, Oñate-Ocaña LF, et al. Gastric cancer in relation to the intake of nutrients involved in one-carbon metabolism among MTHFR 677 TT carriers. European Journal of Nutrition 2009;48:269-76.

263. Oterino A, Valle N, Bravo Y, et al. MTHFR T677 homozygosis influences the presence of aura in migraineurs. CEPHALALGIA 2004;24:491-4.

264. Robitaille J, Hamner HC, Cogswell ME, Yang Q. Does the MTHFR 677C--<GT>T variant affect the Recommended Dietary Allowance for folate in the US population? American Journal of Clinical Nutrition 2009;89:1269-73.

265. Steenweg-de Graaff J, Roza S, Hofman A, Verhutst F, Tiemeier H. Maternal folate status in early pregnancy and child emotional and behavioral problems: the Generation R Study. American Journal of Clinical Nutrition 2012;95:1413-21.

266. Yang QH, Botto LD, Gallagher M, et al. Prevalence and effects of gene-gene and gene-nutrient interactions on serum folate and serum total homocysteine concentrations in the United States: findings from the third National Health and Nutrition Examination Survey DNA Bank. American Journal of Clinical Nutrition 2008;88:232-46.

267. Russell RM. Current framework for DRI development: what are the pros and cons?... reprinted with permission from The Development of DRIs 1994-2004: Lessons learned and new challenges: workshop summary ©2008 by the National Academies of Sciences, courtest of the National Academies Press, Washington, DC, USA. Nutrition Reviews 2008;66:455-8.

268. Murphy SP, Barr SI. Challenges in using the Dietary Reference Intakes to plan diets for groups. Nutrition Reviews 2005;63:267-71.

269. Beaton GH. When is an individual an individual versus a member of a group? An issue in the application of the Dietary Reference Intakes. Nutrition Reviews 2006;64:211-25.

270. Trumbo PR. Challenges with using chronic disease endpoints in setting dietary reference intakes. Nutrition Reviews 2008;66:459-64.

271. Institute of Medicine. Dietary Reference Intakes: Applications in Dietary Assessment. . In. Washington, DC: The National Academies Press; 2000.

272. Abrams SA. Setting Dietary Reference Intakes with the use of bioavailability data: calcium. American Journal of Clinical Nutrition 2010;91:1474S-7.

273. Aggett PJ. Population reference intakes and micronutrient bioavailability: a European perspective. American Journal of Clinical Nutrition 2010;91:1433S-7.

274. Cox CE. Persistent Systemic Inflammation in Chronic Critical Illness... 49th Respiratory Care Journal Conference, "The Chronically Critically Ill Patient," September 2011, Florida. Respiratory Care 2012;57:859-66.

275. Edwards T. Inflammation, pain, and chronic disease: an integrative approach to treatment and prevention. Alternative Therapies in Health & Medicine 2005;11:20-8.

276. Fearing Tornwall R, Chow AK. The association between periodontal disease and the systemic inflammatory conditions of obesity, arthritis, Alzheimer's and renal diseases. Canadian Journal of Dental Hygiene 2012;46:115-23.

277. Gurenlian JR. Inflammation: the relationship between oral health and systemic disease. Dental Assistant 2009;78:8.

278. Holmes C, Cunningham C, Zotova E, et al. Systemic inflammation and disease progression in Alzheimer disease. Neurology 2009;73:768-74.

279. Koelink P, Overbeek S, Braber S, et al. Targeting chemokine receptors in chronic inflammatory diseases: an extensive review. Pharmacology & Therapeutics 2012;133:1-18.

280. Nielsen FH. Magnesium, inflammation, and obesity in chronic disease. Nutrition Reviews 2010;68:333-40.

281. Provinciali M, Cardelli M, Marchegiani F. Inflammation, chronic obstructive pulmonary disease and aging. Current Opinion in Pulmonary Medicine 2012;17:S3-10.

282. Rath E, Haller D. Inflammation and cellular stress: a mechanistic link between immune-mediated and metabolically driven pathologies. European Journal of Nutrition 2011;50:219-33.

283. Roifman I, Beck P, Anderson T, Eisenberg M, Genest J. Chronic inflammatory diseases and cardiovascular risk: a systematic review. The Canadian Journal Of Cardiology 2011;27:174-82.

284. Rountree R. Roundoc Rx: inflammation and functional medicine interventions: part 1---Inflammation and chronic disease. Alternative & Complementary Therapies 2010;16:72-6.

285. Walter RE, Wilk JB, Larson MG, et al. Systemic inflammation and COPD: the Framingham Heart Study. Chest 2008;133:19-25.

286. Watz H, Waschki B, Kirsten A, et al. The metabolic syndrome in patients with chronic bronchitis and COPD: frequency and associated consequences for systemic inflammation and physical inactivity. Chest 2009;136:1039-46.

287. Jones JM. The State of the Science, Port 4-Roles in Inflammation, Insulin Resistance, and Metabolic Syndrome. Nutrition Today 2013;48:101-7.

288. Perry VH. Contribution of systemic inflammation to chronic neurodegeneration. Acta Neuropathologica 2010;120:277-86.

289. Schiff M, Bénit P, Coulibaly A, Loublier S, El-Khoury R, Rustin P. Mitochondrial response to controlled nutrition in health and disease. Nutrition Reviews 2011;69:65-75.

290. Denny A, Stanner S. The role of nutrition in healthy ageing. Practice Nursing 2008;19:225-30.

291. Stanner S, Denny A. Healthy ageing: the role of nutrition and lifestyle -- a new British Nutrition Foundation Task Force Report. Nutrition Bulletin 2009;34:58-63.

292. Chun O, Chung S, Claycombe K, Song W. Serum C-reactive protein concentrations are inversely associated with dietary flavonoid intake in US adults. . J Nutr 2008;138:753-60.

293. Duncan A, Talwar D, McMillan D, Stefanowica F, O'Reilly D. Quantitative data on the magnitude of the systemic inflammatory response and its effect on micronutrient status based on plasma measurements. . Am J Clin Nutr 2012;95:64-71.

294. Pellegrini N, Valtuena S, Ardigo D, et al. Intake of plant lignans matairesinol, secoisolariciresinol, pinoresinol, and lariciresinol in relation to vascular inflammation and endothelial dysfunction in middle age-elderly men and post-menopausal women living in Northern Italy. . Nutr Metab Cardiovasc Dis 2010;20:64-71.

295. Tomkins A. Assessing micronutrient status in the presence of inflammation. J Nutr 2003;133:Suppl:1649S-55S.

296. Pfeiffer CM, Sternberg MR, Schleicher RL. Selected Physiologic Variables Are Weakly to Moderately Associated with 29 Biomarkers of Diet and Nutrition, NHANES 2003-2006. Journal of Nutrition 2013;143:1001S-10.

297. Molica F, Morel S, Kwak B, Rohner-Jeanrenaud F, Steffens S. Adipokines at the crossroad between obesity and cardiovascular disease. Thromb Haemost 2015;113:553-66.

298. Gaggini M, Saponaro C, Gastaldelli A. Not all fats are created equal: adipose vs. ectopic fat, implication in cardiometabolic diseases. Horm Mol Biol Clin Investig 2015;22:7-18.

299. Kim SY, Sharma AJ, Callaghan WM. Gestational diabetes and childhood obesity: what is the link? Current Opinion in Obstetrics & Gynecology 2012;24:376-81.

300. Visioning Report: Moving Forward – A Vision for the Continuum of Dietetics Education, Credentialing and Practice. 2012. (Accessed August, 2013, at http://cdrnet.org/vault/2459/web/files/10369.pdf.)

301. Highlights of the 10 Change Drivers. 2015. (Accessed at http://www.eatrightpro.org/~/media/eatrightpro%20files/leadership/volunteering/committee%20leader%20resources/highlightsofchangedrivers.ashx.)

302. Pagano G, Guida M, Tommasi F, Oral R. Health effects and toxicity mechanisms of rare earth elements-Knowledge gaps and research prospects. Ecotoxicol Environ Saf 2015;115:40-8.

303. Lee D, Jacobs DJ. Hormesis and public health: can glutathione depletion and mitochondrial dysfunction due to very low-dose chronic exposure to persistent organic pollutants be mitigated? J Epidemiol Community Health 2015;69:294-300. .

304. Ha S-D, Park S, Han CY, Nguyen ML, Kim SO. Cellular adaptation to anthrax lethal toxin-induced mitochondrial cholesterol enrichment, hyperpolarization, and reactive oxygen species generation through downregulating MLN64 in macrophages. Molecular And Cellular Biology 2012;32:4846-60.

305. Klohs WD, Steinkampf RW. Possible link between the intrinsic drug resistance of colon tumors and a detoxification mechanism of intestinal cells. Cancer Research 1988;48:3025-30.

306. Li H, Pakstis AJ, Kidd JR, Kidd KK. Selection on the human bitter taste gene, TAS2R16, in Eurasian populations. Human Biology 2011;83:363-77.

307. Mortensen HM, Froment A, Lema G, et al. Characterization of genetic variation and natural selection at the arylamine N-acetyltransferase genes in global human populations. Pharmacogenomics 2011;12:1545-58.

308. van Belkum A, Melles DC, Nouwen J, et al. Co-evolutionary aspects of human colonisation and infection by Staphylococcus aureus. Infection, Genetics And Evolution: Journal Of Molecular Epidemiology And Evolutionary Genetics In Infectious Diseases 2009;9:32-47.

309. Wooding S. Signatures of natural selection in a primate bitter taste receptor. Journal Of Molecular Evolution 2011;73:257-65.

310. Baillie-Hamilton P. Chemical toxins: A hypothesis to explain the global obesity epidemic. JAltCompMed 2002;8:185-92.

311. Pesticides and Food: How the Government Regulates Pesticides (Accessed August, 2013, at http://www.epa.gov/pesticides/food/govt.htm.)

312. Declassifying Confidentiality Claims to Increase Access to Chemical Information. (Accessed August, 2013, at http://www.epa.gov/oppt/existingchemicals/pubs/transparency-charts.html.)

313. Bland JS. Managing biotransformation: introduction and overview. Altern Ther Health Med 2007 13:S85-7.

314. Challem J. Current Controversies in Nutrition: Why Nutrition Should Be Your First-Line Therapy. Alternative & Complementary Therapies 2011;17:319-22.

315. Cummings JH, Antoine J-M, Azpiroz F, et al. PASSCLAIM1—Gut health and immunity. European Journal of Nutrition 2004;43:ii118-ii73.

316. Gonzalez MJMMJR. Metabolic Correction: A Functional Explanation of Orthomolecular Medicine. Journal of Orthomolecular Medicine 2012;27:13-20.

317. Kidd PM. Alzheimer's Disease, Amnestic Mild Cognitive Impairment, and Age-Associated Memory Impairment: Current Understanding and Progress Toward Integrative Prevention. Alternative Medicine Review 2008;13:85-115.

318. Minich D, Bland J. ACID-ALKALINE BALANCE: ROLE IN CHRONIC DISEASE AND DETOXIFICATION. Alternative Therapies in Health & Medicine 2007;13:62-5.

319. Shelton BH. Obesity as an inflammatory disease: Homotoxicology is a valuable answer to control it. Journal of Biomedical Therapy 2004;22:12-.

320. Smith RG. Nutrition and Eye Diseases. Journal of Orthomolecular Medicine 2010;25:67-76.

321. Yaktine AL, Nesheim MC, James CA. Nutrient and contaminant tradeoffs: exchanging meat, poultry, or seafood for dietary protein. Nutrition Reviews 2008;66:113-22.

322. Bales CW, Kraus WE. Caloric Restriction: Implications for human cardiometabolic health. Journal of Cardiopulmonary Rehabilitation & Prevention 2013;33:201-8.

323. Hyman FN, Sempos E, Saltsman J, Glinsmann WH. Evidence for success of caloric restriction in weight loss and control: summary of data from industry. Annals Of Internal Medicine 1993;119:681-7.

324. Le Couteur DG, Sinclair DA. A blueprint for developing therapeutic approaches that increase healthspan and delay death. The Journals of Gerontology: Series A: Biological Sciences and Medical Sciences 2010;65A:693-4.

325. Michalsen A, Riegert M, Ludtke R, et al. Mediterranean diet or extended fasting's influence on changing the intestinal microflora, immunoglobulin A secretion and clinical outcome in patients with rheumatoid arthritis and fibromyalgia: an observational study. BMC Complementary & Alternative Medicine 2005;5:9p.

326. Miladipour AH, Shakhssalim N, Parvin M, Azadvari M. Effect of ramadan fasting on urinary risk factors for calculus formation. Iranian Journal of Kidney Diseases 2012;6:33-8.

327. Pathy R, Mills K, Gazeley S, Ridgley A, Kiran T. Health is a spiritual thing: perspectives of health care professionals and female Somali and Bangladeshi women on the health impacts of fasting during Ramadan. Ethnicity & Health 2011;16:43-56.

328. Peterson S, Nayda R, Hill PC. Muslim person's experiences of diabetes during Ramadan: Information for health professionals. Contemporary Nurse: A Journal for the Australian Nursing Profession 2012;41:41-7.

329. Reed JL, De Souza MJ, Williams NI. Effects of exercise combined with caloric restriction on inflammatory cytokines. Applied Physiology, Nutrition & Metabolism 2010;35:573-82.

330. Reeds DN. Nutrition support in the obese, diabetic patient: the role of hypocaloric feeding. Current Opinion in Gastroenterology 2009;25:151-4.

331. Rochon J, Bales CW, Ravussin E, et al. Design and conduct of the CALERIE study: comprehensive assessment of the long-term effects of reducing intake of energy. The Journals Of Gerontology Series A, Biological Sciences And Medical Sciences 2011;66:97-108.

332. Roth GS. Caloric Restriction and Caloric Restriction Mimetics: Current Status and Promise for the Future. Journal of the American Geriatrics Society 2005;53:S280-S3.

333. Shahzad A. Diabetes in Ramadan. Journal of the Royal Society of Medicine 2003;96:reply 52.

334. Bangasser DA, Valentino RJ. Sex differences in molecular and cellular substrates of stress. Cellular and Molecular Neurobiology 2012;32:709-23.

335. Bland JS. Psychoneuro-nutritional medicine: an advancing paradigm. Alternative Therapies in Health & Medicine 1995;1:22-7.

336. Chandwani K, Ryan J, Peppone L, Janelsins M, Sprod L, Devine K. Cancer-Related Stress and Complementary and Alternative Medicine: A Review. Evidence-based Complementary & Alternative Medicine (eCAM) 2012:1-15.

337. Goldstein DS. Stress, allostatic load, catecholamines, and other neurotransmitters in neurodegenerative diseases. Cellular and Molecular Neurobiology 2012;32:661-6.

338. Grant N, Hamer M, Steptoe A. Social Isolation and Stress-related Cardiovascular, Lipid, and Cortisol Responses. Annals of Behavioral Medicine 2009;37:29-37.

339. Hamer M. Psychosocial stress and cardiovascular disease risk: the role of physical activity. Psychosomatic Medicine 2012;74:896-903.

340. Holloway TJ. The root of the problem: an irritable bowel or an average American lifestyle? Gastrointestinal Nursing 2010;8:31.

341. Jones JD, Tucker CM, Herman KC. Stress and nutrition among African American women with hypertension. American Journal of Health Behavior 2009;33:661-72.

342. Lutgendorf SK, Sood AK, Antoni MH. Host factors and cancer progression: biobehavioral signaling pathways and interventions. Journal of Clinical Oncology 2010;28:4094-9.

343. Peltzer K, Shisana O, Zuma K, Van Wyk B, Zungu-Dirwayi N. Job stress, job satisfaction and stress-related illnesses among South African educators. Stress & Health: Journal of the International Society for the Investigation of Stress 2009;25:247-57.

344. Roepke SK, Grant I. Toward a more complete understanding of the effects of personal mastery on cardiometabolic health. Health Psychology 2011;30:615-32.

345. Shalev AY. Posttraumatic stress disorder and stress-related disorders. Psychiatric Clinics of North America 2009;32:687-704.

346. Shirom A, Toker S, Berliner S, Itzhak S. The Job Demand-Control-Support Model and stress related low-grade inflammatory responses among healthy employees: A longitudinal study. Work & Stress 2008;22:138-52.

347. Wirth SM, Macaulay TE, Winstead PS, Smith KM. Stress-related mucosal disease: considerations of current medication prophylaxis. Orthopedics 2007;30:1010-4.

348. Alternative Farming Systems Information Center. (Accessed 1/8, 2016, at http://afsic.nal.usda.gov/community-supported-agriculture-3.)

349. D. A. Re-conceptualising holism in the contemporary nursing mandate: From individual to organisational relationships. Soc Sci Med 2014;119C:131-8.

350. Sanchez-Menegay C, Stalder H. Do physicians take into account patients' expectations? J Gen Intern Med 1994;9:404-6.

34404183R00168

Made in the USA
Lexington, KY
22 March 2019